Recent Advances in Tonsils and Mucosal Barriers of the Upper Airways

Advances in Oto-Rhino-Laryngology

Vol. 72

Series Editor

G. Randolph Boston, Mass.

Proceedings of the 7th International Symposium on Tonsils and Mucosal Barriers of the Upper Airways, July 7–9, 2010, Asahikawa, Japan

Recent Advances in Tonsils and Mucosal Barriers of the Upper Airways

Volume Editor

Yasuaki Harabuchi Asahikawa

Co-Editors

Tatsuya Hayashi Asahikawa
Akihiro Katada Asahikawa

43 figures, 18 in color, and 17 tables, 2011

KARGER

Basel · Freiburg · Paris · London · New York · New Delhi · Bangkok · Beijing · Tokyo · Kuala Lumpur · Singapore · Sydney

Yasuaki Harabuchi
Department of Otolaryngology- Head and Neck Surgery
Asahikawa Medical University
Midorigaoka Higashi 2-1-1-1
Asahikawa, Hokkaido 078-8510 (Japan)

Tatsuya Hayashi
Department of Otolaryngology- Head and Neck Surgery
Asahikawa Medical University
Midorigaoka Higashi 2-1-1-1
Asahikawa, Hokkaido 078-8510 (Japan)

Akihiro Katada
Department of Otolaryngology- Head and Neck Surgery
Asahikawa Medical University
Midorigaoka Higashi 2-1-1-1
Asahikawa, Hokkaido 078-8510 (Japan)

Library of Congress Cataloging-in-Publication Data

International Symposium on Tonsils and Mucosal Barriers of Upper Airways (7th : 2010 : Asahikawa-shi, Japan)
Recent advances in tonsils and mucosal barriers of the upper airways : proceedings of the 7th International Symposium on Tonsils and Mucosal Barriers of the Upper Airways, July 7-9, 2010, Asahikawa, Japan / volume editor, Yasuaki Harabuchi ; co-editors, Tatsuya Hayashi, Akihiro Katada.
p. ; cm. -- (Advances in oto-rhino-laryngology, ISSN 0065-3071 ; v. 72)
Includes bibliographical references and index.
ISBN 978-3-8055-9722-7 (hard cover : alk. paper) -- ISBN 978-3-8055-9723-4 (e-ISBN)
1. Tonsils--Congresses. 2. Tonsils--Diseases--Congresses. 3. Immunity--Congresses. 4. Respiratory infections--Congresses. I. Harabuchi, Yasuaki. II. Hayashi, Tatsuya, 1961- III. Katada, Akihiro. IV. Title. V. Series: Advances in oto-rhino-laryngology ; v. 72. 0065-3071
[DNLM: 1. Palatine Tonsil--Congresses. 2. Immunity, Mucosal--Congresses. 3. Respiratory Tract Infections--drug therapy--Congresses. WV 430]
RF481.I58 2010
616.3'14--dc22

2011010431

Bibliographic Indices. This publication is listed in bibliographic services, including Current Contents®.

Drug Dosage. The authors and the publisher have exerted every effort to ensure that drug selection and dosage set forth in this text are in accord with current recommendations and practice at the time of publication. However, in view of ongoing research, changes in government regulations, and the constant flow of information relating to drug therapy and drug reactions, the reader is urged to check the package insert for each drug for any change in indications and dosage and for added warnings and precautions. This is particularly important when the recommended agent is a new and/or infrequently employed drug.

www.karger.com
Printed in Switzerland on acid-free and non-aging paper (ISO 9706) by Reinhardt Druck, Basel
ISSN 0065–3071
ISBN 978–3–8055–9722–7
e-ISBN 978–3–8055–9723–4

Contents

Preface

As a president of the 7th International Symposium on Tonsils and Mucosal Barriers of the Upper Airways (ISTMB), I had the great pleasure and honor to organize the symposium held in Asahikawa City, Japan, July 7–9, 2010. I am sure that the 7th symposium was extremely fruitful and successful for all of the participants.

Over the past few decades, since the 1st meeting of this symposium held in Kyoto in 1987, the various aspects of tonsils and mucosal immunity of upper airways have kept attracting both researchers and clinicians from all over the world. The symposium was designed to provide updates on information concerning tonsils and mucosal immunity as well as to build good friendships among all the participants.

In this 7th symposium, we had 154 presentations and over 250 participants from all over the world. This was twice the number of the past symposium and was highest of all the symposiums held so far. The topics extended widely to both basic and clinical research areas of tonsils and upper airways such as: (1) immunology and mucosal defense systems, (2) bacteriology and virology, (3) mucosal vaccine for upper airway infections, (4) MALT, NALT and LALT, (5) clinical manifests and pathogenesis of tonsil-related diseases such as IgA nephropathy, palmoplantal pustulosis, reactive arthritis, and other diseases, (6) association of tonsils with otitis media, (7) allergic diseases in the upper airways, (8) obstructive sleep apnea syndrome, and (9) medical and surgical treatments of tonsillar diseases. These proceedings mark the summary of topics presented in the 7th ISTMB. I am sure that the proceedings will provide new interests in this area.

Finally, I wish to sincerely express my appreciation to all of the participants, members of the organizing committee, and my colleagues at the Department of Otolaryngology- Head and Neck Surgery, Asahikawa Medical University. The 8th symposium will be organized by Professor David Nadal and held in Zürich, Switzerland, in 2013. I hope that basic and clinical scientists in this area from all over the world will join the meeting.

Yasuaki Harabuchi
President, 7th International Symposium on Tonsils and Mucosal Barriers of the Upper Airways (ISTMB)
Professor and Chairman, Department of Otolaryngology- Head and Neck Surgery, Asahikawa Medical University

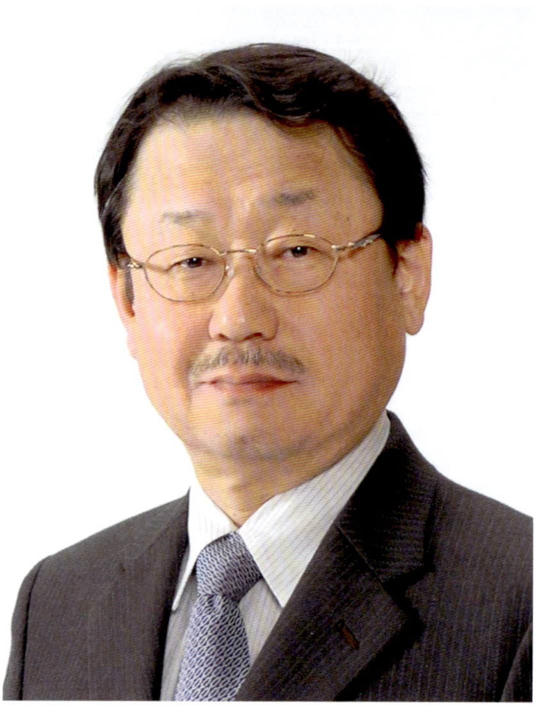

President

Yasuaki Harabuchi, MD, PhD

1982	Graduated from Asahikawa Medical University, Asahikawa, Japan
1985–1986	Research fellow, Department of Virology, Cancer Institute, School of Medicine, Hokkaido University, Sapporo, Japan
1990–1993	Research Instructor, Division of Infectious Diseases, Department of Pediatrics, State University of New York at Buffalo, USA
1998	Professor and Chairman, Department of Otolaryngology- Head and Neck Surgery, Asahikawa Medical University, Asahikawa, Japan

Symposium Organization

President
Yasuaki Harabuchi Asahikawa, Japan

Honorary Presidents
Desiderio Passàli Siena, Italy
Noboru Yamanaka Wakayama, Japan

Executive Advisory Council
Akikatsu Kataura Sapporo, Japan
Atsushi Komatsuzaki Tokyo, Japan
Ginichiro Ichikawa Tokyo, Japan

Scientific Advisory Council
Luisa Bellussi Siena, Italy
Per Brandtzaeg Oslo, Norway
David E. Briles Birmingham, Ala., USA
Pasquale Cassano Foggia, Italy
Paul B. van Cauwenberge Ghent, Belgium
Luiza Hayashi Endo São Paulo, Brazil
Howard Faden Buffalo, N.Y., USA
Shigeharu Fujieda Fukui, Japan
Roberto P. Garofalo Galveston, Tex., USA
Naoyuki Hasebe Asahikawa, Japan
Yoshiyuki Hiki Toyoake, Japan
Tetsuo Himi Sapporo, Japan
Osamu Hotta Sendai, Japan
Hajime Iizuka Asahikawa, Japan
Edward L. Kaplan Minneapolis, Minn., USA
Hideyuki Kawauchi Shimane, Japan
Michio Kimura Osaka, Japan
Hiroshi Kiyono Tokyo, Japan
Yuichi Kurono Kagoshima, Japan
Jennelle M. Kyd Rockhampton, Australia
Kar Neng Lai Hong Kong, China
David J. Lim Los Angeles, Calif., USA
Hirofumi Makino Okayama, Japan
Yu Masuda Okayama, Japan
Jiri Mestecky Birmingham, Ala., USA
Timothy F. Murphy Buffalo, N.Y., USA
David Nadal Zurich, Switzerland
Jan Novak Birmingham, Ala., USA
Pearay L. Ogra Buffalo, N.Y., USA
Ken Okamoto Seki, Japan
Gaetano Paludetti Rome, Italy
Keehyun Park Suwon, Korea
Ruby Pawankar Tokyo, Japan
Noriyuki Sato Sapporo, Japan
Norimasa Sawada Sapporo, Japan
Anne G. M. Schilder Utrecht, Netherlands
Jaroslav Slipka Plzen, Czech Republic
Jaroslav Slipka Jr. Plzen, Czech Republic
Masashi Suzuki Oita, Japan
Yusuke Suzuki Tokyo, Japan
Hiroshi Takenaka Osaka, Japan
Masatoshi Tateno Asahikawa, Japan
Yasmin M. Thanavala Buffalo, N.Y., USA
Helgi Valdimarsson Reykjavík, Iceland
Michael R. Wessels Boston, Mass., USA
Toshio Yamashita Osaka, Japan
Shunpei Yokota Yokohama, Japan

Program Committee
Hirofumi Akagi Okayama, Japan
Keiji Fujihara Wakayama, Japan

Tatsuya Hayashi Asahikawa, Japan
Susan K. Hollingshead Birmingham, Ala., USA
Muneki Hotomi Wakayama, Japan
Satomi Kobayashi Tokyo, Japan
Shigeto Kobayashi Tokyo, Japan
Miki Takahara Asahikawa, Japan
Hiroshi Tsubota Sapporo, Japan

Local Organizing Committee
Masaru Aoyagi Yamagata, Japan
Hideo Edamatsu Tokyo, Japan
Satoshi Fukuda Sapporo, Japan
Mitsuru Furukawa Kanazawa, Japan
Nobuhiko Furuya Maebashi, Japan
Kiyofumi Gyo Toon, Ehime, Japan
Akira Hara Tsukuba, Japan
Tamotsu Harada Kurashiki, Japan
Shinichi Haruna Shimotsuga, Tochigi, Japan
Katsuhiro Hirakawa Hiroshima, Japan
Yasuo Hisa Kyoto, Japan
Hiroshi Hosoi Nara, Japan
Masamitsu Hyodo Nangoku, Kochi, Japan
Keiichi Ichimura Shimotsuke, Tochigi, Japan
Masahiro Iida Isehara, Kanagawa, Japan
Yukiko Iino Saitama, Japan
Katsuhisa Ikeda Tokyo, Japan
Minoru Ikeda Tokyo, Japan
Akira Inokuchi Saga, Japan
Hidenori Inohara Osaka, Japan
Hideki Hirabayashi Shimotsuga, Tochigi, Japan
Kazuo Ishikawa Akita, Japan
Yasuhiro Kase Iruma, Saitama, Japan
Seiji Kishimoto Tokyo, Japan
Hiroya Kitano Yonago, Japan
Izumi Koizuka Kawasaki, Kanagawa, Japan
Naoyuki Kono Mitaka, Tokyo, Japan
Fumiyo Kudo Chiba, Japan
Kiyonori Kuki Arita, Wakayama, Japan
Sachiko Matsutani Sendai, Japan
Hiroyuki Mineta Hamamatsu, Japan
Takaki Miwa Kanazawa, Japan
Soichiro Miyazaki Otsu, Japan
Nozomu Mori Kida, Kagawa, Japan
Keisuke Masuyama Chuo, Yamanashi, Japan
Shingo Murakami Nagoya, Japan
Kensei Naito Toyoake, Aichi, Japan
Takashi Nakagawa Fukuoka, Japan
Tadashi Nakashima Kurume, Japan
Tsutomu Nakashima Nagoya, Japan
Kenichi Nibu Kobe, Japan
Shinichi Nishi Niigata, Japan
Kazunori Nishizaki Okayama, Japan
Kaoru Ogawa Tokyo, Japan
Yoshitaka Okamoto Chiba, Japan
Toshio Okoshi Tokyo, Japan
Koichi Omori Fukushima, Japan
Masafumi Sakagami Nishinomiya, Japan
Hiroaki Sato Morioka, Japan
Fumiaki Shido Tomakomai, Japan
Takeshi Shimizu Otsu, Japan
Hideichi Shinkawa Hirosaki, Japan
Akihiro Shiotani Tokorozawa, Japan
Harumi Suzaki Tokyo, Japan
Mamoru Suzuki Tokyo, Japan
Kenji Suzuki Nagoya, Japan
Hideaki Suzuki Kitakyushu, Japan
Mikio Suzuki Nakagami, Okinawa, Japan
Sugata Takahashi Niigata, Japan
Haruo Takahashi Nagasaki, Japan
Kazuhiko Takeuchi Tsu, Japan
Koichi Tomoda Moriguchi, Osaka, Japan
Tetsuya Tono Miyazaki, Japan
Shinichi Usami Matsumoto, Japan
Kensuke Watanabe Koshigaya, Japan
Yukio Watanabe Toyama, Japan
Hideaki Yamabe Hirosaki, Japan
Hideo Yamane Osaka, Japan
Hiroshi Yamashita Ube, Japan
Tatsuya Yamasoba Tokyo, Japan
Toshio Yoshihara Tokyo, Japan
Tomokazu Yoshizaki Kanazawa, Japan
Nobuyuki Yoshizawa Chofu, Tokyo, Japan

Harabuchi Y (ed): Recent Advances in Tonsils and Mucosal Barriers of the Upper Airways.
Adv Otorhinolaryngol. Basel, Karger, 2011, vol 72, pp 1–5

Clinical Manifestations and Pathogenesis of Tonsillar Focal Diseases: IgA Nephropathy and Palmoplantar Pustulosis

Yasuaki Harabuchi

Department of Otolaryngology- Head and Neck Surgery, Asahikawa Medical University, Asahikawa, Hokkaido, Japan

Abstract

Tonsillar focal disease is defined as clinical disorders in the distant organ from the tonsil that are caused by the tonsils without any symptoms of the tonsil itself. Palmoplantar pustulosis and IgA nephropathy are known typical tonsillar focal diseases. In this paper, the clinical outcome of tonsillectomy and the etiological evidence of related diseases are reviewed.

In 400 BC, Hippocrates already described an association between rheumatoid arthritis and oral disease. Before the 20 century, tonsillar focal diseases were thought to be inflammatory diseases due to bacterial infection or toxins arising from focal tonsillitis, leading to poststreptococcal infectious diseases such as glomerulonephritis, endocarditis, and myocarditis. However, the concept of the disease has changed due to a decline in the frequency of poststreptococcal infectious diseases. It is now thought that these diseases are autoimmune diseases due to a novel immune response of the focus tonsil, including skin disease such as palmoplantar pustulosis (PPP), psoriasis, etc., osteo-arthal diseases such as sternocostoclavicular hyperostosis, rheumatoid arthritis and reactive arthritis, and renal diseases like IgA nephropathy (IgAN). Systemic autoimmune diseases such as Behcet's disease and inflammatory bowel diseases are sometimes though to be in this category as tonsillectomy is reported to be effective for their treatment.

PPP is characterized by symmetrical, erythematous, scaly plaques with numerous, sterile nonbacterial, pinpoint pustules restricted to the palms and soles. PPP is known to be a typical tonsillar focal disease, because a dramatic effectiveness of tonsillectomy for improvement of the skin lesion has been shown in over 80% of PPP patients in previous reports (table 1).

IgAN is the most common form of glomerulonephritis characterized by glomerular IgA-immune complex deposits. 30–40% of the patients progress to renal failure and require renal replacement therapy at around 20 years after developing the disease. Tonsillitis often induces exacerbation of hematuria and/or proteinuria. Therefore, IgAN is known to be a typical tonsillar focal disease. Table 2 shows results from other studies on the clinical outcome of tonsillectomy in IgAN patients. Every study with an observation period of over 5 years reported that clinical remission and renal survival rates are better in the tonsillectomy group than in the non-tonsillectomy group. Recently, tonsillectomy combined with steroid pulse therapy has been reported to be more effective and has thus become the standard treatment for IgAN in Japan.

Table 1. Effects of tonsillectomy for PPP

Author	Year	Therapy	Number of cases	Observation period, months	Disappearance rates, %	Improvement rates, %
Ono	1977	tonsillectomy non-tonsillectomy	73 24	>3	52 11	84* 39
Hashiguchi	1992	tonsillectomy	33	12–120	55	94
Tsubota	1994	tonsillectomy	289	3–60	54	88
Fujihara	1999	tonsillectomy non-tonsillectomy	181 77	3–144 (median 21)	43 25	81 66
Kidera	2000	tonsillectomy	50	1–3	8	88
Yamakita	2004	tonsillectomy non-tonsillectomy	23 57	18	13 0	61* 18
Harabuchi	2008	tonsillectomy	103	6–50 (median 12)	40	89
Hashimoto	2006	tonsillectomy	27	>3		90
Fujihara	2009	tonsillectomy	42	18		91
Yamakita	2009	tonsillectomy non-tonsillectomy	26 37	18	46 15	85* 35
Our results	2010	tonsillectomy	27	12	40	93

Disappearance rate = Percentage of the cases in whom skin rash disappeared; improvement rate = percentage of the cases in whom skin rash was improved over 50%. $*p < 0.01$.

The characteristics of tonsillar mononuclear cells (TMC) taken from cases with tonsillar focal diseases are as follows:

1 The numbers of CD25 or HLA class II-positive T cells increased in tonsils from PPP patients. The expression of CTLA-4 mRNA, a co-stimulatory molecule inhibiting T cell activation, decreased and the expression of Smad7 mRNA and protein, an inhibitor of TGF-β signaling, increased in tonsillar T cells from PPP patients. These data suggest that tonsillar T cells may be more activated in PPP patients and that CTLA-4 and Smad7 may take part in the activation of tonsillar T cells [1].

2 Expressions of the skin homing receptor CLA, CC chemokine receptor 6 (CCR6) and β_1-integrin in PPP patients and of T cell receptor (TCR) V beta 6 and CXCR3 in IgAN patients were significantly increased on both tonsillar and peripheral T cells. In vitro stimulus with α-streptococcal antigens or *Haemophilus parainfluenzae* antigens significantly enhanced the expression on tonsillar T cells from PPP and IgAN patients (fig. 1). The expressions on peripheral T cells decreased after tonsillectomy in PPP and IgAN patients. In the PPP skin or IgAN renal lesions, E-selectin (ligand of CLA), CCL20 (ligand of CCR6), vascular cell adhesion molecule-1 (ligand for β_1-integrin) and IP-10 (ligand of CXCR3) were highly expressed. These data suggest that tonsillar T cells from PPP and IgAN patients show a hyper-immune response to α-streptococci

Table 2. Clinical outcome of tonsillectomy in IgAN patients

Author	Year	Therapy	Number of cases	Average of observation period, months	Clinical outcome: clinical remission, %	Clinical outcome: renal survival, %	Remark
Tomioka	1996	tonsillectomy	104	>60	38		
Hotta	2001	tonsillectomy + steroid	191	82	60*		serum Cr ≤ 1.4 mg/dl
		steroid	34		35		
Sato	2003	tonsillectomy + steroid pulse	30	70		87*	serum Cr ≥ 1.5 mg/dl
		steroid	25			44	
		others	15			27	
Akagi	2004	tonsillectomy	41	158	24	95*	
		others	30		13	73	
Nishi	2004	tonsillectomy	46	206		89*	
		others	74	191		74	
Komatsu	2005	tonsillectomy	104	62	32*	88*	
		others	133		17	64	
Miyazaki	2007	tonsillectomy + steroid pulse	75	60	70*		uric protein/day ≥ 1 g
		steroid pulse	18		39		
Chen	2007	tonsillectomy	54	130	46*	96	uric protein/day ≥ 1 g
		others	58		28	88	

*Presence of statistical difference.

or *H. parainfluenzae*, resulting in increased expressions of CLA, CCR6 and TCRV beta 6. Such T cells recruit to PPP skin lesions or the glomerulus in IgAN through the blood circulation, resulting in tissue damage [2–5].

3 In IgAN, in vitro stimulation with CpG-oligodeoxynucleotides (CpG-ODN), which consists of specific 6-base sequences commonly observed in bacterial and virus DNAs, significantly enhanced the production of IgA, IFN-γ and B cell activation factor (BAFF) of TMC. IFN-γ stimulation also significantly enhanced the BAFF production of TMC (fig. 2). These data suggest that a hyper-immune response to microbial DNA may lead to hyperproduction of BAFF upregulated by IFN-γ of TMC, resulting in the hyperproduction of IgA in IgAN patients [6].

On the basis of our data, we now propose the pathogenesis of tonsillar focal diseases to be as follows (fig. 3): The healthy human, because of his immunological tolerance, does not show an immune response to indigenous organisms such as α-streptococci, *H. parainfluenzae* or microbial DNA. However, since patients with tonsillar focal diseases may have a derangement of this immunological tolerance, TMC shows a hyper-immune response to such organisms. Thus, tonsillar T cells expressing homing receptors to skin and kidney are activated and move into the blood circulation, resulting in recruitment to PPP skin lesions and IgAN glomeruli. Moreover, tonsillar B cells produce high amounts of IgA autoantibody, resulting in deposition of the IgA immune complex in the IgAN glomerulus.

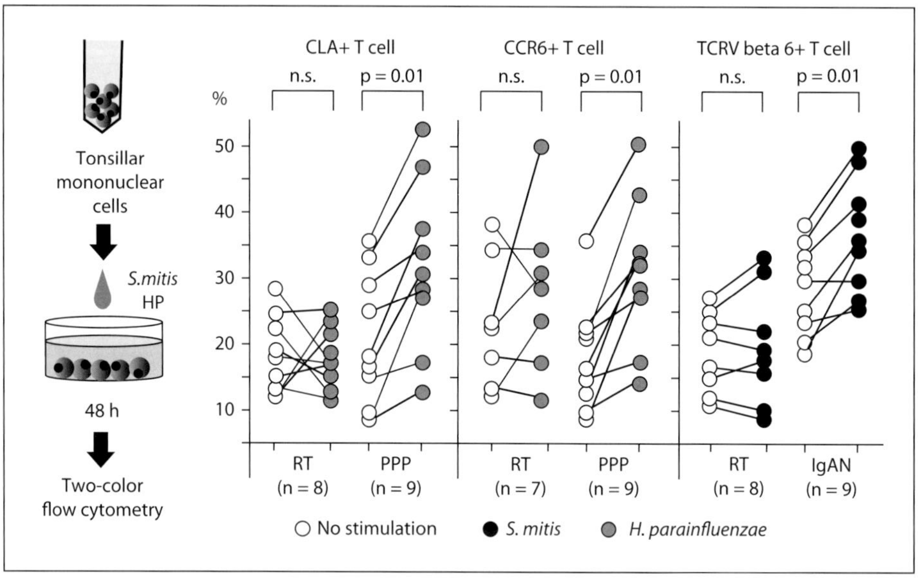

Fig. 1. Changes in expressions of CLA, CCR6 and TCRV beta 6 on tonsillar T-cells stimulated with α-streptococcal and *H. parainfluenzae* antigens in vitro. The numbers of CLA and CCR6-positive tonsillar T cells significantly increased by stimulation of *S. mitis* in PPP patients, but the percentages did not change in recurrent tonsillitis (RT) patients. Similarly, the number of TCRV beta 6-positive tonsillar T cells significantly increased by stimulation of *H. parainfluenzae* in IgAN patients, but did not change in RT patients.

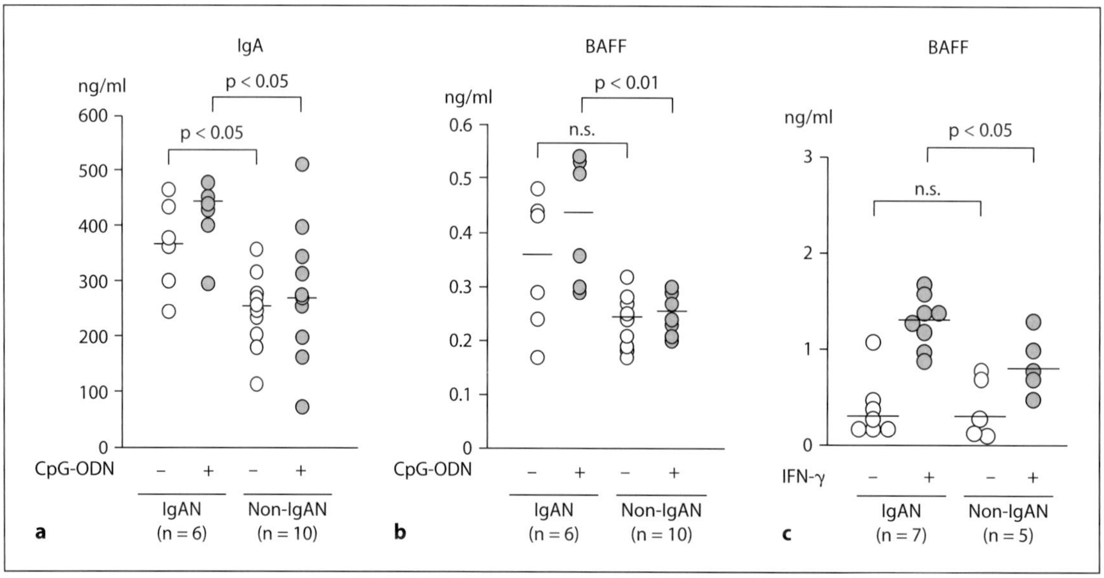

Fig. 2. Production of IgA (**a**) and BAFF (**b**) stimulated with CpG-ODN, and BAFF (**c**) stimulated with IFN-γ by tonsillar mononuclear cells (TMC). The IgA and BAFF production by TMC with stimulation of CpG-ODN was significantly higher in IgAN patients than in non-IgAN patients. BAFF production by TMC with stimulation of IFN-γ was also significantly higher in IgAN patients than in non-IgAN patients.

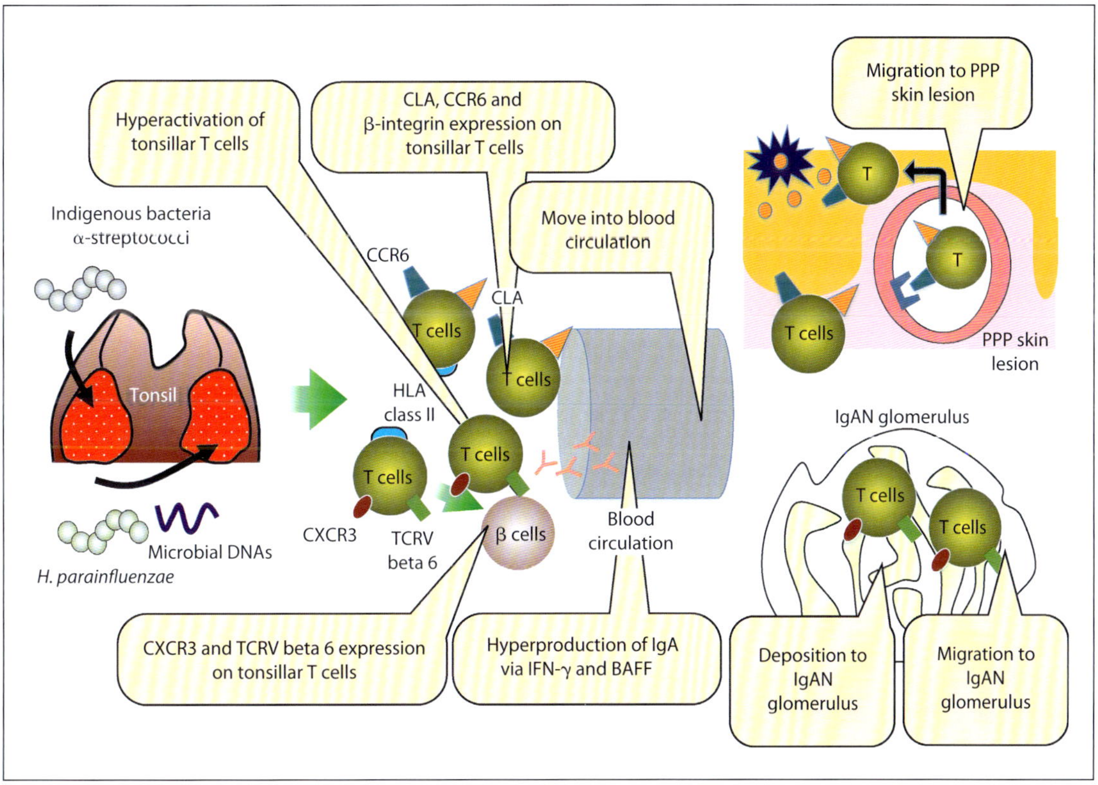

Fig. 3. Pathogenesis of tonsillar focal diseases.

References

1 Takahara M, Kishibe K, Nozawa H, Harabuchi Y: Increase of activated T-cells and up-regulation of Smad7 without elevation of TGF-beta expression in tonsils from patients with pustulosis palmaris et plantaris. Clin Immunol 2005;115:192–199.

2 Nozawa H, Kishibe K, Takahara M, Harabuchi Y: Expression of cutaneous lymphocyte-associated antigen (CLA) in tonsillar T-cells and its induction by in vitro stimulation with alpha-streptococci in patients with pustulosis palmaris et plantaris (PPP). Clin Immunol 2005;116:42–53.

3 Yoshizaki T, Bandoh N, Ueda S, Nozawa H, Goto T, Kishibe K, Takahara M, Harabuchi Y: Up-regulation of CC chemokine receptor 6 on tonsillar T cells and its induction by in vitro stimulation with a-streptococci in patients with pustulosis palmaris et plantaris. Clin Exp Immunol 2009;157:71–82.

4 Nozawa H, Takahara M, Yoshizaki T, Goto T, Bandoh N, Harabuchi Y: Selective expansion of T cell receptor (TCR) V beta 6 in tonsillar and peripheral blood T cells and its induction by in vitro stimulation with *Haemophilus parainfluenzae* in patients with IgA nephropathy. Clin Exp Immunol 2008;151:25–33.

5 Ueda S, Takahara M, Tohtani T, Yoshizaki T, Kishibe K, Harabuchi Y: Up-regulation of beta 1 integrin on tonsillar T cells and its induction by in vitro stimulation with alpha-streptococci in patients with pustulosis palmaris et plantaris. J Clin Immunol 2010;in press.

6 Goto T, Bandoh N, Yoshizaki T, Nozawa H, Takahara M, Ueda S, Hayashi T, Harabuchi Y: Increase in B-cell-activation factor (BAFF) and IFN-gamma productions by tonsillar mononuclear cells stimulated with deoxycytidyl-deoxyguanosine oligodeoxynucleotides (CpG-ODN) in patients with IgA nephropathy. Clin Immunol 2008;126: 260–269.

Yasuaki Harabuchi
Department of Otolaryngology- Head and Neck Surgery, Asahikawa Medical University
Midorigaoka E2–1–1–1
Asahikawa, Hokkaido, 078-8510 (Japan)
Tel. +81 166 68 2554, E-Mail hyasu@asahikawa-med.ac.jp

Harabuchi Y (ed): Recent Advances in Tonsils and Mucosal Barriers of the Upper Airways.
Adv Otorhinolaryngol. Basel, Karger, 2011, vol 72, pp 6–19

Moving Towards a New Era in the Research of Tonsils and Mucosal Barriers

Noboru Yamanaka

Professor and Chairman, Department of Otolaryngology, Head and Neck Surgery, Director, Infection and Immunity Research Center, Wakayama Medical University, Wakayama, Japan

Abstract

The palatine and nasopharyngeal tonsils (adenoids) are lymphoepithelial tissues located in strategic anatomical areas of the oral pharynx and nasopharynx. These immunocompetent tissues represent the first line of defense against ingested or inhaled foreign proteins such as bacteria, viruses, or food antigens. Accompanying the advances being made in the field of medicine today, the role of the tonsils in immunocompetence is becoming extremely important. Upper respiratory tract infections such as acute otitis media, acute rhinosinusitis and acute pharyngo-tonsillitis are diseases that occur with extremely high frequency, and the antimicrobial agents used to treat these diseases account for a large proportion of health care costs. The increasingly refractory nature of upper respiratory tract infections caused by drug-resistant bacteria has become a major worldwide concern. The elucidation of the immune functions of the tonsils and mucosal membranes of the upper respiratory tract is considered to have important significance. The tonsils are also considered to play an important role as one of the causes of sleep apnea syndrome, and have been reported to be intimately involved in the manifestation of IgA nephropathy and palmoplantar pustulosis, a kind of skin disorder. Interest has continued to grow in this symposium with each session ever since it was first held in Kyoto, Japan in 1987. Since then, the symposium has been held every 3–4 years; in Pavia in 1991, in Sapporo in 1995, in Ghent in 1999, in Wakayama in 2003, and in Siena in 2006. Since the 5th symposium in Wakayama, the topics were extended to mucosal barriers of upper airways including the mucosal immune system, innate immunity, and mucosal vaccine. Recent fine technologies and information on molecular biological approaches for upper airways will continue to advance our understanding of epidemiology, etiology, pathogenesis, diagnosis and management of tonsil-related disorders and various upper respiratory tract infections such as otitis media and rhinosinusitis. Moreover, in the era of drug-resistant microbes, we should exert more effort to develop powerful and effective mucosal vaccines against pathogens in upper airways.

The palatine and nasopharyngeal tonsils (adenoids) are lymphoepithelial tissues located in strategic anatomical areas of the oral pharynx and nasopharynx. These immunocompetent tissues represent the first line of defense against ingested or inhaled foreign proteins such as bacteria, viruses or food antigens. Accompanying the advances being made in the field of medicine today, the role of the tonsils in immunocompetence is becoming extremely important.

Upper respiratory tract infections such as acute otitis media, acute rhinosinusitis and acute pharyngo-tonsillitis are diseases that occur with extremely high frequency, and the antimicrobial agents used to treat these diseases account for a large proportion of health care costs. The increasingly refractory nature of upper respiratory tract infections caused by drug-resistant bacteria has been becoming a major worldwide concern. The elucidation of the immune functions of the tonsils and mucosal membranes of the upper respiratory tract is considered to have important significance.

The tonsils are also considered to play an important role as one of the causes of sleep apnea syndrome, and have been reported to be intimately involved in the manifestation of IgA nephropathy and palmoplantar pustulosis, a kind of skin disorder. Interest has continued to grow in this symposium with each session ever since it was first held in Kyoto, Japan in 1987. Since then, the symposium has been held every 3–4 years, in Pavia in 1991, in Sapporo in 1995, in Ghent in 1999, in Wakayama in 2003, and in Siena in 2006. Since the 5th symposium in Wakayama, the topics were extended to mucosal barriers of upper airways including mucosal immune system, innate immunity, mucosal vaccine, and so on. In every symposium, a prestigious scientific committee and faculty of invited speakers and young scientists treated the main topics in different areas and have brought a tremendous achievement to this field.

Topics in Microbiology of Upper Airways

Bacterial Density of Streptococcus pneumoniae in the Nasopharynx of Children

The nasopharyngeal bacterial flora establishes during the first year of life in children [1–3]. The nasopharynx is then densely colonized with a broad array of microorganisms including commensal bacteria as well as potential pathogens. *S. pneumoniae* is one of the normal inhabitants in the human nasopharynx and also becomes a causative pathogen responsible for upper respiratory infections (URIs) including acute otitis media (AOM) and acute rhinosinusitis (ARS). *S. pneumoniae* colonizes as many as 54% of children by 1 year of age [2]. However, the colonization with pneumococci is asymptomatic in most cases. When the mucosal defence is deteriorated by viral infections, the pathogen may invade adjacent sites such as middle ear cavity or paranasal sinuses causing AOM or ARS, respectively. The presence of *S. pneumoniae* in the nasopharynx will be dramatically changed during the clinical course of URIs. An increase of pneumococci and a parallel decrease of commensal flora in the nasopharynx are found during episodes of AOM among children younger than 3 years of age [4]. In addition, pneumococcal colonization causes horizontal spread of this pathogen in children attending day-care centers and among siblings. Although a few data are available on age-related changes of pneumococcal colonization and serotype distribution of *S. pneumoniae* among healthy children, quantitative changes in bacterial load may reflect the maintenance of nasopharyngeal colonization with pneumococci and the development of URIs.

We investigated the differences of nasopharyngeal density of *S. pneumoniae* between children with URIs and healthy children. In this study, not only the detection rates of *S. pneumoniae* but also the density of *S. pneumoniae* in the nasopharynx was increased in children with URIs (fig. 1). Faden et al. [4] reported the increasing prevalence of causative pathogens in the nasopharynx during episodes of AOM. *S. pneumoniae* carriage during healthy conditions was reported to be lower at 13–43% compared to those at 97–100% during pneumococcal AOM episodes. The heavy colonization by potential pathogens in the nasopharynx is associated with the high incidence of AOM among children.

Thus, quantitative changes in nasopharyngeal colonization by pneumococci would reflect a development of URIs.

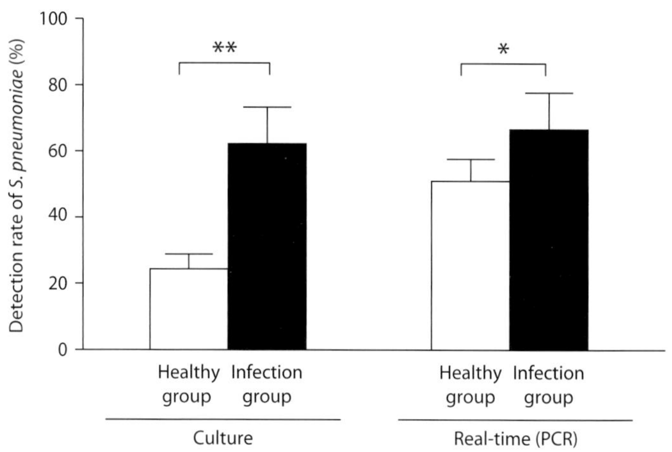

Fig. 1. Differences in nasopharyngeal colonization of pneumococci between the healthy group and the infection group. ** $p < 0.01$ and * $p < 0.05$ by Fisher's exact test.

Distribution of Fibronectin-Binding Protein Genes and Streptococcal Pyrogenic Exotoxins Genes among Streptococcus pyogenes in Japan

S. pyogenes is a major etiological agent causing various infectious diseases among both noninvasive diseases such as acute otitis media (AOM) and pharyngo-tonsillitis and invasive diseases such as toxic shock syndrome, bacteremia, arthritis, rheumatic fever, and necrotizing fasciitis [5]. Although *S. pyogenes* has long been considered an extracellular pathogen that adheres to human mucosal epithelium, some isolates possess an invasive capacity for cultured human epithelial cells [6]. Penicillins were reported to fail to eradicate *S. pyogenes* in up to 30% of patients with pharyngo-tonsillitis. Intracellular localization of *S. pyogenes* is a good explanation for the antimicrobial treatment failures of *S. pyogenes* infections [7].

Surface proteins have been considered as virulence factors of *S. pyogenes* and more than a dozen surface proteins may be involved in adherence and intracellular invasion of this pathogen. Fibronectin-binding proteins encoded by *prtF1* and *prtF2* genes have been shown to be important adhesins for binding to the extracellular matrix of respiratory epithelial cells that result in promoting entry of *S. pyogenes* into the cells. Although the *prtF1* gene was shown to be prevalent among *S. pyogenes* strains persisting among asymptomatic carriers, a recent study showed no association between the *prtF1* gene and source of isolates such as invasive disease and throat swabs from asymptomatic carriers. In Japan, about 77.3% of *S. pyogenes* isolates from throat swabs of patients with pharyngitis were reported to harbor the *prtF1* gene. Prevalence of the *prtF2* gene was also not different among strains from both sources. Streptococcus pyrogenic exotoxins, a family of highly mitogenic proteins encoded by *spe* genes, were secreted by a vast majority of *S. pyogenes,* have very potent activities as super antigens, and play key roles in the disease manifestation [8].

Binding to extracellular matrix proteins supports the persistent colonization of *S. pyogenes* on mucosal surfaces. The *prtF1* gene was highly identified at 77.3% in strains from patients with pharyngitis [8]. The proportion of isolates carrying the *prtF1* gene is higher among strains from noninvasive infections than strains from invasive infections in our study (table 1), although the prevalence of isolates with *prtF1* gene among strains from invasive infections varied between 50 and 65% in other studies. In contrast, the carriage rate of the *prtF2* gene was comparable to the proportion generally reported by other studies. The isolates carrying *prtF1* and *prtF2* genes simultaneously were prevalent among strains from noninvasive infections than strains from invasive infections. The genomic analysis for *prtF1* and *prtF2* genes showed that both genes inherited either within a potential pathogenicity island in the serotype M12 or at another loci of the genome of serotypes M3 and M18 as a potential consequence of genome-scale recombination events. The isolates with *prtF1* gene form noninvasive infections had more repeats than the isolates from invasive infections. However, the repeat numbers in the *prtF1* gene was unrelated to the ability to bind fibronectin. Repeat variations may alter *S. pyogenes* to escape the immune system during binding to epithelial cells such as the repeat variations in M-protein of *emm* type 6. Furthermore, *S. pyogenes* isolates harboring *speA*, and *speZ* were more frequent among strains without *prtF1* and *prtF2* genes, as opposite of *speC*. The streptococcal pyrogenic exotoxins cause potent inflammatory responses and tissue damage. The *speA* or *smeZ* were considered to be correlated with the development of severe complications of diseases. In contrast, there is no difference regarding the distribution *sil* gene among *prtF1*- and *prtF2*-positive isolates. These finding suggested that the *prtF1* and *prtF2* genes may mainly contribute to binding of *S. pyogenes* to the extracellular matrix of host cell rather than disease complications. Although a previous study supported that internalization has a potential role in the early stages of invasive diseases, recent studies have demonstrated that invasive isolates internalized less efficiently than strains derived from patients with skin or throat infections. However, the biological significance of internalization of *S. pyogenes* is not clear. The strains bearing *prtF1* and/or *prtF2* gene might be better colonizers of the human host.

Internalization of Nontypeable Haemophilus influenzae into Epithelial Cells Plays an Important Role in Prolonged and Recurrent Respiratory Infections
H. influenzae is a common commensal organism of the human nasopharynx [9, 10]. The bacterium also becomes an important causative pathogen for both localized and systemic invasive infectious diseases [11]. Nonencapsulated, nontypeable *H. influenzae* (NTHi) accounts for the majority of localized infectious disease including otitis media, sinusitis, bronchitis, and conjunctivitis, while encapsulated serotype B strains are responsible for over 95% of invasive diseases such as septicemia and meningitis [12, 13].

It is widely recognized that the diseases caused by *H. influenzae* begin with the colonization on the nasopharyneal epithelium followed by either contiguous spread within the respiratory tract or invasion of the bloodstream. Although several factors are responsible for nasopharyngeal colonization, the characteristics of *H. influenzae* that promote its survival in the nasopharynx remain poorly defined. Intimate association of NTHi with respiratory tract epithelia might be a necessary prerequisite factor for infection. Following their adhesion onto epithelial cells, some NTHi can internalize into epithelial cells in vitro, although the pathogen has been traditionally regarded as an extracellular bacterium [14, 15]. The ability of NTHi to internalize into epithelial cells by micropinocytosis has been reported [16–18]. In addition, NTHi adheres to and enters into the human bronchial epithelial cells via the interaction of lipo-oligosaccharides with platelet-activating factor [19]. Furthermore, NTHi resides and multiplies intracellularly in macrophage-like cells found in human adenoid tissue [20].

The relatively high frequency of persistent infections, occurring in spite of intensive therapy, would be consistent with the notion that NTHi could facultatively exist intracellularly and thereby evade both host defenses, in particularly circulating antibodies, and the effects of antibiotic

Table 1. Prevalence of fibronectin-binding protein genes depending on the source of the isolates

Source	Number of isolates	*prtF 1* gene						*prtF 2* gene		
		frequencies of RD2 repeats					total	frequencies of FBRD repeats		
		1	2	3	4	6		1	2	3
Invasive	13	2				0	2 (15.4%)	1	1	1
Noninvasive	259	11	10	10	23	0	54 (20.8%)	4	23	8
Total	272						56 (20.6%)			

treatment. Although most ß-lactams are sensitive to extracellular bacterium, these antimicrobial reagents do not transport into the cytoplasm [15]. Azithromycin shows better phagocytic penetration and transport into cells [21–23]. Thus, the antibiotic azithromycin still remains attractive for the treatment of intracellular pathogens like NTHi.

We attempted to gain insight into the mechanisms by which *H. influenzae* attaches to and persists within the nasopharynx. We examined the interactions between clinical isolates of *H. influenzae* from acute otitis media (AOM) patients and cultured human epithelial cells. In the process, we evaluated the invasion and transcytosis of NTHi into human epithelial cells and also used in vitro adherence and internalization models to study the bacteriological efficacy of azithromycin against NTHi under a variety of conditions. A small number of NTHi were capable of entering into the epithelial cells. Pictures taken via SEM, TEM and CLSM showed internalization of NTHi into epithelial cells by the process of micropinocytosis (fig. 2). The number of surface antigens associated with the adherence of NTHi to epithelial cells has been reported, however, less information is available concerning changes in antimicrobial susceptibilities relative to the adherence of bacteria to the epithelial cells. Although ceftriaxone, which is frequently prescribed for treatment of respiratory tract infections, has been shown to exhibit bactericidal efficacy against NTHi in vitro, the antimicrobial reagent could not kill the NTHi associated with HEp-2 cells (fig. 3a, 4). In contrast to these antibiotics, azithromycin can kill both cell-associated and planktonic NTHi (fig. 3b, 4). The following two probabilities can help explain how NTHi evades antimicrobial killing.

Our study showed a wide spectrum in the level of NTHi adherence, internalization and penetration. The possibility that NTHi could enter mammalian cells and thereby escape the local immune system suggests that the host cells act as a reservoir for NTHi. This might be a feasible explanation for the recurrent or prolonged clinical course of infections with NTHi that are typical in some patients. Azithromycin showed a marked bacteriological efficacy in that had NTHi adhered to, internalized into, and penetrated through cultured human epithelial cells. These data suggested that azithromycin might be therapeutically significant against prolonged respiratory tract infections due to NTHi.

Novel Scoring System for the Management of Acute Pharyngo-Tonsillitis [24]

Sore throat is one of the commonest respiratory symptoms in general practice and the vast majority of adults presenting sore throat have acute pharyngitis. Acute tonsillitis also accompanies

	prtF 1 and *prtF 2* genes									Absent
	prtF 1 gene					*prtF 2* gene				
total	frequencies of RD2 repeats					frequencies of FBRD repeats			total	
	1	2	3	4	6	1	2	3		
3 (23.1%)	2	0	0	0	0	2	0	0	2 (15.4%)	6 (46.2%)
35 (13.5%)	45	24	15	47	0	26	105	0	131 (50.5%)	39 (15.2%)
38 (13.9%)									133 (49.0%)	45 (16.5%)

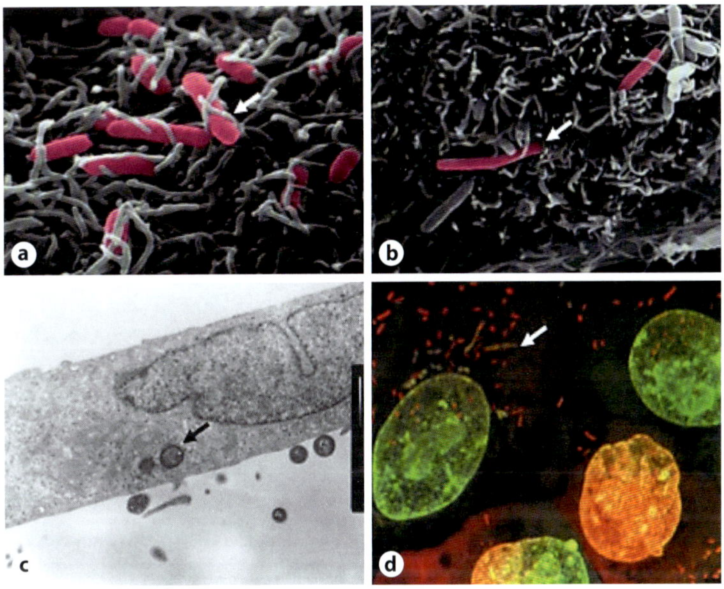

Fig. 2. Interaction of NTHi with HEp-2 cells evaluated by scanning electron microscopy, transmission electron microscopy, and confocal laser scanning microscopy. **a, b** Scanning electron microscopy. **c** Transmission electron microscopy. **d** Confocal laser scanning microscopy.

acute pharyngitis and is obvious from the typical appearance of the tonsils as crypts studded with purulent material or purulent exudations covering the palatine tonsils [26, 27].

The management of acute pharyngo-tonsillitis is an important issue for quality of care because this infectious disease is frequent in the outpatients setting. Most cases are caused by viral infections and are self-limiting only by symptomatic treatment. Approximately 5–15% of cases in adults are caused by *S. pyogenes* and the patients are prescribed antimicrobial agents. In contrast to the rationale of managements for pharyngo-tonsillitis, antibiotics are actually prescribed to a majority of adult patients at approximately 75% [25]. The best way to manage adult patients with pharyngo-tonsillitis is still controversial among countries. Optimal management depends on both the

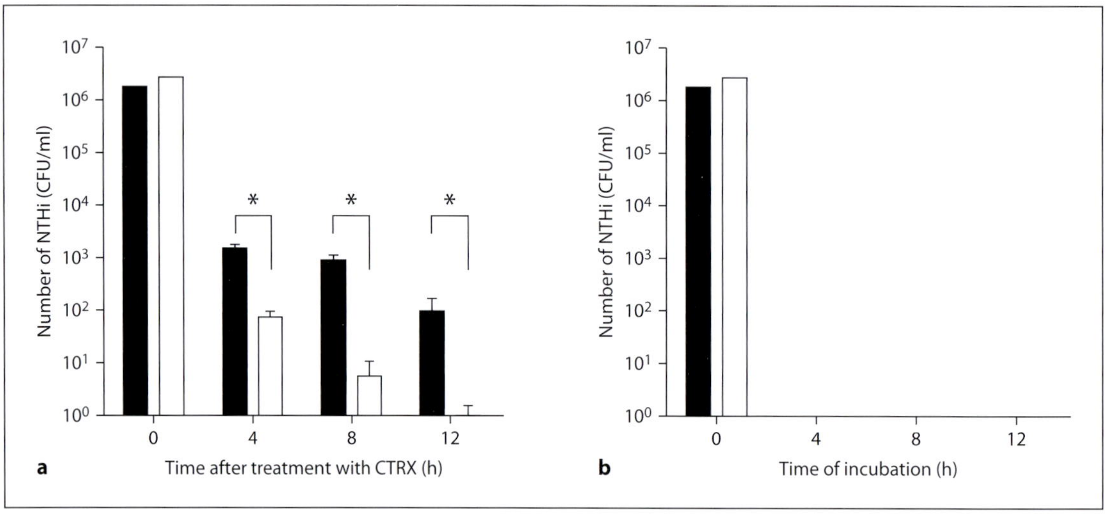

Fig. 3. **a** Bacteriological effects of antimicorbial agaents on NTHi interacted with HEp-2 cells and planktonic organism. **a** Ceftriaxone (2 × MIC). **b** Azithromycin (1 × MIC).

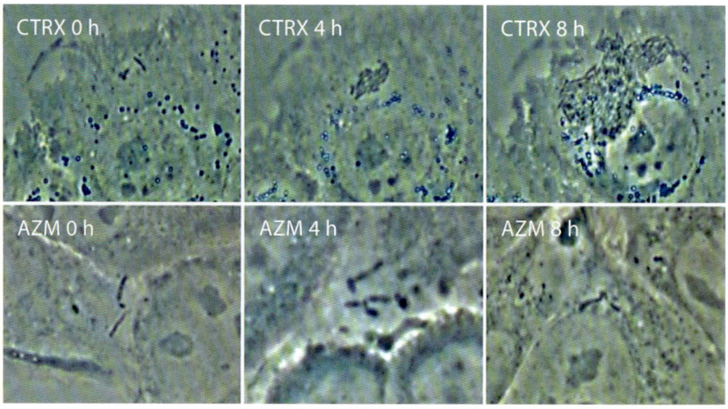

Fig. 4. Morphological changes of NTHi adhered to and internalized into HEp-2 cells after the treatment with antimicrobial agents. Upper picture: ceftriaxone (CTRX); lower picture: azithromycin (AZM).

clinical likelihood of infections with *S. pyogenes* and the relative importance assigned to the criteria to avoid overuse and/or underuse of antibiotics to prevent complications. It is important to develop a clinical scoring system that is easy to use and to assess accurate clinical features of acute pharyngo-tonsillitis with special emphasis on infections with *S. pyogenes* in adults [26, 27].

We organized a nationwide prospective surveillance study group (Pharyngo-tonsillitis Study Group: PhaTONS) in Japan during 2004 to 2005. The aims of this prospective study were to evaluate the causative pathogens of adult acute pharyngo-tonsillitis in comparison with clinical features. An appropriate scoring system was also developed and applied for evaluating severities and clinical course of acute pharyngo-tonsillitis.

Determinations of infections due to *S. pyogenes* have been an important issue for studying acute pharyngo-tonsillitis. Several clinical findings have a discriminative value in distinguishing

Table 2. A Clinical scoring system for acute pharyngo-tonsillitis

	Clinical scores		
	0	1	2
Symptoms			
Difficulties in daily life	not so annoying	annoying, but can work	absence from work
Sore throat/swallowing pain	discomfort	sore, but can swallow	difficult to swallow
Fever	<37.5°C	37.6–38.5°C	<38.6°C
Pharyngo–tonsillar findings			
Pharyngeal erythema or swelling	mild	moderate	marked
Tonsillar erythema or swelling	mild	moderate	marked
Presence of exudates or plugs in tonsils	none	scattered	whole tonsil

S. pyogenes from other causes of acute pharyngo-tonsillitis. The ability of experienced physicians to predict positive throat cultures of *S. pyogenes* is moderate with estimated sensitivity and specificity in the range of 55–74 and 58–76%, respectively. In an attempt to improve clinical sensitivity and specificity, investigators have developed clinical decision rules based on constellation of physical signs and symptoms. The Centor score has been the most reliable predictor for estimating the likelihood of infections of *S. pyogenes* in a patients presenting with sore throat [27]. The score is calculated by determining how many of the following four clinical features are present: history of fever, tonsillar exudates, anterior cervical adenopathy, and absence of cough. In the usual clinical setting, the majority of primary care physicians prescribe antimicrobial agents and painkillers based on the severity of illness. Although the Center score is useful to infer *S. pyogenes*, the score is not valuable for diagnosis of the severity of the illness. A rapid antigen detection kit for *S. pyogenes* using a latex agglutination method is also applied to determine infections with *S. pyogenes*. The test showed a negative predicting value at 95% and a relatively lower positive predicting value at 62%. There has been a general consensus that negative rapid antigen tests for *S. pyogenes* GAS (group a Streptococcus) should be confirmed by the culture test. However, recent guidelines have suggested that confirmation of negative rapid antigen test results for *S. pyogenes* GAS in adults is either not necessary or only needed if the sensitivity of the rapid antigen test is <80%. The rapid antigen test has a lower sensitivity compared to a well-performed culture. Therefore, the importance of rapid identification of *S. pyogenes* is still controversial.

We applied a scoring system based on symptoms and clinical findings to diagnose the severity of acute pharyngo-tonsillitis (table 2). The scoring system reflected that severities of illness correlated well with number of WBCs and CRP levels. Although we could not find any correlations between identification of *S. pyogenes* detected in 13.6% and severity of disease, identification of *S. pyogenes* clearly correlated with number of WBCs (fig. 5) and CRP levels (fig. 6). Regarding antibiotic treatment, it is important to discriminate causative agents such as bacterial and/or virus infection in acute pharyngo-tonsillitis. However, it is sometimes difficult to discriminate them in the usual clinical setting. The current study was also designed to evaluate correlation among clinical parameters such as clinical scores, WBC, and CRP. Viruses were identified in only 21 (9.8%) patients and there was no correlation between

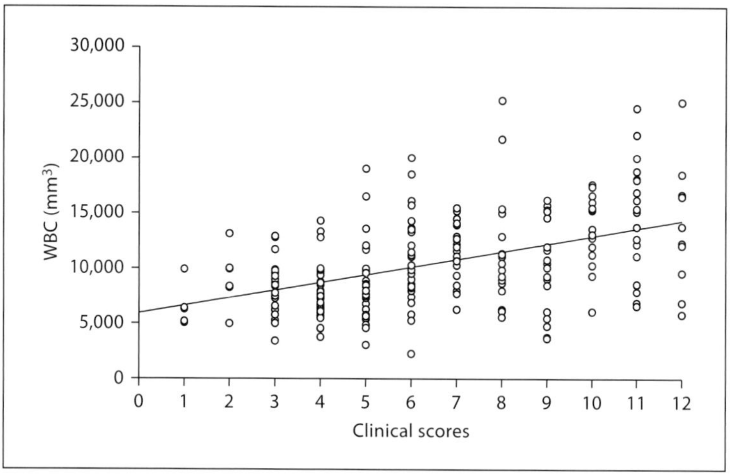

Fig. 5. Correlation between number of white blood counts and PhaTONS score.

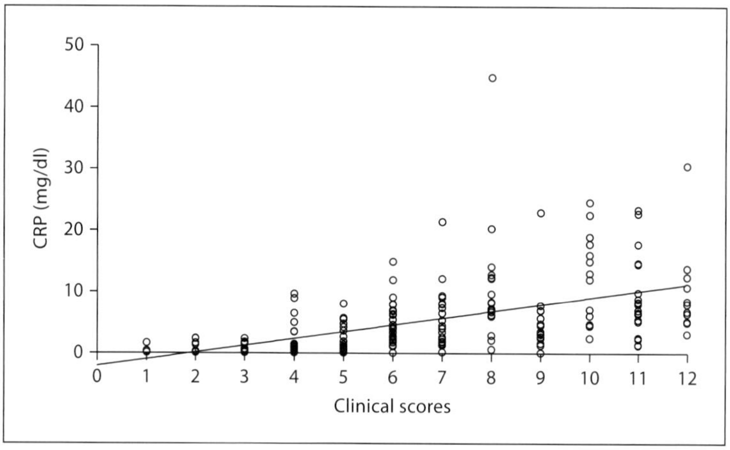

Fig. 6. Correlation between serum levels of CRP and PhaTONS score β.

identification of viruses and number of WBCs or CRP levels. In contrast, the number of total WBCs and the CRP levels at the first visit were significantly higher in cases with *S. pyogenes,* indicating the importance of *S. pyogenes* as the causative pathogen for acute pharyngo-tonsillitis. Thus, the clinical scoring system and blood test could discriminate the possible bacterial infections from virus infections. The current findings strongly suggest that the clinical scoring system will be valuable to determine the severity of the disease.

Tonsillar Focal Infections: An Autoimmune Disease Related to Tonsils

Pustulosis palmaris et plantaris (PPP) is an intractable chronic disease of the skin that causes pustules, erythema, and cornification of the palms of the hands and the soles of the feet. Andrews and colleagues first reported the success of tonsillectomy in treating PPP in 1935. The effectiveness of tonsillectomy on this skin disease has since been reported, and this procedure has become the first-line of therapy for PPP in Japan [28–31]. Based on those

Table 3. Pathogens identified in PhaTONS study

Pathogens		Numbers of isolates/cases	%
Bacteria	*S. pyogenes*	29/214	13.6
	Haemolytic streptococci	35/214	16.4
	β-Hemolytic streptococcus	6/214	
	Group C streptococcus	8/214	
	Group G streptococcus	6/214	
	S. agalactiae	11/214	
	H. influenzae	52/214	24.3
	H. haemolyticus	23/214	10.7
	S. pnuemoniae	11/214	5.1
	M. catarrhalis	8/214	3.7
	S. aureus	71/214	33.2
	Others	13/214	6.1
Virus	Adenovirus	10/205	4.9
	Influenza virus	6/205	2.9
	RS virus	2/191	1.0
	Human metapneumo virus	13/206	6.3

findings, many studies proposed focal tonsillar infection in the pathogenesis of PPP. However, a definite conclusion on the immunologic mechanism by which the tonsillar infection causes skin eruption on the hands and feet has yet to be clarified.

Recent progress in molecular immunology has shown evidence on the close relationship between oral cavity infections and chronic systemic diseases. This relation has been explained mainly by molecular mimicry between bacterial and host antigens. Heat shock protein (HSP) is one of the most possible candidates for cross-reactivity and immunologic response in chronic inflammatory diseases.

HSPs exist both in prokaryotic and eukaryotic cells, and physical as well as chemical stress induces their expression in order to protect the cells from lethal damage. Protein structure is highly conserved between different species and microbial flora or pathogenic bacteria in the oral cavity are also shown to have HSPs. The amino acid sequence of HSP65 (GroEL) from *Porphyromonas gingivalis*, Gram-negative anaerobic bacilli residing in the oropharynx, shows a 49% identity to that of human HSP60 [32]. Bacterial HSPs have a highly immunogenic potential to provoke T cell activation and antibody production [33]. The antibodies and T cells against bacterial Hsp60 and Hsp70 also recognize mammalian Hsp60 and Hsp70, respectively, as a result of cross-reactivity [34]. Activation of T cells and anti-Hsp antibodies may cause inflammatory reactions and injury of tissues. Therefore, Hsp60 and Hsp70 have been implicated in the pathogenesis of a number of autoimmune diseases and inflammatory conditions such as Takayasu's arteritis, Kawasaki disease, atherosclerosis, and chronic arthritis.

We developed an experimental animal model for PPP disease [35, 36]. SCID mice were transplanted with skin grafts and tonsillar/blood lymphocytes from PPP patients or control groups. In this model, it is feasible to investigate the role of various parameters on the pathogenesis of PPP including origin of lymphocytes, interaction

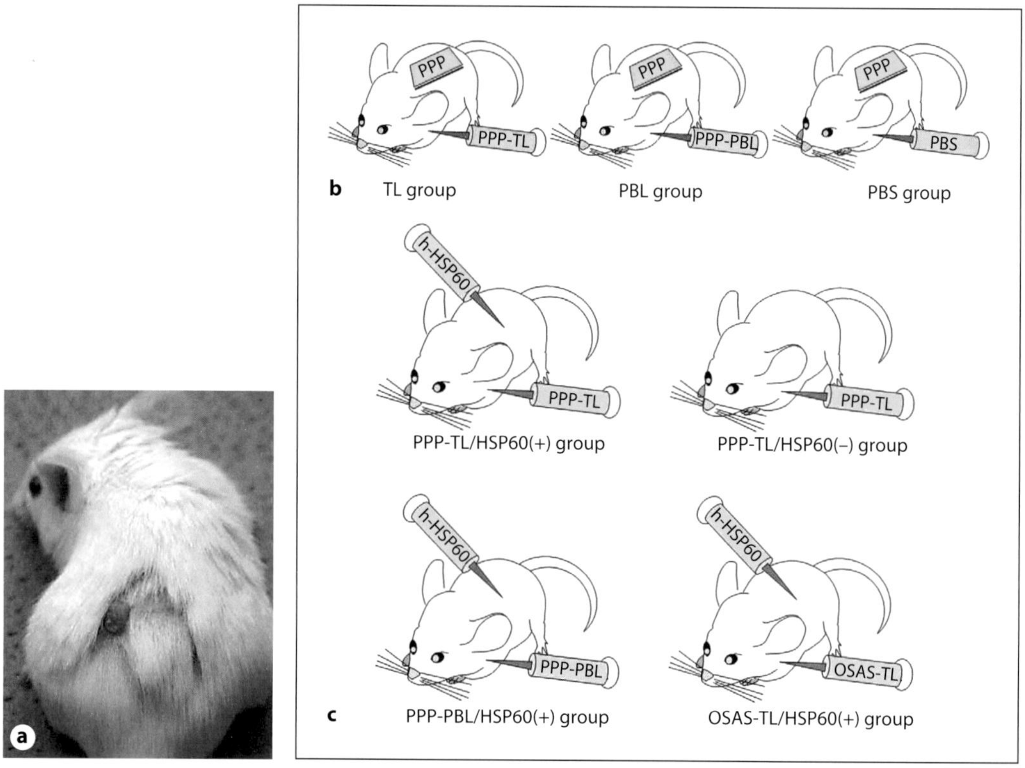

Fig. 7. Establishment of human lymphocyte/PPP skin/SCID mouse chimeras. **a** Final view of skin-grafted SCID mouse after exposure of skin-graft outside. **b** SCID mice groups developed in experiment 1. TL = The group of mice transplanted with tonsillar lymphocytes and skin grafts harvested around the PPP lesions (PPP skin); PBL = the mice group transplanted with peripheral blood lymphocytes and PPP skin; PBS = the control group with PBS injection and PPP-skin grafting. **c** SCID mice groups developed in experiment 4; PPP-TL = the mice group transplanted with tonsillar lymphocytes (TL) of PPP patients with/without HSP60 injection; PPP-PBL =: the mice group transplanted with peripheral blood lymphocytes of PPP patients + HSP60 injection; OSAS-TL = the mice group transplanted with TL of OSAS patients + HSP60 injection.

between lymphocytes, and skin grafts or external antigenic stimulus (fig. 7).

By using that model, we showed that the main source of CD4+ lymphocytes in skin lesions would be palatine tonsil tissue (fig. 8a). Our results are also consistent with those in the previous study of SCID mice model. Takahara et al. [37] displayed expansion of T cell nodules in tonsillar tissues of PPP patients compared with OSAS. These findings indicate the role of the tonsils as secondary lymphoid organs in the immune response related to PPP and may explain the improvement of skin lesions after tonsillectomy in PPP patients.

Previously, the expression level of HSP60 was reported to increase in skin and mucosal lesions of SLE and Behçet's disease, although HSP60 is expressed to some degree in normal skin or mucous membranes of the oral cavity. In this study, we also found a strong expression of HSP60 in the epidermal layer of skin lesions from PPP patients, which implied the role of HSP in the pathogenesis of disease (fig. 8b). We observed that anti-HSP65 antibody levels had a nonsignificant tendency to be

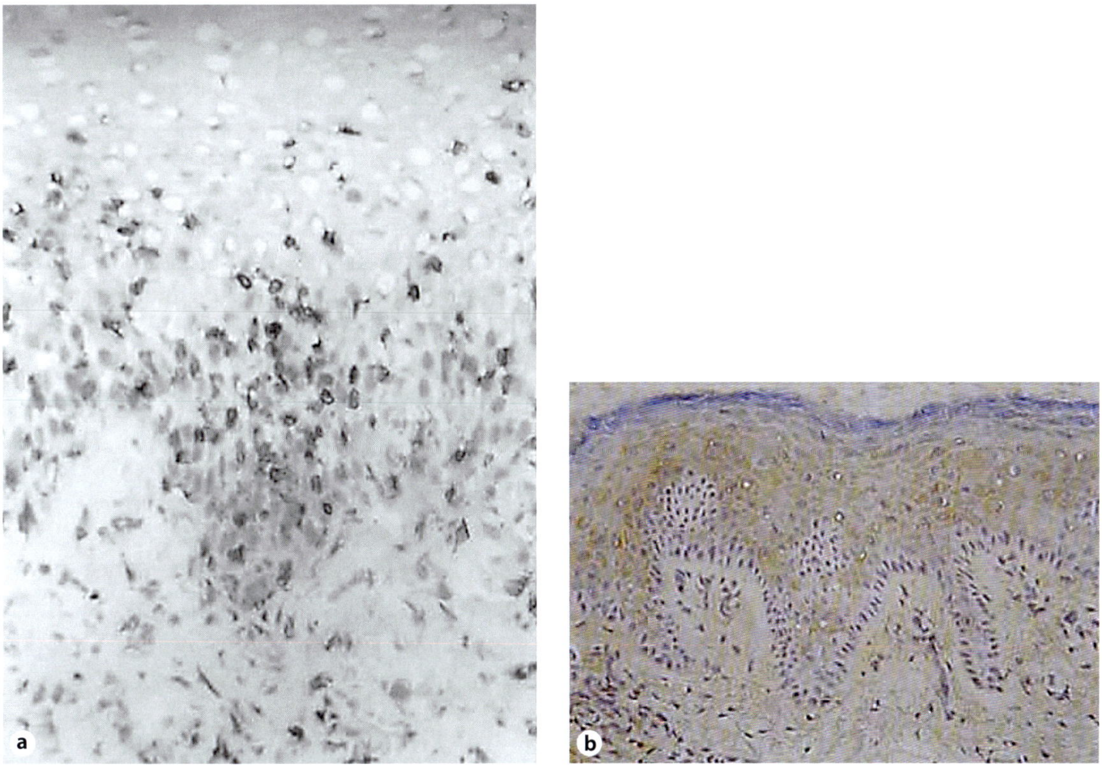

Fig. 8. **a** Immunohistochemical analysis of grafts of TL/PPP skin/SCID mice; CD4+ T lymphocytes infiltrated the area around papillary dermis in great numbers. ×400. **b** Diffuse cytoplasmic immunoreactivity of basal and suprabasal keratinocytes with human HSP60 in the skin graft. ×400.

higher in sera of SCID mice grafted with skin and tonsillar lymphocytes of PPP patients than those grafted with skin and blood lymphocytes. These findings imply that HSP65 antigen expressed by various microbial agents including intraoral flora or pathogens may serve as an antigenic stimulus for T cells of tonsil in PPP. Concerning the relationship between HSPs and PPP, only a few studies exist in the literature. Izaki et al. [38] showed significantly high anti-HSP65 IgG levels in sera of PPP patients with tonsillar or periodontal infection. Another study also observed similar findings and a decrease in anti-HSP65 antibody levels after the treatment of periodontal infection in PPP patients [39].

Interestingly, we found that anti-HSP65 antibody levels in the serum significantly correlated with CD4+ cell infiltration in the skin grafts of TL/PPP skin SCID mice. Furthermore, anti-HSP65 antibody levels showed close correlation to IL-6 and IFN-γ levels in sera of the same SCID mice group. These results are in accordance with immunologic characteristics of HSP, which are potent activators of the innate immune system and are capable of inducing the production of pro-inflammatory cytokines. All these findings indicate the active role of anti-HSP65 antibodies in the inflammation process of PPP.

Finally, it is important to clarify whether self HSP60 plays a role as an antigenic target in PPP. When we injected recombinant human HSP60 in SCID mice transplanted with TL, anti-HSP65 antibody levels were significantly higher compared to the control group without the HSP60 stimulation. These findings may indicate that preactivated tonsillar lymphocytes against bacterial HSP65 could recognize human HSP60 as the same target and shows a reaction as anti-HSP65 antibody production in PPP. Moreover, anti-HSP65 antibody levels were also significantly higher in the group of mice transplanted with tonsillar lymphocytes of PPP patients than those of OSAS patients. These data support our hypothesis that tonsillar lymphocytes but not blood lymphocytes might have been prestimulated with HSP65 from oral bacteria in PPP patients.

In conclusion, we demonstrated that tonsillar lymphocytes have been sensitized by HSP65 from oral bacteria to produce antibodies. Furthermore, we found that human HSP60 was also able to trigger the immune response of these lymphocytes against bacterial HSP65, which may indicate immune cross-reactivity between HSP60/65 in PPP. Future studies focused on cellular and humoral immune responses to specific epitopes of HSP60 and HSP65 would be essential to clarify the exact pathogenesis of PPP.

Conclusions

Recent fine technologies and information on molecular biological approaches for upper airways infections will continue to advance our understanding of the epidemiology, etiology, pathogenesis, diagnosis and management of tonsil-related disorders and various upper respiratory tract infections such as otitis media, rhinosinusitis and pharyngo-tonsillitis. Moreover, in the era of drug-resistant microbes, we should exert more effort to develop powerful and effective mucosal vaccines against pathogens in upper airways. I sincerely hope that the International Symposium on Tonsils and Mucosal Barriers of the Upper Airways will forward a great breakthrough on the pathogenesis of various diseases of the upper airways and contribute tremendously to the development in the prevention, diagnosis and treatment of infectious diseases.

References

1. Ogami M, Hotomi M, Togawa A, Yamanaka N. A comparison of conventional and molecular microbiology in detecting differences in pneumococcal colonization in healthy children and children with upper respiratory illness. Eur J Pediatr 2010;169:1221–1225.
2. Faden H, Duffy L, Williams A, et al: Epidemiology of nasopharyngeal colonization with non typeable *Haemophilus influenzae* in the first two years of life. J Infect Dis 1995;172:132–135.
3. Faden H, Stanievich J, Brodsky L, et al: Changes in nasopharyngeal flora during otitis media of childhood. Pediatr Infect Dis J 1990;9:623–626.
4. Faden H, Waz MJ, Bernstein JM, et al: Nasopharyngeal flora in the first three years of life in normal and otitis-prone children. Ann Otol Rhinol Laryngol 1991;100:612–615.
5. Hotomi M, Billal SD, Togawa A, et al: Distribution of fibronectin-binding genes (prtF1 and prtF2) and streptococcal pyrogenic exotoxin genes (*spe*) among *Streptococcus pyogenes* in Japan. J Infect Chemother 2009;15: 367–373.
6. Bisno AL, Brito MO, Collins CM: Molecular basis of group A streptococcal virulence. Lancet Infet Dis 2003;3:191–200.
7. Hanski E, Caparon M: Protein F, a fibronectin-binding protein, is an adhesion of the group A streptococcus *Streptococcus pyogenes*. Proc Natl Acad Sci USA 1992;89:6172–6176.
8. Schmitz FJ, Beyer A, Charpentier E, et al: Toxin-gene profile heterogeneity among endemic invasive European group A streptococcus isolates. J Infect Dis 2003;188:1578–1586.
9. Hotomi M, Arai J, Billal SD, et al: Non-typeable *Haemophilus influenzae* isolated from intractable acute otitis media internalized into cultured human epithelial cells. Auris Nasus Larynx 2010;37:137–144.
10. Faden H, Duffy L, Williams A, Krystofik DA, Wolf J: Epidemiology of nasopharyngeal colonization with nontypeable *Haemophilus influenzae* in the first 2 years of life. J Infect Dis 1995;172:132–135.
11. Turk DC: The pathogenicity of *Haemophilus influenzae*. J Med Microbiol 1982;18:1–16.
12. Murphy TF, Apicella MA: Nontypeable *Haemophilus influenzae*: a review of clinical aspects, surface antigens and the human response to infection. Rev Infect Dis 1987;9:1–15.

13 Murphy TF: Respiratory infections caused by nontypeable *Haemophilus influenzae*. Curr Opin Infect Dis 2003;16:129–134.
14 St Geme JW III, Falkow S: *Haemophilus influenzae* adhered to and enters cultured human epithelial cells. Infect Immun 1990;58:4036–4044.
15 St Geme JW III: Nontypeable *Haemophilus influenzae* disease: epidemiology, pathogenesis and prospects prevention. Infect Agents Dis 1993;2:1–16.
16 St Geme JW III, Falkow S: Loss of capsule expression by *Haemophilus inlufenzae* type b results in enhanced adherence to and invasion of human cells. Infect Immun 1991;59:1325–1333.
17 Ahren IL, Williams DL, Rice PJ, Forsgren A, Riesbeck K: The importance of a ß-glucan receptor in the nonopsonic entry of nontypeable *Haemophilus influenzae* into human monocytic and epithelial cells. J Infect Dis 2006;184:150–158.
18 Ketterer MR, Shao JQ, Hornick DB, Buscher B, Bandi VK, Apicella MA: Infection of primary human bronchial epithelial cells by *Haemophilus influenzae*: macropinocytosis as a mechanism of airway epithelial cell entry. Infect Immun 1999;67:4161–4170.
19 Swords WE, Ketterer MR, Shao J, Campbell CA, Weiser JN, Apicella MA: Binding of the non-typeable *Haemophilus influenzae* lipooligosaccharide to the PAF receptor initiates host cell signalling. Cell Microbiol 2001;3:525–536.
20 Forsgren J, Samuelson A, Ahlin A, Jonasson J, Rynnel-Dagoo B, Lindberg A: *Haemophilus influenzae* resides and multiplies intracellularly in human adenoid tissue as demonstrated by in situ hybridization and bacterial viability assay. Infect Immun 1994;62:673–679.
21 Wildfeuer A, Laufen H, Zimmermann T: Uptake of azithromycin by various cells and its intracellular activity under in vitro conditions. Antimicrob Agents Chemother 1996;40:75–79.
22 Lode H: The pharmacokinetics of azithromycin and their clinical significance. Eur. J. Clin Microbiol Infect Dis 1991;10:808–812.
23 Alder JD, Ewing PJ, Nilius AM, Mitten M, Tovcimak A, Oleksijew A, Jarvis K, Paige L, Tanaka SK: Dynamics of clarithromycin and azithromycin efficacies against experimental *Haemophilus influenzae* pulmonary infection. Antimicrob Agents Chemother 1998;42:2385–2390.
24 Suzumoto M, Hotomi M, Billal SD, Fujihara K, Harabuchi Y, Yamanaka N: A scoring system for management of acute pharyngo-tonsillitis in adults. Auris Nasus Larynx 2009;36:314–320
25 Bisno AL, Gerber MA, Gwaltney JM, Kaplan EL, Schwartz RH. Practice guidelines for the diagnosis and management of group A streptococcal pharyngitis. Clin Infect Dis 2002;35:113–125.
26 Breese BB: A simple scorecard for the tentative diagnosis of streptococcal pharyngitis. Am J Dis Child 1977;131:514–517.
27 Centor RM, Witherspoon JM, Dalton HP, Brody CE, Link K: The diagnosis of strep throat in adults in the emergency room. Med Decis Making 1981;1:239–249.
28 Hayashi M, Fujihara K, Beder LB, et al: Pathogenic role of tonsillar lymphocytes in associated with HSP60/65 in pustulosis palmaris et plantaris. Auris Nasus Larynx 2009;36:578–585.
29 Yokoyama M, Hashigucci K, Yamasaki Y: Effect of tonsillectomy in patients with pustulosis palmaris et plantaris. Acta Otolaryngol 2004;124:1109–1110.
30 Kuki K, Kimura T, Hayashi Y, Tabata T: Focus tonsils and skin diseases with special reference to palmoplantar pustulosis. Adv Otorhinolaryngol 1992;47: 196–202.
31 Yamanaka N, Shido F, Kataura A: Tonsillectomy-induced changes in antikeratin antibodies in patients with pustulosis palmaris et plantaris: a clinical correlation. Arch Otorhinolaryngol 1989;246:109–112.
32 Hotokezaka H, Hayashida H, Ohara N, et al: Cloning and sequencing of the groESL homologue from *Porphyromonas gingivalis*. Biochim Biophys Acta 1994;1219:175–178.
33 Zugel U, Kaufmann SH: Immune response against heat shock proteins in infectious diseases. Immunobiology 1999;201:22–35.
34 Kiessling R, Gronberg A, Ivanyi J, et al: Role of hsp60 during autoimmune and bacterial inflammation. Immunol Rev 1991;121:91–111.
35 Yamanaka N, Yamamoto Y, Kuki K: Engraftment of tonsillar mononuclear cells in human skin/SCID mouse chimera – validation of a novel xenogeneic transplantation model for autoimmune diseases. Microbiol Immunol 2001;45:507–514.
36 Yamamoto Y, Kuki K, Hayashi Y, Yamanaka N: A study of the pathogenesis of tonsillar focal infection – transplantation of human tonsillar lymphocytes and human skin into SCID mice. Nippon Jibiinkoka Gakkai Kaiho 2000;103:796–802.
37 Takahara M, Kishibe K, Nozawa H, Harabuchi Y: Increase of activated T-cells and up-regulation of Smad7 without elevation of TGF-beta expression in tonsils from patients with pustulosis palmaris et plantaris. Clin Immunol 2005;115:192–199.
38 Izaki S, Goto Y, Kaburagi Y, Kitamura K, Nomaguchi H: Antibody production to heat shock proteins with M_r 65 kD (HSP65) in cutaneous inflammation: a possible relation to focal infection. Acta Otolaryngol Suppl 1996;523:197–200.
39 Ishihara K, Ando T, Kosugi M, et al: Relationships between the onset of pustulosis palmaris et plantaris, periodontitis and bacterial heat shock proteins. Oral Microbiol Immunol 2000;15: 232–237.

Noboru Yamanaka, MD, PhD
Department of Otolaryngology,
Head and Neck Surgery, Wakayama Medical University
811–1 Kimiidera
Wakayama 641-8509 (Japan)
Tel. +81 73 441 0651, E-Mail ynobi@wakayama-med.ac.jp

Harabuchi Y (ed): Recent Advances in Tonsils and Mucosal Barriers of the Upper Airways.
Adv Otorhinolaryngol. Basel, Karger, 2011, vol 72, pp 20–24

Immune Functions of Nasopharyngeal Lymphoid Tissue

Per Brandtzaeg

Laboratory for Immunohistochemistry and Immunopathology, Centre for Immune Regulation, University of Oslo, and Department of Pathology, Oslo University Hospital, Rikshospitalet, Oslo, Norway

Abstract

This brief review will focus on nasopharynx-associated lymphoid tissue as a unique inductive immune site for B cell responses and plasma cell generation. The anatomical and immunological characteristics of Waldeyer's lymphoid ring should make the nasal route for vaccine administration highly relevant in future clinical trials to stimulate both mucosal and systemic immunity. In this context, the potential immunological consequences of removing both the tonsils and the adenoids have to be considered.

The unpaired nasopharyngeal tonsil (also called the adenoids) and the palatine and lingual tonsils constitute most of Waldeyer's ring. These lymphoepithelial structures appear functionally comparable to the nasopharynx-associated lymphoid tissue (NALT) in rodents, which is a lymphoid organ present on both sides of the nasopharyngeal duct dorsal to the cartilaginous soft palate [1, 2]. Waldeyer's ring is strategically located to generate regional immunity because all of its elements are exposed to both airborne and alimentary antigens. However, although Waldeyer's ring functions as part of mucosa-associated lymphoid tissue (MALT), it also shows similarities with lymph nodes and may, in addition, participate as effector organs of local systemic type as well as mucosal secretory type of adaptive humoral immunity.

Activation of B Cells in Germinal Centers

Primary follicles of secondary lymphoid organs such as the tonsils contain mainly recirculating naïve B cells positive for surface IgD and IgM (sIgD+sIgM+) – both co-expressed isotypes exhibiting the same specificity for antigen. Germinal centers (GCs) are hallmarks of secondary follicles generated after stimulation of naïve B cells immediately outside the follicles through cognate help from activated CD4+ T cells [3]. These helper T (T_H) cells have received processed foreign antigen from dendritic cells (DCs) in the context of class II molecules of the major histocompatibility complex (MHC) – in humans also called HLA class II molecules such as HLA-DR. The stimulated B cells can then colonize the follicles and act as 'founder cells' for GCs.

The GCs can be divided into various more or less well-defined morphological compartments [3]. B cell stimulation in the dark zone results in exponential growth revealed by proliferation. The generated centroblasts hypermutate their *Ig V-region* genes and give rise to centrocytes; these cells will die by apoptosis in the light zone unless they are selected by high affinity binding to antigens on the surface of follicular DCs (FDCs). These B cells next take up such antigens and process and present them via HLA class II molecules to follicular T_H (T_{FH}) cells, which can be identified by their high level of CXCR5 expression.

Cognate interaction between T_{FH} cells, which express the costimulatory CD40 ligand (C40L, CD154), and B cells, which express CD40, appears to be an important event in the GC reaction [3]. The same is true for the expression of *bcl-2 gene* products following immune activation of centrocytes to prevent their apoptosis. Indeed, if the CD40L–CD40 interaction is experimentally blocked, GCs are not formed. Importantly, this costimulatory interaction promotes switching of the Ig heavy chain constant *(C_H) genes* of B cells from C_μ (IgM) to downstream isotypes, as well as differentiation to plasmablasts and plasma cells (PCs) producing high-affinity antibody. A prerequisite for cognate interaction between B and T_{FH} cells, is that the former express costimulatory B7 (CD80/CD86) molecules, which can bind to the CD28 receptor on T cells. Classical memory B cells (sIgD–sIgM+) with strong B7 expression are also found extrafollicularly related to the crypt epithelium where they also may exert an antigen-presenting function.

Expression of the *J-chain gene* occurs in a variable subset of tonsillar plasmablasts [4]. This gene encodes a 15-kDa peptide, the J (joining) chain, which is a crucial structural part of dimers and trimers of IgA (collectively called polymeric IgA, pIgA) as well as pentameric IgM. The J chain facilitates the binding of pIgs to the epithelial pIg receptor (pIgR), also called membrane secretory component (SC). The pIg-pIgR interaction is a central step in the formation and export of secretory IgA (SIgA) and secretory IgM (SIgM) antibodies [5].

Induction of Secretory Immunity in Tonsils

The cytokine profiles and other microenvironmental factors determining isotype differentiation and coexpression of J chain in B cells remain obscure [3]; it appears that clonal maturation in the course of several proliferative cycles results in reduced J-chain expression, thus promoting monomer production by IgA+ PCs. Whereas downstream *C_H gene* switching in GCs of healthy tonsils gives rise to a relatively high fraction of extrafollicular IgA+J-chain+ PCs (~50% of total IgA+ PCs), most extrafollicular IgG+ PCs show little or no J-chain expression (~2%). The fact that tonsillar IgA+ PCs are mainly of the IgA1 isotype (at least >95%), along with the presence of relatively many IgD+ PCs, supports the notion that tonsillar B cell differentiation takes place mainly through classical downstream *C_H gene* switching together with some nonclassical switching to IgD [6].

It may be envisioned that only a fraction of the pIgA-expressing plasmablasts that exit from GCs, will terminate their differentiation as extrafollicular PCs; instead, many of them may home to regional secretory effector sites for terminal differentiation to pIgA-producing PCs there (fig. 1). The adenoids possess, in addition, a local secretory immune system because patches of the crypt epithelium express pIgR/SC [2]. This is not the case in the palatine tonsils where only passive paracellular transfer of IgG and IgA takes place through the reticular crypt epithelium. Because this epithelium is of squamous type in the palatine tonsils, it is additionally protected by its production of the antimicrobial peptide calprotectin [7]. Therefore, topical surface protection differs between the two lymphoid organs.

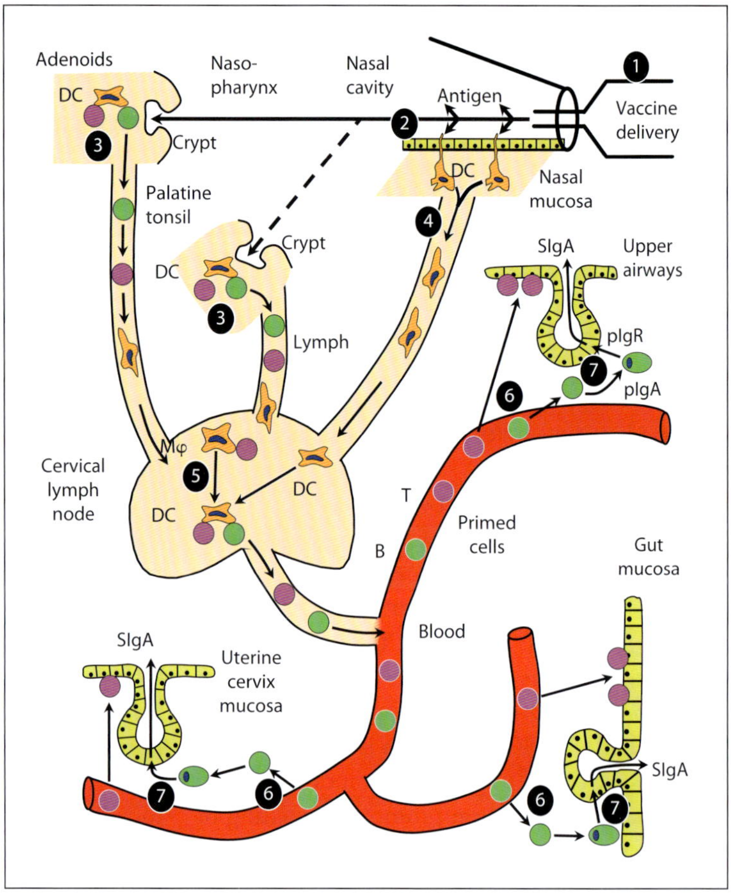

Fig. 1. Model for T (violet) and B (green) cell induction after nasal vaccine administration, followed by generation of secretory IgA (SIgA) antibodies. (1) Delivery device for nasal vaccine administration (nasal spray, drops or OptiMist®). (2) Adjuvanted uptake of vaccine antigen through nasal mucosa. (3) Immune induction in adenoids and palatine tonsils (human NALT). (4) Antigen targeting and migration of mucosal dendritic cells (DCs). (5) Immune induction and amplification in regional (cervical) lymph nodes. (6) Compartmentalized homing/extravasation of NALT-induced T and B cells to secretory effector sites in airways, gut and uterine cervix. (7) Epithelial expression of polymeric Ig receptor (pIgR) mediating external transport of dimeric IgA (pIgA) to generate SIgA. As discussed in the text, NALT-derived B cells preferentially extravasate at regional effector sites and in systemic lymphoid organs, while showing only poor homing capacity for the small intestinal lamina propria.

Dissemination of Activated Tonsillar B Cells

Nasal and bronchial mucosae, as well as salivary and lacrimal glands, contain an IgA1+ and IgD+ PC distribution similar to that of the extrafollicular tonsillar compartment [3, 8]. This fact supports the notion that regional secretory tissues are seeded by GC-derived B cell blasts from Waldeyer's ring [6, 7]. Its immune-inductive function would hence be similar to that of rodent NALT [1]. A possible minor blast contribution to the airways from bronchus-associated lymphoid tissue (BALT) remains uncertain, because organized lymphoid follicles do not regularly exist in the healthy human lung [8]. It has also been documented in many studies that nasal immunization of humans induces specific IgA antibodies in nasopharyngeal secretions, in addition to enhancing systemic immunity [3].

Attempts have been made to track directly the dissemination of B cell blasts from Waldeyer's ring by means of molecular markers. Using a DNA marker, namely a deletion of the IgM C_H *gene*, we showed that activated tonsillar B cells undergoing a so-called nonclassical switch to IgD+J-chain+ plasmablasts preferentially home through cervical lymph nodes to the upper airways and associated glands [9]. The extravasation of activated memory/effector B and T cells into effector tissues takes place through the local microvascular endothelium and is controlled in a site-specific manner [8]. This process is better defined for the intestinal lamina propria than for other secretory tissues. Thus, a B-cell homing dichotomy between the gut and the upper aerodigestive tract has a molecular basis in terms of adhesion molecules and chemokines. Endothelial MAdCAM-1 is expressed throughout the gut lamina propria, where it binds gut-associated lymphoid tissue (GALT)-derived memory/effector T and B cell blasts with high surface levels of the integrin α4β7 [3].

Homing to the small intestine is, in addition, determined by the chemokine receptor CCR9 which interacts with its ligand TECK (CCL25) produced preferentially by the epithelium in that part of the gut. Conversely, homing to the colonic lamina propria is fine-tuned by CCR10 interacting with MEC (CCL25). The latter molecular pair is apparently also important for homing of tonsillar B cell blasts to the upper airway mucosa [8, 9]. These cells show poor gut-homing properties due to low levels of surface α4β7 but express, instead, CD62L (L-selectin). This adhesion molecule enables such NALT-derived cells to enter not only regional secretory tissues related to the airways but also peripheral lymph nodes and to some extent the uterine cervix mucosa [3, 9]. Integration of mucosal immunity induced in Waldeyer's ring with systemic immunity is further enhanced by the expression of CD62L and CCR7 on tonsillar B cell blasts.

Effect of Adenotonsillectomy on Immunity

The above information provides strong support for the notion that Waldeyer's ring functions as inductive NALT in humans and supply secretory effector sites of the upper aerodigestive region with activated pIgA precursor cells (fig. 1). To evaluate clinically this notion, it is important to study the effect of adenotonsillectomy on the regional SIgA levels. The pioneer report by Ogra [10] showed that combined tonsillectomy and adenoidectomy in children reduced the level of IgA antibody to poliovirus 3- to 4-fold in their nasopharyngeal secretions and delayed or abrogated their local SIgA response to subsequent live oral poliovaccine. Notably, however, this result could merely have reflected the abolished local secretory immune function due to removal of the adenoids rather than lack of regional immune-inductive capacity after the operation.

There is a need for more extensive immunological studies focusing collectively on the adenoids and palatine tonsils. Considerable redundancy of inductive lymphoid tissue in Waldeyer's ring might mask a potentially unwanted immunological effect of adenotonsillectomy. This possibility is supported by studies that have reported reduced SIgA levels in saliva from children with pharyngitis involving recurrent tonsillitis or adenoid hyperplasia, perhaps reflecting decreased global pIgA induction in Waldeyer's ring due to inflammation-induced downregulation of J-chain expression as seen in recurrent tonsillitis [11].

Nasal Vaccination

The potential advantage of nasal immunization is illustrated by the protection achieved against influenza. Many studies in experimental animals and humans have demonstrated that nasal vaccination gives rise to cross-protection against drifted influenza virus strains. With an available live attenuated influenza vaccine for intranasal administration (FluMist), good protection was achieved despite the fact that the epidemic strain was not part of the vaccine [12].

Recent reports have documented the efficacy and effectiveness of the trivalent, live attenuated nasal spray influenza vaccine (CAIV-T), both in healthy children and adults. Although nasal vaccination also efficiently induces systemic immunity, a combination of intranasal and parenteral immunization may be preferable for optimal protection when an inactivated influenza vaccine is used [12]. Alternatively, the effect of subunit vaccines applied topically can be enhanced by incorporation into liposomes or with the addition of a nontoxic mucosal adjuvant such as Eurocine®.

References

1 Fukuyama S, Hiroi T, Yokota Y, Rennert PD, Yanagita M, Kinoshita N, Terawaki S, Shikina T, Yamamoto M, Kurono Y, Kiyono H: Initiation of NALT organogenesis is independent of the IL-7R, LTβR, and NIK signaling pathways but requires the Id2 gene and CD3–CD4+CD45+ cells. Immunity 2002;17:31–40.

2 Brandtzaeg P: Immune functions and immunopathology of palatine and nasopharyngeal tonsils; in Bernstein JM, Ogra PL (eds): Immunology of the Ear. New York, Raven Press, 1987, pp 63–106.

3 Brandtzaeg P, Johansen F-E: Mucosal B cells: phenotypic characteristics, transcriptional regulation, and homing properties. Immunol Rev 2005;206:32–63.

4 Korsrud FR, Brandtzaeg P: Immunohistochemical evaluation of J-chain expression by intra- and extra-follicular immunoglobulin-producing human tonsillar cells. Scand J Immunol 1981;13:271–280.

5 Brandtzaeg P, Prydz H: Direct evidence for an integrated function of J chain and secretory component in epithelial transport of immunoglobulins. Nature 1984;311:71–73.

6 Brandtzaeg P, Baekkevold ES, Farstad IN, Jahnsen FL, Johansen F-E, Nilsen EM, Yamanaka T: Regional specialization in the mucosal immune system: what happens in the microcompartments? Immunol Today 1999;20:141–151.

7 Brandtzaeg P: Immunological functions of adenoids; in van Cauwenberge P, Wang D-Y, Ingels K, Bachert C (eds): The Nose. The Hague, Kugler Publications, 1998, pp 233–246.

8 Brandtzaeg P: Function of mucosa-associated lymphoid tissue in antibody formation. Immunol Invest 2010;39:303–355.

9 Johansen F-E, Baekkevold ES, Carlsen HS, Farstad IN, Soler D, Brandtzaeg P: Regional induction of adhesion molecules and chemokine receptors explains disparate homing of human B cells to systemic and mucosal effector sites: dispersion from tonsils. Blood 2005;106:593–600.

10 Ogra PL: Effect of tonsillectomy and adenoidectomy on nasopharyngeal antibody response to poliovirus. N Engl J Med 1971;284:59–64.

11 Korsrud FR, Brandtzaeg P: Influence of tonsillar disease on the expression of J-chain by immunoglobulin-producing cells in human palatine and nasopharyngeal tonsils. Scand J Immunol 1981;13:281–287.

12 Brandtzaeg P: Induction of secretory immunity and memory at mucosal surfaces. Vaccine 2007;25:5467–5484.

Prof. Per Brandtzaeg
Department of Pathology, Oslo University Hospital, Rikshospitalet
PO Box 4950 Nydalen
NO–0424 Oslo (Norway)
Tel. +47 23 07 27 43, E-Mail per.brandtzaeg@medisin.uio.no

Harabuchi Y (ed): Recent Advances in Tonsils and Mucosal Barriers of the Upper Airways.
Adv Otorhinolaryngol. Basel, Karger, 2011, vol 72, pp 25–27

Elicitation of Mucosal Immunity by Proteins of *Streptococcus pneumoniae*

David E. Briles[a] · Eliane Miyaji[b] · Yoshiko Fukuyama[a] · Daniela M. Ferreira[b,c] · Kohtaro Fujihashi[a]

[a]University of Alabama at Birmingham, Birmingham, Ala., USA; [b]Instituto Butantan, São Paulo, Brazil; [c]Liverpool School of Tropical Medicine, Liverpool, UK

Abstract

Pneumococcal diseases such as otitis media, pneumonia, and meningitis are invariably preceded by nasopharyngeal colonization, and herd immunity against pneumococcal disease requires protection against colonization. An early study in mice demonstrated that mucosal immunization with cholera toxin B subunit as adjuvant could elicit solid mucosal immunity. Recent data from several laboratories provides support for three different mechanisms by which adaptive immunity can provide protection against colonization. (1) IL-17-dependent T cell immunity can recruit PMN to sites of colonization. This IL-17-dependent immunity can be elicited by immunization with antigen plus a mucosal adjuvant, or can be elicited by colonization itself. (2) Immunity against colonization can be mediated by mucosal IgA and at the mucosal surface passive mucosal IgA antibody provides much better protection against carriage than passive IgG antibody. (3) Complement-fixing IgG antibody can protect against colonization and may act by protecting against colonization of bacteria.

Protection against colonization by *Streptococcus pneumoniae* is critical for preventing transmission of pneumococci to others. Thus, the protection against colonization is an important attribute of useful present and future pneumococcal vaccines. Moreover, since the development of otitis media, pneumonia, and meningitis caused by *S. pneumoniae* is invariably preceded by colonization, a vaccine that can protect against colonization can also protect from subsequent disease.

During colonization pneumococci exist as two separate sub-populations. One of these populations is of the transparent phase (thin capsule) and is recovered by nasal wash of the colonized mice. The other, generally much larger population is of the opaque phase (thick capsule) and is probably associated with the infected tissue surface since it is only released by homogenization of the nasal tissue [1]. During colonization pneumococci are dividing [2] but their numbers of CFU remain relatively constant [2, 3]. It is also known that colonizing pneumococci cause local (subclinical) inflammation [1, 4] making interactions between the host immune mechanisms and the colonizing bacteria inevitable. It seems likely that the relatively constant numbers of pneumococci during colonization is at least in part the result of immunity compensating for the continual bacterial growth.

In 1997, it was shown that mucosal immunization with killed pneumococci, full-length pneumococcal protein A (PspA), or a polysaccharide protein conjugate, along with cholera toxin B subunit as adjuvant could elicit mucosal immunity against colonization [3, 5]. The mechanism by which this immunity acted was not readily apparent. Data from several laboratories now provides support for three different mechanisms by which adaptive immunity can protect against colonization in mice.

IL-17-dependent T cell immunity can recruit PMN to sites of nasal colonization. This immunity can be elicited by intranasal immunization with several pneumococcal antigens and killed whole pneumococci using cholera toxin as adjuvant [6, 7]. Similarly natural colonization in mice elicits IL-17-dependent immunity which also acts to resolve colonization [8]. The cytokine IL-17 results in recruitment of PMN, which probably protect against colonization by attacking the pneumococci that are closely associated with the mucosal tissue.

More recently, it has been shown that by mucosal immunization with pneumococcal surface protein A (PspA), with plasmid DNA encoding Flt3 as adjuvant, elicits very high levels of mucosal secretory (S)-IgA antibody to PspA that can elicit virtually complete protection against acquisition of colonization [9]. Moreover, if the S-IgA antibody to PspA from the nasal wash of an immunized mouse was used to coat pneumococci prior nasal infection the subsequent colonization was largely prevented. If IgG antibody was similarly used to coat the pneumococci no protection was seen. These results suggest that S-IgA can in fact prevent colonization with pneumococci and the mechanism probably does not involve protection by phagocytes, which would have worked well with the IgG coated bacteria. It seem likely that S-IgA antibody to PspA may bind the pneumococci to the flowing nasal mucus, thus facilitating their clearance and preventing them from ever being able to attach to the nasal tissue.

Finally it has been observed that in the mouse, serum IgG2, but not IgG1 antibody can protect against nasal colonization with pneumococci [10]. IgG2 antibody is known to activate complement and to bind Fc-receptors better than IgG1 antibody [11]. One or both of these properties may explain why mouse serum IgG2 but not serum IgG1 is able to protect against nasal colonization with pneumococci. It seems likely that the site of action of the IgG2 antibodies is at the surface of the nasal tissue where the bulk of the colonizing pneumococci are present and cause inflammation. In man antibodies of subclasses IgG1, IgG2, and IgG3, all activate complement efficiently; only IgG4 does not. Thus, in the case of man it is likely that most serum immune responses to proteins or polysaccharides will elicit strong complement-activating antibody responses. Thus, the observation that serum IgG2 antibody in the mouse can protect against nasal colonization with pneumococci may explain how it is that intramuscular immunization of humans with conjugate vaccines has been able to protect against colonization with *S. pneumoniae* and *Haemophilus influenzae*.

The discovery that immunity to colonization can be elicited by IL-17 T cells, mucosal IgA, and complement activating antibody, gives vaccine makers at least three different effector mechanisms to exploit as they engineer their pneumococcal vaccines to elicit immunity to colonization. The fact that PspA was able to elicit protection via mucosal S-IgA and serum IgG2 antibodies may however be dependent on the fact that PspA is one of the most common proteins expressed on the pneumococcal surface.

References

1 Briles DE, Novak L, Hotomi M, van Ginkel FW, King J: Nasal colonization with *Streptococcus pneumoniae* includes subpopulations of surface and invasive pneumococci. Infect Immun 2005;73:6945–6951.

2 Balachandran P, Brooks-Walter A, Virolainen-Julkunen A, Hollingshead SK, Briles DE: The role of pneumococcal surface protein C (PspC) in nasopharyngeal carriage and pneumonia and its ability to elicit protection against carriage of *Streptococcus pneumoniae*. Infect Immun 2002;70:2526–2534.

3 Wu H-Y, Virolainen A, Mathews B, King J, Russell M, Briles DE: Establishment of a *Streptococcus pneumoniae* nasopharyngeal colonization model in adult mice. Microb Pathog 1997;23:127–137.

4 Beisswenger C, Lysenko ES, Weiser JN: Early bacterial colonization induces toll-like receptor-dependent transforming growth factor beta signaling in the epithelium. Infect Immun 2009;77:2212–2220.

5 Wu H-Y, Nahm M, Guo Y, Russell M, Briles DE: Intranasal immunization of mice with PspA (pneumococcal surface protein A) can prevent intranasal carriage, pulmonary infection, and sepsis with *Streptococcus pneumoniae*. J Infect Dis 1997;175:839–846.

6 Basset A, Thompson CM, Hollingshead SK, et al: Antibody-independent, CD4+ T cell-dependent protection against pneumococcal colonization elicited by intranasal immunization with purified pneumococcal proteins. Infect Immun 2007;75:5460–5464.

7 Lu YJ, Gross J, Bogaert D, et al: Interleukin-17A mediates acquired immunity to pneumococcal colonization. PLoS Pathog 2008;4:e1000159.

8 Zhang Z, Clarke TB, Weiser JN: Cellular effectors mediating Th17-dependent clearance of pneumococcal colonization in mice. J Clin Invest 2009;119:1899–1909.

9 Fukuyama Y, King JD, Kataoka K, et al: Secretory-IgA antibodies play an important role in the immunity to *Streptococcus pneumoniae*. J Immunol 2010;185:1755–1762.

10 Ferreira DM, Oliveira ML, Moreno AT, Ho PL, Briles DE, Miyaji EN: Protection against nasal colonization with *Streptococcus pneumoniae* by parenteral immunization with a DNA vaccine encoding PspA (pneumococcal surface protein A). Microb Pathog 2010;48:205–213.

11 Pleass RJ, Behnke JM: B-cells get the T-cells but antibodies get the worms. Trends Parasitol 2009;25:443–446.

David E. Briles
Department of Microbiology, University of Alabama at Birmingham
658 Beville Biomedical Research Building
Birmingham, AL 35294–2170 (USA)
Tel. +1 205 595 9250, E-Mail dbriles@uab.edu

Harabuchi Y (ed): Recent Advances in Tonsils and Mucosal Barriers of the Upper Airways.
Adv Otorhinolaryngol. Basel, Karger, 2011, vol 72, pp 28–30

Mucosal Immune Barrier and Antigen-Presenting System in Human Nasal Epithelial Cells

Tetsuo Himi[a] · Ken-ichi Takano[a] · Noriko Ogasawara[a] · Mitsuru Go[a] · Makoto Kurose[a] · Jun-ichi Koizumi[a] · Ryuta Kamekura[a] · Atsushi Kondo[a] · Tsuyoshi Ohkuni[a] · Tomoyuki Masaki[a] · Takashi Kojima[b] · Norimasa Sawada[b] · Hiroyuki Tsutsumi[c]

Departments of [a]Otolaryngology, [b]Pathology and [c]Pediatrics, Sapporo Medical University School of Medicine, Sapporo, Japan

Abstract

The upper respiratory tract including the nasal cavity, which is the first site of invading antigen exposure, plays a crucial role in host defense via the mucosal immune response. The epithelium of nasal mucosa forms a continuous barrier against a wide variety of exogenous antigens. The epithelial barrier function is regulated in large part by the apical-most intercellular junction, referred to as the tight junction. Antigen-presenting cells, particularly dendritic cells (DCs), are known to play an important role in human nasal mucosa. Recently, the author and colleagues discovered a new mechanism for pathogen uptake in the nasal mucosa, by which DCs open the tight junctions between epithelial cells and send dendrites outside the epithelium to directly sample the pathogen. In order to preserve the integrity of the epithelial barrier and penetrate beyond well-developed epithelial tight junctions, DCs express tight junction proteins. We also found that these DCs are activated by nasal epithelial-derived TSLP induced by stimuli such as cytokines and Toll-like receptor ligands. In this lecture, I will talk about the novel mechanisms in host defense in terms of innate immunity of the nasal mucosa from the point of view of the mucosal barrier function.

Tight Junctions in Human Nasal Mucosa

The upper respiratory tract, which is the first site of invading antigen exposure, plays a crucial role in host defense via the mucosal immune response. The epithelium of upper respiratory tissues such as nasal mucosa forms a continuous barrier against a wide variety of exogenous antigens. The epithelial barrier function is regulated in large part by the apical-most intercellular junction, referred to as the tight junction. In human nasal mucosa with or without allergic rhinitis, the tight junction protein expression, structures, and function of the epithelial tight junctions were well maintained [1].

Analysis in regulation systems of tight junction barrier in human nasal epithelium is helpful in protection from allergen invasion or in increased susceptibility to antigen sensitization. For example, when human nasal epithelial cells (HNECs) were treated with TGF-β, which is associated with nasal polyposis, upregulation of claudin-4 was observed, without a change of barrier function [2]. Activation of protein kinase C by 12-O-tetradeca noylophorbol-13-acetate increased transepithelial electrical resistance, together with up-regulation of tight junction proteins at the transcriptional level [3]. Furthermore, it affected the subcellular localization of the tight junction proteins and the numbers of tight junction strands. The peroxisome proliferator-activated (PPAR)-γ agonists also enhanced the barrier function of HNECs together with the upregulation of tight junction molecules at the transcriptional level [4]. A significant increase of tight junction strands was also observed after treatment with rosiglitazone [4]. These findings could be novel drugs for protection against inhaled substances and pathogens in the airway epithelium of human nasal mucosa.

Antigen Sampling or Uptake in Nasal Mucosa

Dendritic cells (DCs) are considered to be the most powerful antigen-presenting cells and play a central role in antigen sensitization and the initiation of primary immune responses. In human nasal epithelium with allergic rhinitis, HLA-DR and CD11c-positive DCs expressed tight-junction protein claudin-1 and penetrated beyond the apical-most tight-junction protein occludin to minimize the increase in permeability of the epithelial barrier [1]. In mature DCs that has elongated dendrites, JAM-A are significantly increased compared to the monocytes [5]. PPARγ agonists prevented the elongation of dendrites but not upregulation of JAM-A in mature DCs [5]. These suggest that the induction of JAM-A occurred during differentiation of human THP-1 DCs and was independent of PPARγ and the p38 MAPK pathway.

Epithelial Cells as a Source of Pro-Allergic Cytokine

Epithelial-derived thymic stromal lymphopoietin (TSLP) triggers DC-mediated Th2-type inflammatory responses and is a master switch for allergic inflammatory diseases. High expression of TSLP was found in the epithelium from patients with allergic rhinitis with recruitment and infiltration of DCs [6]. TSLP rapidly enhances the barrier function of cultured HNECs, together with an increase of tight junction proteins. The nasal epithelial-derived TSLP not only activates DCs but also preserves the epithelial barrier via the up-regulation of tight-junction proteins, thereby regulating antigen sensitization during the early stage of allergic rhinitis [6]. Furthermore, TSLP induces expression of tight junction protein claudin-7 in DCs via NF-κB as well as via toll-like receptors and may control tight junctions of DCs to preserve the epithelial barrier during allergic inflammation [7].

Conclusion

Epithelial cells possess well-developed tight junctions and also have regulatory mechanisms of antigen sampling. During immune responses, nasal epithelial cells release specific cytokines regarding the trigger and maintenance of allergic diseases. Nasal epithelial cell-derived cytokines also interact with intraepithelial DCs and subepithelial DCs to alter the ability of DCs to skew Th2 polarization. Nasal epithelial cells regulate the adaptive immune response by expression of soluble and cell-surface molecules that alter the function of DC, T cell and B cell. Thus, the nasal epithelium is central role to the pathogenesis in allergy.

References

1 Takano K, Kojima T, Go M, Murata M, Ichimiya S, Himi T, Sawada N: HLA-DR- and CD11c-positive dendritic cells penetrate beyond well-developed epithelial tight junctions in human nasal mucosa of allergic rhinitis. J Histochem Cytochem 2005;53:611–619.

2 Kurose M, Kojima T, Koizumi J, Kamekura R, Ninomiya T, Murata M, Ichimiya S, Osanai M, Chiba H, Himi T, Sawada N: Induction of claudins in passaged hTERT-transfected human nasal epithelial cells with an extended life span. Cell Tissue Res 2007;330:63–74.

3 Koizumi J, Kojima T, Ogasawara N, Kamekura R, Kurose M, Go M, Harimaya A, Murata M, Osanai M, Chiba H, Himi T, Sawada N: Protein kinase C enhances tight junction barrier function of human nasal epithelial cells in primary culture by transcriptional regulation. Mol Pharmacol 2008;74:432–442.

4 Ogasawara N, Kojima T, Go M, Ohkuni T, Koizumi J, Kamekura R, Masaki T, Murata M, Tanaka S, Fuchimoto J, Himi T, Sawada N: PPARgamma agonists upregulate the barrier function of tight junctions via a PKC pathway in human nasal epithelial cells. Pharmacol Res 2010;61:489–498.

5 Ogasawara N, Kojima T, Go M, Fuchimoto J, Kamekura R, Koizumi J, Ohkuni T, Masaki T, Murata M, Tanaka S, Ichimiya S, Himi T, Sawada N: Induction of JAM-A during differentiation of human THP-1 dendritic cells. Biochem Biophys Res Commun 2009;389:543–549.

6 Kamekura R, Kojima T, Koizumi J, Ogasawara N, Kurose M, Go M, Harimaya A, Murata M, Tanaka S, Chiba H, Himi T, Sawada N: Thymic stromal lymphopoietin enhances tight-junction barrier function of human nasal epithelial cells. Cell Tissue Res 2009;338:283–293.

7 Kamekura R, Kojima T, Takashima A, Koizumi J, Ogasawara N, Go M, Takano K, Murata M, Tanaka S, Ichimiya S, Himi T, Sawada N: Thymic stromal lymphopoietin induces tight junction protein claudin-7 via NF-kappaB in dendritic cells. Histochem Cell Biol 2010;133:339–348.

Tetsuo Himi, MD, PhD
Department of Otolaryngology
Sapporo Medical University School of Medicine
S1. W17.
Sapporo 060-8556 (Japan)
Tel. +81 11 611 2111, E-Mail himi@sapmed.ac.jp

Harabuchi Y (ed): Recent Advances in Tonsils and Mucosal Barriers of the Upper Airways.
Adv Otorhinolaryngol. Basel, Karger, 2011, vol 72, pp 31–36

Craniofacial Mucosal Immune System: Importance of Its Unique Organogenesis and Function in the Development of a Mucosal Vaccine

Kazunari Okada[a,b] · Tatsuya Yamasoba[b] · Hiroshi Kiyono[a]

Division of Mucosal Immunology, Department of Microbiology and Immunology, Institute of Medical Science, and [b]Department of Otorhinolaryngology and Head and Neck Surgery, Division of Surgical Science, The Graduate School of Medicine, University of Tokyo, Tokyo, Japan

Abstract

Mucosa-associated lymphoid tissues (MALT) play a critical role as inductive sites for the initiation of antigen-specific protective immunity against pathogens penetrating the mucus membranes. Nasopharynx-associated lymphoid tissue (NALT), situated at the bottom of the rodent nasal cavity, is thought to be an important site for the induction of antigen-specific immune response to inhaled antigens. In addition, we have recently shown that tear duct-associated lymphoid tissue (TALT), present in the murine tear duct bridging the ocular and nasal cavities, is involved in the induction and regulation of both nasal and ocular immunity. Interestingly, cellular requirements for the organogenesis of NALT and TALT are quite different from those of other MALT (e.g. Peyer's patches; PPs) and peripheral lymphoid tissues. Moreover, mucosal imprinting molecules of NALT and TALT inducer cells are totally independent of currently known chemokines and adhesion molecules in PPs and lymph nodes, such as the CXCR5-CXCL13, α4β1 integrin-vascular cell adhesion molecule-1 (VCAM1), and CCR9-CCL25 axes. NALT and TALT lymphocytes are also independent of these tissue-specific migration molecules. Together with already-characterized conjunctiva-associated lymphoid tissue (CALT), which has been demonstrated to play a critical role in ocular defense, the MALT associated with the head region seems to be coordinately organizing the unique craniofacial mucosal immune system of the ocular, nasal, oral-pharynx mucus membranes. Clarification of the immunological network of this unique craniofacial immune system will facilitate the development of a safe and effective mucosal vaccine against respiratory and ocular infections.

Mucosal Immune System

The mucosal immune system is an essential arm of host defense, especially at sites of invasion by bacterial and viral pathogens, such as the aero-digestive and reproductive tract mucosa [1]. In contrast, the systemic immune system provides protective immunity via the elimination of pathogens that have invaded peripheral tissues. Mucosa-associated lymphoid tissue (MALT), a member of the secondary lymphoid tissue family, develops immediately beneath the mucus membrane in the aero-digestive tract. It has been shown to play a key role in the initiation of antigen-specific mucosal immunity [1] (fig. 1). The mucosal surface of MALT is generally covered with follicle-

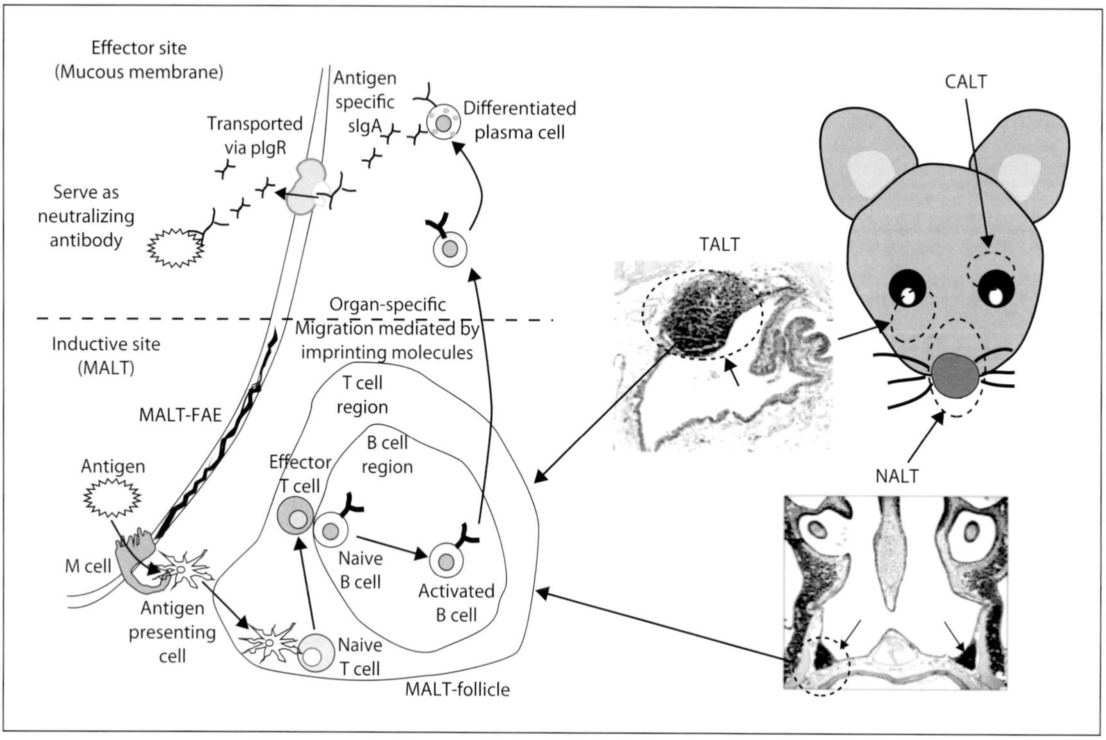

Fig. 1. Induction mechanism of antigen-specific mucosal immunity and overview of the murine craniofacial immune system. Left half: Antigens are taken up by M cells at MALT-FAE, the inductive site. APCs process these antigens, followed by migration to MALT T cell region to stimulate naive T cells. Activated effector T cells encounter and activate naive B cells. Activated antigen specific IgA$^+$ B cells migrate to mucus membrane, the effector site. Imprinting molecules mediate this kind of organ-specific migration. Then B cells differentiate into plasma cells to produce antigen specific sIgAs. These sIgAs are transported to mucosal surface, with help of pIgRs expressed on epithelial cells. SIgAs serve as neutralizing antibodies. Right half: NALT, TALT and CALT are an indispensable part of the murine craniofacial immune system. NALT at the bottom of the nasal cavity, TALT at the lacrimal sac, and CALT at the conjunctiva. Human craniofacial immune system is similar, including tonsils of Waldeyer's ring instead of NALT.

associated epithelium (FAE) containing professional antigen-sampling M cells. These M cells actively take up antigens and transfer them to antigen-presenting cells (APCs), such as dendritic cells (DCs) and macrophages [1]. Following antigen capturing and processing, these stimulated APCs migrate to the T cell regions of the MALT-draining lymph nodes for priming and activation of naive T cells to become effector subsets. Some of these activated helper T (Th) cells encounter naïve B cells and selectively induce class switch recombination from IgM to IgA [1]. These IgA$^+$ B cells and effector T cells encounter their mucosal imprinting molecules and adopt their antigen-specificity in MALT. For example, Peyer's patch (PP) DCs have been shown to induce the expression of gut imprinting molecules (e.g. CCR9 and $\alpha 4\beta 7$ integrin) on activated Th cells and IgA$^+$ B cells by producing retinoic acid. Imprinting by retinoic acid results in the preferential migration of the activated Th and IgA$^+$ B cells to effector sites in the distant intestinal lamina propria region [2]. PP-derived Th cells and IgA$^+$ B cells interact with mucosal DCs and epithelial cells for the induction of secretory IgA (sIgA) [1]. Dimeric (or polymeric) forms of IgA antibodies, produced by plasma cells that have differentiated from IgA^+ B cells in the lamina propria region, bind to polymeric Ig receptors (pIgR) expressed by epithelial cells to form sIgA. This sIgA is then transported into the gut lumen, leading to the creation of the first line of defense offered by the humoral arm of mucosal immunity.

Evidences for the Presence of Craniofacial Mucosal Immune System

Induction and regulation of intestinal mucosal immunity have been extensively elucidated. Parts of gut-associated lymphoid tissue (GALT), such as PPs, play a central role as the inductive tissue responsible for the initiation of an antigen-specific IgA response [3]. In contrast, the respiratory mucosal immune system is less well understood due to the complexity of immunological defenses of the upper and lower respiratory tracts. In general, the upper respiratory tract has been shown to be predominantly protected by mucosal immunity, and the lower respiratory tract protected by a mixture of both mucosal and systemic immunity, respectively. NALT has been identified as a pair of bell-shaped lymphoid tissues situated at the bottom of the nasal cavity in rodents [4, 5] (fig. 1). Although NALT has not been anatomically located in the adult human nasal cavity, a previous report has indicated that NALT-like structures are found only in human infants [6]. Although tonsils are seen in humans and not rodents [7], and the anatomical location of NALT is different for rodents and humans, Waldeyer's ring (seen in humans) is believed to be an analog of murine NALT [8]. The NALT epithelium contains M cells [9]. As NALT B cells express activation-induced cytidine deaminase (AID), class switch recombination from μ to α heavy chains can be induced [10]. Thus, NALT has been shown to be the site for the generation of memory-type IgA^+ B cells. Th1/Th2-type cells and cytotoxic T cells are also induced in NALT after nasal immunization or infection [4]. These findings suggest that NALT fulfils the necessary immunological criteria as an inductive tissue for the upper respiratory tract against inhaled antigens.

In addition to NALT, we have recently reported that an organized lymphoid structure of TALT was found in the murine lacrimal sac, adjacent to the tear duct [11] (fig. 1). Although TALT has also been identified in the human tear duct which connects the ocular and nasal cavities [12], its function is still unclear. Extensive analysis of murine TALT has been done to elucidate its role in the induction and regulation of antigen-specific immune responses against ocular antigens. TALT possesses FAE, which contains M cells and is distinct from the lacrimal mucus membrane. B cells and DCs accumulate in the subepithelial dome lesion, forming lymphoid follicle like PPs and NALT. As we have shown, mice were immunized by administering eye drops containing cholera toxin (CT), both the formation of germinal centers for IgA^+ B cell responses and the induction of antigen-specific Th cells were observed in TALT [11]. Furthermore, ocular immunization resulted in the initiation of antigen-specific T and B cell responses in NALT due to the traveling of the antigen from the ocular surface to the nasal cavity via the tear duct [11]. Thus, our results suggest that TALT plays an important role for not only ocular, but also nasal immune responses, and that ocular immunization induces antigen-specific IgA response via both TALT- and NALT-mediated mucosal immune systems. Another type of lymphoid tissue believed to be involved in the induction of protective immunity for the ocular surface is the conjunctiva-associated lymphoid tissue (CALT) which develops in mammals other than rodents as a small lymphoid follicle in the conjunctiva [13]. Yet another member of the craniofacial immune system is the tubal tonsil located at the entrance of the Eustachian tube, and thought to be associated with the middle ear mucosa and hence, ear

Table 1. Unique organogenesis programs of the craniofacial mucosal immune system – comparing with PPs

	PPs	NALT	TALT
Chronological development	prenatal	postnatal	
CXCR5-CXCL13 CCR9-CCL25 (chemokine)	dependent	independent	
LTα1β2-LTβR IL7-IL7R (cytokine)	dependent	independent	
α4β1 integrin-VCAM1 (adhesion molecule)	dependent	independent	
RORγt (transcription factor)	dependent	independent	
Id2 (gene)	dependent		independent

immunity. Thus, it is natural and logical to consider the mucosal immune system regulated by these different MALTs situated in the craniofacial area, such as NALT, TALT, CALT, and Waldeyere's ring tonsils, as an organized craniofacial immune system.

Uniqueness in the Development of Craniofacial Mucosal Immune System

The major organized lymphoid structures of the craniofacial mucosal immune system, such as NALT and TALT, have been shown to possess a unique organogenesis program when compared with other secondary lymphoid tissues such as the PPs (table 1) [5, 11]. Chronological examination of tissue development revealed that genesis of most of the secondary lymphoid tissues, including PPs and peripheral lymph nodes (pLNs), was initiated during the prenatal stage [14]. In contrast, the development of NALT and TALT started only after birth [5, 11]. In addition, essential organogenesis molecules required for the development of PPs and other lymphoid tissues were all found to be dispensable for the formation of NALT [5] and TALT [11]. For example, retinoic orphan receptor RORγt, a molecule associated with the transcription machinery and found to be indispensable for the development of PPs and pLNs [14], is not required for the development of NALT and TALT [5, 11]. Similarly, neither the IL-7/IL-7R cytokine family nor the LTα1β2-LTβR signaling pathways, which are involved in the genesis of PPs and pLNs, have been found to be essential for NALT and TALT genesis. Interestingly, even Id2, another well-known transcriptional molecule for lymphoid tissue genesis that is essential for the development of PPs, pLNs, and NALT, is dispensable for TALT genesis. RORγt serves as the master regulator of gut immunity (in terms of chemokine expression) [15], and of the generation of regulatory T and Th17 cells [16]. We expect that such molecules must be involved in the regulation of the craniofacial mucosal immune system operated by NALT and TALT, but that they have not yet been identified.

Craniofacial Immune System and Vaccine Development: A New Type of Mucosal Vaccine

As many pathogens are transmitted via the mucosal surfaces of the respiratory route, it is desirable to develop an effective vaccine that can provide a first-line defense against respiratory pathogens. Vaccines administered via the mucosal route are ideal as they can induce both systemic and mucosal immune responses, resulting in the induction of two layers of protection. Nasal vaccines have been shown to be effective for the induction of viral antigen-specific immunity for the craniofacial immune system [17, 18]. FluMist®, derived from cold-adapted influenza virus, is currently available as a nasal vaccine [19]. Our laboratory has recently reported a new nanotechnology-based, nasal vaccine antigen delivery system for a subunit vaccine [20]. Nanogel is a nanometer-sized hydrogel which can be fused with a protein antigen and act as an artificial chaperone for the delivery of the native form of the vaccine antigen to epithelial cells and APCs, such as DCs, when given via the nasal route. It should be noted that a cationic form of nanogel enhances the longevity of its adhesion to the nasal epithelium, leading to effective vaccine antigen delivery to mucosal dendritic cells in the nasal cavity for the initiation of antigen-specific immune response. Nasal cationic-nanogels containing vaccine antigens (e.g. *Clostridium botulium* toxoid and tetanus toxoid) have thus been shown to be effective in the induction of antigen-specific systemic IgG and nasal IgA responses without the co-administration of adjuvants. This vaccine antigen delivery system can avoid the transmission of the vaccine component to the central nervous system through the olfactory epithelium [21].

Our understanding of the ocular immune system, including TALT, led us to consider the development of an ocular or eye drop vaccine. Although effectively able to induce mucosal and systemic immunity, our ocular vaccine is still undergoing preclinical safety evaluation and is not yet ready for clinical use. A better understanding of the craniofacial immune system will facilitate the development of novel mucosal vaccines, which can contribute to the prevention and control of respiratory and ocular infectious diseases.

References

1 Mestecky J, Blumberg R, Kiyono H, McGhee JR: Fundamental Immunology, ed 5. San Diego, Academic Press, 2003, pp 965–1020.

2 Mora J, Iwata M, Eksteen B, Song S, Junt T, Senman B, Otipoby KL, Yokota A, Takeuchi H, Ricciardi-Castagnoli P, Rajewsky K, Adams DH, Andrian UH: Generation of gut-homing IgA-secreting B cells by intestinal dendritic cells. Science 2006;314:1157–1160.

3 Kiyono H, Fukuyama S: Nalt- versus Peyer's-patch-mediated mucosal immunity. Nat Rev Immunol 2004;4: 699–710.

4 Yanagita M, Hiroi T, Kitagaki N, Hamada S, Ito H, Shimauchi H, Murakami S, Okada H, Kiyono H: Nasopharyngeal-associated lymphoreticular tissue (NALT) immunity: fimbriae-specific Th1 and Th2 cell-regulated IgA responses for the inhibition of bacterial attachment to epithelial cells and subsequent inflammatory cytokine production. J Immunol 1999;162:3559–3565.

5 Fukuyama S, Hiroi T, Yokota Y, Rennert P, Yanagita M, Kinoshita N, Terawaki S, Shikina T, Yamamoto M, Kurono Y: Initiation of NALT organogenesis is independent of the IL-7R, LTβR, and NIK signaling pathways but requires the Id2 gene and $CD3^-CD4^+CD45^+$ cells. Immunity 2002;17:31–40.

6 Debertin AS, Tschernig T,Tönjes H, Kleemann WJ, Tröger HD, Pabst R: Nasal-associated lymphoid tissue (NALT): frequency and localization in young children. Clin Exp Immunol 2003;134:503–507.

7 Kuper CF, Koornstra PJ, Hameleers DM, Biewenga J, Spit BJ, Duijvestijn AM, van Breda Vriesman PJ, Sminia T: The role of nasopharyngeal lymphoid tissue. Immunol Today 1992;13:219–224.

8 Kuper C, Hameleers D, Bruijntjes J, Ven I: Lymphoid and non-lymphoid cells in nasal-associated lymphoid tissue (NALT) in the rat. Cell Tissue Res 1990;259:371–377.

9 Park H, Francis K, Yu J, Cleary PP: Membranous cells in nasal-associated lymphoid tissue: a portal of entry for the respiratory mucosal pathogen group A Streptococcus. J Immunol 2003;171:2532–2537.

10 Shimoda M, Nakamura T, Takahashi Y: Isotype-specific selection of high affinity memory B cells in nasal-associated lymphoid tissue. J Exp Med 2001;194: 1597–1607.

11 Nagatake T, Fukuyama S, Kim D-Y, Goda K, Igarashi O, Sato S, Nochi T, Sagara H, Yokota Y, Jetten AM, Kaisho T, Akira S, Mimuro H, Sasakawa C, Fukui Y, Fujihashi K, Akiyama T, Inoue J-i, Penninger JM, Kunisawa J, Kiyono H: Id2-, RORγt-, and LTβR-independent initiation of lymphoid organogenesis in ocular immunity. J Exp Med 2009;206:2351–2364.

12 Knop E, Knop N: Lacrimal drainage-associated lymphoid tissue (LDALT): a part of the human mucosal immune system. Invest Ophthalmol Vis Sci 2001;42:566–574.

13 Cain C, Phillips T: Developmental changes in conjunctiva-associated lymphoid tissue of the rabbit. Invest Ophthalmol Vis Sci 2008;49:644–649.

14 Eberl G, Marmon S, Sunshine M, Rennert P, Choi Y, Littman D: An essential function for the nuclear receptor RORγt in the generation of fetal lymphoid tissue inducer cells. Nat Immunol 2003;5:64–73.

15 Iwata M, Hirakiyama A, Eshima Y, Kagechika H, Kato C, Song SY: Retinoic acid imprints gut-homing specificity on T cells. Immunity 2004;21:527–538.

16 Zhou L, Lopes J, Chong M, Ivanov I, Min R, Victora G, Shen Y, Du J, Rubtsov Y, Rudensky A: TGF-β-induced Foxp3 inhibits Th17 cell differentiation by antagonizing rorγt function. Nature 2008;453:236–240.

17 Imaoka K, Miller C, Kubota M, McChesney MB, Lohman B, Yamamoto M, Fujihashi K, Someya K, Honda M, McGhee JR, Kiyono H: nasal immunization of nonhuman primates with simian immunodeficiency virus p55gag and cholera toxin adjuvant induces Th1/Th2 help for virus-specific immune responses in reproductive tissues. J Immunol 1998;161:5952–5958.

18 Kurono Y, Yamamoto M, Fujihashi K, Kodama S, Suzuki M, Mogi G, McGhee J, Kiyono H: Nasal Immunization Induces *Haemophilus influenzae*-specific Th1 and Th2 responses with mucosal IgA and systemic IgG antibodies for protective immunity. J Infect Dis 1999;180:122–132.

19 Jackson LA, Holmes SJ, Mendelman PM, Huggins L, Cho I, Rhorer J: Safety of a trivalent live attenuated intranasal influenza vaccine, FluMist, administered in addition to parenteral trivalent inactivated influenza vaccine to seniors with chronic medical conditions. Vaccine 1999;17:1905–1909.

20 Nochi T, Yuki Y, Takahashi H, Sawada S, Mejima M, Kohda T, Harada N, Kong I, Sato A, Kataoka N, Tokuhara D, Kurokawa S, Takahashi Y, Tsukada H, Kozaki S, Akiyoshi K, Kiyono H: Nanogel antigenic protein-delivery system for adjuvant-free intranasal vaccines. Nat Mater 2010;9:572–578.

21 Mutsch M, Zhou W, Rhodes P, Bopp M, Chen R, Linder T, Spyr C, Steffen R: Use of the inactivated intranasal influenza vaccine and the risk of Bell's Palsy in Switzerland. N Engl J Med 2004;350:896–903.

Hiroshi Kiyono
Division of Mucosal Immunology, Department of Microbiology and Immunology
Institute of Medical Science, University of Tokyo
4–6–1 Shirokanedai, Minato-ku, Tokyo 108-8639 (Japan)
Tel. +81 3 5449 5271, E-Mail kiyono@ims.u-tokyo.ac.jp

Harabuchi Y (ed): Recent Advances in Tonsils and Mucosal Barriers of the Upper Airways.
Adv Otorhinolaryngol. Basel, Karger, 2011, vol 72, pp 37–39

Tonsillectomy with Steroid Pulse: A Curative Therapy for IgA Nephropathy

Osamu Hotta

Department of Nephropathy, Sendai Shakaihoken Hospital, Sendai, Japan

Abstract

IgA nephropathy (IgAN), the most common form of primary glomerulonephritis progressing to end-stage renal disease (ESRD), has been regarded as an incurable disease. However, in recent years, it has been demonstrated that combined tonsillectomy with steroid pulse (TS) therapy, if administrated in the relatively early stage of the disease, can yield clinical remission in patients with IgAN. However, clinical remission is no longer obtained when the same treatment is administrated in cases with more advanced disease and/or a longer duration of nephropathy. Thus, the paradigm of managing IgAN patients is shifting in Japan from 'slowing the progression and the delaying the onset of ESRD' (by conventional therapy using a RAS inhibitor and/or corticosteroids at low doses in selected patients with advanced IgAN) to 'achieving remission' by the TS therapy in patients with early disease. In the new paradigm aimed at clinical remission, the principle for initiation of TS therapy should be 'the earlier, the better'.

IgA nephropathy (IgAN) is the most common form of primary glomerulonephritis worldwide, and is also one of the most important causes of end-stage renal failure necessitating kidney replacement therapy [1].

IgAN is still regarded as an incurable chronic kidney disease (CKD) in countries other than Japan. However, in recent years, it has been demonstrated in Japan that combined tonsillectomy with steroid pulse (TS) therapy, especially if undertaken in the relatively early stage of the disease, can yield clinical remission in patients with IgAN (fig 1) [2–4]. Thus, TS therapy has come to be adopted as the first-line treatment to achieve clinical remission in cases of IgAN in Japan.

Since 1988, about 1500 patients with IgAN have been treated by TS therapy at Sendai Shakaihoken Hospital. In this paper, mainly based on our data, I shall focus on the optimal timing of TS therapy to achieve clinical remission.

Effects of Tonsillectomy with Steroid Pulse Therapy in IgA Nephropathy

Clinical remission, defined as both negative proteinuria and hematuria by urinary dipstick tests, was obtained in over 80% of patients with IgAN of mild histological grade. Although disappearance of hematuria was obtained in more than 80% of patients regardless of the histological grade of IgAN, the rate of disappearance of proteinuria decreased in tandem with an increasing histological grade [5]. Moreover, a repeat biopsy study showed that the glomerular vasculitis was

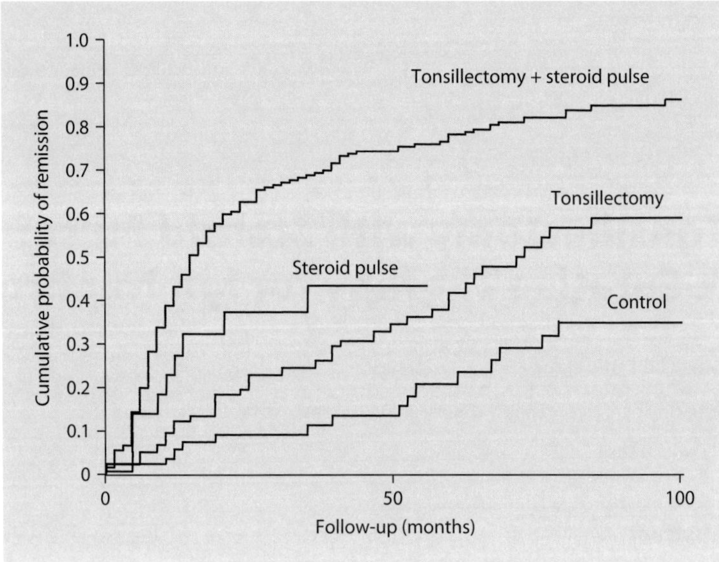

Fig. 1. Cumulative probability of clinical remission by treatment group.

no longer present and the mesangial proliferation had significantly regressed in second renal biopsies obtained a long interval (mean 77.1 months) after the TS therapy [6].

Worthy of particular mention is that in those patients with a short duration of nephropathy (≤3years), the remission rate was 87.1% (230/264), whereas in those with a longer duration of nephropathy (>3 years), the remission rate was much lower at 54.3% (63/116) [7].

Recently, Komatsu et al. [3] conducted a prospective controlled study in which they noted a higher likelihood of clinical remission following steroid pulse therapy combined with tonsillectomy than with steroid pulse therapy alone.

Optimal Timing of Tonsillectomy with Steroid Pulse Therapy

The primary goal of treatment for IgAN has conventionally been slowing of the disease progression, like for any other CKD such as diabetic nephropathy or hypertensive nephrosclerosis. However, if remission or cure of the disease can be achieved, then 'remission or cure of the nephropathy' should obviously be aimed for rather than 'slowing of disease progression'.

In the early stage of the disease, the major contributory factor to the progression of IgAN to end-stage renal disease is the glomerular vasculitis itself, which is usually smoldering in nature. However, as the chronic kidney injury progresses, various other factors, such as glomerular hypertension, protein-loading tubulointerstitial injury and ischemic kidney injury rather than glomerular vasculitis become the major contributory factors for progressive nephron loss. Thus, TS therapy may be expected to be effective only if it is undertaken at a relatively early stage of IgAN, as the target of this combination therapy is the smoldering glomerular vasculitis.

In the course of IgAN, there are two important points that must be borne in mind in relation to treatment, namely the 'point of no remission' and the 'point of no slowing'. If TS therapy is undertaken before the 'point of no remission', the likelihood of clinical remission is high, whereas

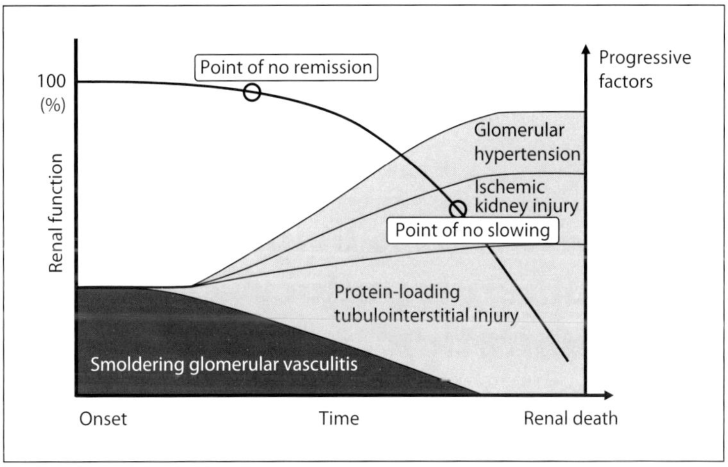

Fig. 2. Clinical course of IgAN and factors contributing to progressions. There are two important points; the 'point of no remission' and the 'point of no slowing'.

if the treatment is initiated after this point, clinical remission may no longer occur, while slowing of the disease progression may be expected. However, after the stage of the 'point of no slowing', no beneficial effect whatsoever may be expected and, on the contrary, the treatment may even accelerate the disease progression (fig. 2). Thus, to obtain clinical remission, IgAN must be detected at an early stage (i.e. prior to the 'point of no remission') and for this purpose, annual mass screening by urinalysis is very effective and important.

References

1 Schena FP: A retrospective analysis of the natural history of primary IgA nephropathy worldwide. Am J Med 1990;89:209–215.

2 Hotta O, Miyazaki M, Furuta T, et al: Tonsillectomy and steroid pulse therapy significantly impact in patients with IgA nephropathy. Am J Kidney Dis 2001;38:736–742.

3 Komatsu H, Fujimoto S, Hara S, et al: Effect of tonsillectomy plus steroid pulse therapy on clinical remission of IgA nephropathy: a controlled study. Clin J Am Soc Nephrol 2008;3:1301–1307.

4 Kawaguchi T, Ieiri N, Yamazaki S, et al: Clinical effectiveness of steroid pulse therapy combined with tonsillectomy in patients with immunoglobulin A nephropathy presenting glomerular haematuria and minimal proteinuria. Nephrology 2010;15:116–123.

5 Hotta O: Use of corticosteroids, other immunosuppressive therapies, and tonsillectomy in the treatment of IgA nephropathy. Semin Nephrol 2004;24:244–255.

6 Hotta O, Furuta T, Chiba S, et al: Regression of IgA nephropathy: a repeat biopsy study. Am J Kidney Dis 2002;39:493–502.

7 Ieiri N, Hotta O, Taguma Y: Impact of annual urine health check-up system to obtain clinical remission in patients with IgA nephropathy. Contrib Nephrol. Basel, Karger, 2007, vol 157, pp 104–108.

Osamu Hotta, MD
Department of Nephrology, Sendai Shakaihoken Hospital
Tsutsumimachi 3-16-1
Aoba-ku, Sendai 981-8501 (Japan)
Tel. +81 22 275 3111, ext. 358, E-Mail hottao@remus.dti.ne.jp

Harabuchi Y (ed): Recent Advances in Tonsils and Mucosal Barriers of the Upper Airways.
Adv Otorhinolaryngol. Basel, Karger, 2011, vol 72, pp 40–44

Recent Advances in IgA Nephropathy – The Glomerulopodocytic-Tubular Communication

Kar Neng Lai · Sydney C.W. Tang · Joseph C.K. Leung

Department of Medicine, Queen Mary Hospital, University of Hong Kong, Hong Kong, SAR, China

Abstract

IgA nephropathy (IgAN) is characterized by mesangial deposition of pathogenic polymeric IgA1 with rare deposits in the tubular epithelial cells (TEC). Recently, a novel mechanism involving a glomerulopodocytic-tubular cross-talk in the development of tubulointerstitial damage in IgAN has been revealed. Podocytes are positioned strategically along the glomerulotubular axis and plays an important role in mediating the glomerulo-tubular cross-talk. In IgAN, podocyte markers are reduced in the glomeruli. In vitro study implicates humoral factors (predominantly tumor necrosis factor-α and transforming growth factor-β) released from mesangial cells alter the glomerular permeability in the event of proteinuria and tubulointerstitial injury in IgAN. These mediators released from mesangial cells after IgA deposition further activate TEC leading to subsequent inflammatory changes in the renal tubulointerstitium.

Risk of IgAN progressing to renal failure is now well recognized. Notably, the renal progression correlates closely with the severity of tubulointerstitial lesions than that of the glomerular lesions.

Mechanisms for Tubulointerstitial Injury in IgAN

In IgAN, mesangial IgA deposition induces local release of cytokines, complements and angiotensin II (Ang II) leading to glomerular inflammation [1]. It remains unclear how mesangial IgA deposition leads to tubulointerstitial injury in IgAN. There are four possible pathogenetic mechanisms that may operate independently or synergistically: monocyte/macrophage infiltration, proteinuria, direct inflammatory effect of IgA, and a glomerulopodocytic-tubular communication.

The involvement of infiltrating inflammatory cells in the tubulointerstitium is important in mediating tubular injury and renal fibrosis. As a consequence, resident kidney cells become activated during the inflammatory process. In recent years, much attention has focused on the role of tubular epithelial cells (TEC) in orchestrating the infiltration of inflammatory cells and the renal fibrosis via production of inflammatory mediators upon activation. Mediators released by infiltrating cells are directly responsible for the activation of TEC which in turn may amplify the inflammatory cascade by local production of chemotactic mediators that attract even more inflammatory competent cells. The outcome of such a chain reaction is the generation of a positive feedback loop of activation that may lead to the overproduction of extracellular matrix components resulting in fibrosis and ultimately renal failure. Therefore, a cytokine 'cross-talk' network between TEC and interstitial immunocompetent cells can be envisaged to be the major driving force of tubulointerstitial injury in most kidney disease including IgAN. Data from the literature have clearly demonstrated the ability of TEC in producing a wide variety of inflammatory mediators [2]. Proteinuria is the major stimulus of TEC activation and subsequent chemotaxis of infiltrating immunocompetent cells in most glomerular diseases [3, 4]. However, proteinuria may only be one of the several contributory factors in tubulointerstitial injury in IgAN as heavy or nephrotic range proteinuria is uncommon. The other contributory factor is the direct toxic effect following tubular binding of IgA. IgAN patients have increased urinary IgA concentration that correlates with serum creatinine concentration and the urinary protein excretion [5]. IgA deposits are rarely detected in the tubulointerstitium. We demonstrated that there is minimal binding of IgA from IgAN patients to cultured TEC [6]. Failing to demonstrate a specific binding of IgA to TEC and the infrequent occurrence of high-grade proteinuria in IgAN, we postulate a new mechanism of glomerulopodocytic-tubular communication that subsequently leads to tubulointerstitial injury in IgAN.

Podocytes in the Glomerulo-Tubular Axis

Podocytes are highly differentiated cells that play a key role in maintaining the integrity of the glomerular filtration barrier. Podocytes hold a strategic position regulating the trafficking between glomeruli and tubules. A defect in podocyte proteins or injury to podocytes leads to proteinuria, and glomerulosclerosis. A number of podocyte proteins have been identified and genetic mutations of these podocyte proteins are associated with congenital nephrosis. Recently, studies of podocytes in other acquired glomerular diseases such as focal segmental glomerulosclerosis, HIV nephropathy and diabetic nephropathy are emerging. Lately, podocytes are shown to fully express the renin-angiotensin system (RAS) with apoptosis induced by Ang II [7].

Podocyte in IgAN

Podocytes did not express mRNA for any known functional IgA receptors [8]. Importantly, histological demonstration of distinctly separate immunostaining of IgA and nephrin with no colocalization further confirms no direct binding of IgA to podocytes [8]. The most intriguing question is how injury occurs when there is no podocytic binding of IgA in IgAN.

We hypothesized that a glomerulopodocytic cross-talk existed in IgAN based on podocyte culture experiments using conditioned medium from human mesangial cells (HMC) preincubated with different IgA preparations that simulated the in vivo glomerulopodocytic communication via humoral factors. It was postulated that these humoral factors/mediators from mesangial cells first activated the podocytes before reaching the tubulointerstitium either by glomerular filtration or by transportation via the postglomerular capillaries. Upon reaching the tubular compartment, these mediators stimulate tubular epithelial cells to produce cytokines and chemokines that eventually led to tubular damage, interstitial mononuclear cells infiltration and fibrosis [6]. We showed that TNF-α produced by mesangial cells following stimulation by polymeric IgA from IgAN patients led to increased synthesis of TNF-α by podocytes in an autocrine fashion [8].

TNF-α receptor-1 (TNF-R1) and receptor-2 (TNF-R2) are constitutively present in normal podocytes. TNF-R1 promotes systemic immune response and renal T cell apoptosis while intrinsic cell TNF-R2 regulates complement-dependent tissue injury [9]. Both receptors are significantly upregulated in podocytes of IgAN patients [8]. Despite these receptors are not inducible with polymeric IgA isolated from patients with IgAN in vitro, their expression is readily upregulated by IgA-HMC conditioned medium from patients with IgAN or exogenous TNF-α. In vitro study suggests two functional roles played by the TNF-R1 in podocytes following stimulation by IgA-HMC conditioned medium from patients with IgAN: IL-6 synthesis and apoptosis. IL-6 regulates the tubular angiotensin II receptor subtype-1 (ATR1) expression and enhances tubular Ang II production in IgAN [10]. Interaction of Ang II and early expressed ATR1 will activate the protein kinase C (PKC) and mitogen-activated protein kinase (MAPK) pathways, leading to inflammatory responses in TEC. Upregulation of TNF-R1 in podocytes incubated with IgA-HMC conditioned medium may favor apoptotic cell death. The upregulation of TNF-R2 observed in our in vitro study [8] suggests that podocytes are in a chronic pro-inflammatory state in IgAN.

We also found a reduction in nephrin and ezrin in renal tissues from patients with mild IgAN [11]. Nephrin has a crucial role in the filtration barrier of the glomerular podocyte. Podocin serves as a scaffolding molecule to localize nephrin while synaptopodin is associated with the cytoskeleton of parietal podocytes. Ezrin is a glomerular epithelial cell marker of podocyte injury (podocytopathy). Such downregulation of podocyte markers was reproducible in podocyte culture experiments with IgA-HMC conditioned medium from patients with IgAN. Culturing podocytes with recombinant TNF-α or transforming growth factor-β (TGF-β) resulted in similar downregulation of these podocyte markers. Furthermore, these downregulatory changes can be abolished with specific neutralizing antibodies suggesting that both TNF-α and TGF-β play a crucial role in mediating the inflammatory injury along the glomerulo-podocyte axis in IgAN.

It appears that downregulation of podocyte markers by mediators released by mesangial cells following IgA deposition alters the glomerular permeability. This will facilitate mesangial-derived humoral factors/mediators to reach the tubulointerstitium that eventually leads to tubular damage, interstitial mononuclear cells infiltration and fibrosis. The exact mechanism by which these podocyte proteins are downregulated in IgAN has not been examined but transcriptional suppression of nephrin by TNF-α via activation of the phosphatidylinositol-3-kinase/Akt pathway is a likely possibility [12]. The clinical significance is suggested by the finding that the gene expression of nephrin, erzin, podocin but not synaptopodin correlated with the degree of proteinuria, the rise of serum creatinine and the fall in creatinine clearance [11].

A Glomerulotubular Cross-Talk in IgAN via Humoral Factors

Renal tubular epithelial cells do not expressed known functional IgA receptors [10]. Inflammatory cytokines including Ang II are released from mesangial cells following binding to IgA in IgAN [1]. These mediators alter the glomerular barrier pore size allowing the passage of these inflammatory mediators to the tubular lumen. These mediators then activate the TEC which in turn may amplify the inflammatory cascade by local production of chemotactic mediators that attract even more inflammatory competent cells [13]. The mesangial-derived mediators induce an increased proliferation and enhanced expression of inflammatory mediators by TEC including IL-6, TNF-α, TGF-β, soluble intercellullar adhesion molecule-1, and Ang II [10]. This glomerulotubular cross-talk will generate a positive feedback loop of activation in the renal tubules leading to the overproduction of extracellular matrix components that result in fibrosis and renal failure.

Renal Expression of Ang II Subtype-1 Receptor and Ang II Subtype-2 Receptor

Ang II plays a pivotal role as a mediator of glomerular hemodynamic adaptation and also immunologic injury. Ang II subtype-1 receptor (ATR1) and Ang II subtype-2 receptor (ATR2) are present in podocyte of glomerular epithelial cells [14] and TEC [10]. Similar to the findings of Wagner et al. [15], we found a reduction of mesangial ATR1 expression after the acute exposure to pIgA from IgAN patients [16], supporting a local downregulation of ATR1 in IgAN resulting from the negative feedback due to enhanced intraglomerular RAS and, hence, Ang II activity [17, 18]. Interestingly, such adaptive changes are lost gradually with prolonged exposure of mesangial cells to pIgA in IgAN. Hence, the failure to suppress the ATR1 expression continuously in the presence of defective ATR2 activation is likely to permit the development of proliferative and inflammatory processes in the glomerular mesangium that may perpetuate a glomerulotubular cross-talk which finally leads to progression of renal deterioration in IgAN. In the tubular lumen, mesangial-derived TNF-α first increases IL-6 production that, in turn, increases the ATR1 expression and Ang II production. The interaction of Ang II and early expressed ATR1 will activate the PKC and MAPK pathways, leading to inflammatory responses. The early phase of ATR1-dependent inflammation is followed by upregulation of ATR2 expression with continued release of Ang II. The interaction between Ang II and ATR2 leads to apoptosis through downregulation of the MAPK pathway, and this will counterbalance the ATR1-induced MAPK activation.

Acknowledgment

The study was supported by the Research Grant Committee (Hong Kong, SAR) [HKU 7678/07M]. J.C.K. Leung is supported by the L&T Charitable Foundation and the House of INDOCAFE.

References

1 Lai KN, Tang SC, Guh JY, et al: Polymeric IgA1 from IgA nephropathy upregulates synthesis and signal transduction of transforming growth factor-β in human mesangial cell via the renin-angiotensin system. J Am Soc Nephrol 2003;14:3127–3137.

2 van Kooten C, Daha MR, van Es LA: Tubular epithelial cells: A critical cell type in the regulation of renal inflammatory processes. Exp Nephrol 1999;7:429–437.

3 Tang SC, Leung JCK, Abe K, et al: Albumin stimulates interleukin-8 expression in proximal tubular epithelial cells: an in vitro and in vivo study. J Clin Invest 2003;111:515–527.

4 Lai KN, Leung JCK, Chan LY, Tang SC: Interaction between proximal tubular epithelial cells and infiltrating monocytes/T cells in the proteinuric state. Kidney Int 2007;71:526–538.

5 Galla JH, Spotswood MF, Harrison LA, Mestecky J: Urinary IgA in IgA nephropathy and Henoch-Schoenlein purpura. J Clin Immunol 1985;5:298–306.

6 Chan LY, Leung JCK, Tsang AW, et al: Activation of tubular epithelial cells by mesangial-derived TNF-alpha: glomerulotubular communication in IgA nephropathy. Kidney Int 2005;67:602–612.

7 Shankland SJ: The podocyte's response to injury: role in proteinuria and glomerulosclerosis. Kidney Int 2006;69:2131–2147.

8 Lai KN, Leung JC, Chan LY, et al: Activation of podocytes by mesangial-derived TNF-α: glomerulo-podocytic communication in IgA nephropathy. Am J Physiol Renal Physiol 2008;294:F945–F955.

9 Vielhauer V, Stavrakis G, Mayadas TN: Renal cell-expressed TNF receptor 2, not receptor 1, is essential for the development of glomerulonephritis. J Clin Invest 2005;115:1199–1209.

10 Chan LY, Leung JC, Tang SC, et al: Tubular expression of angiotensin II receptors and their regulation in IgA nephropathy. J Am Soc Nephrol 2005;16:2306–2317.

11 Lai KN, Leung JC, Chan LY, et al: Podocyte injury induced by mesangio-derived cytokines in IgA nephropathy. Nephrol Dial Transplant 2009;24:62–72.

12 Takano Y, Yamauchi K, Hayakawa K, et al: Transcriptional suppression of nephrin in podocytes by macrophages: role of inflammatory cytokines and involvement of the P13K/Akt pathway. FEBS Lett 2007;581:421–426.
13 Tam KY, Leung JC, Chan LY, et al: In vitro enhanced chemotaxis of CD25+ mononuclear cells in patients with familial IgA nephropathy through glomerulotubular interactions. Am J Physiol Renal Physiol 2010;299:F359–368.
14 Wang L, Flannery P, Spurney RF: Characterization of angiotensin II-receptor subtypes in podocytes. J Lab Clin Med 2003;142:313–321.
15 Wagner J, Gehlen F, Ciechanowicz A, Ritz E: Angiotensin II receptor type 1 gene expression in human glomerulonephritis and diabetes mellitus. J Am Soc Nephrol 1999;10:545–551.
16 Lai KN, Chan LYY, Tang SC, et al. Mesangial expression of angiotensin II receptor in IgA nephropathy and its regulation by polymeric IgA1. Kidney Int 2004;66:1403–1416.
17 Makita N, Iwai N, Inagami T, Badr K: Two distinct pathways in the down-regulation of type-1 angiotensin II receptor gene in rat glomerular mesangial cells. Biochem Biophys Res Commun 1992;185:142–146.
18 Chansel D, Bizet T, Vandermeersch S, et al: Differential regulation of angiotensin II and losartan binding sites in glomeruli and mesangial cells. Am J Physiol 1994;266:F384–F393.

Prof. K.N. Lai
Department of Medicine, Room 409, Professorial Block,
Queen Mary Hospital, University of Hong Kong
Hong Kong, SAR (China)
Tel. +852 22554251, E-Mail knlai@hkucc.hku.hk

Harabuchi Y (ed): Recent Advances in Tonsils and Mucosal Barriers of the Upper Airways.
Adv Otorhinolaryngol. Basel, Karger, 2011, vol 72, pp 45–49

Immunomodulatory Agents against IgA Nephropathy

Sydney C.W. Tang · Joseph C.K. Leung · Kar Neng Lai

Department of Medicine, Queen Mary Hospital, University of Hong Kong, Hong Kong SAR, China

Abstract

Synthesis of aberrant IgA molecules as the key pathogenetic mechanism of immunoglobulin A nephropathy (IgAN) apparently forms a potential scientific rationale for applying immunomodulatory agents in the treatment of IgAN. There is evidence that corticosteroids can steadily reduce proteinuria and slow down renal progression. Evidence that pulse steroid plus intravenous or oral cyclophosphamide can retard the rate of progression of advanced IgAN was provided by several groups worldwide. Cyclosporin is generally not used to treat IgAN. The efficacy of azathioprine is equivocal. Mycophenolate mofetil reduces proteinuria by up to 30% and favorably impacts renal survival in Chinese patients with mild histologic lesions, but these results were not achieved in Caucasians with more advanced disease. In conclusion, the choice of immunomodulatory therapy remains controversial. We advocate the use of immunomodulatory agents as an adjunctive therapy in patients with proteinuria >1 g/day despite achieving target blood pressure with full renin-angiotensin blockade. More aggressive therapy should be reserved for patients with nephrotic-range proteinuria, crescentic lesions and/or rapidly progressive renal failure.

The predominant glomerular deposition of abnormally glycosylated polymeric IgA (pIgA) and the frequently elevated circulating IgA levels in up to a third of patients with primary immunoglobulin A nephropathy (IgAN) [1] suggest a pathogenetic role for structurally aberrant IgA synthesis. This, coupled with the recent observation of the role of the ubiquitin-proteasome pathway [2], forms a scientific rationale for applying immunomodulatory agents in the treatment of IgAN.

To date, there is a lack of large randomized controlled trials that provide a definitive immunosuppressive protocol for IgAN. A recent meta-analysis [3] of 13 randomized controlled trials involving a total of 623 patients concluded that immunosuppressive agents are a promising strategy and that this approach should be investigated further. Research in this area, as in many other renal diseases, is hampered by the slowly progressive nature of the disease, with 10-year renal survival rates exceeding 85%, marked patient heterogeneity, and the lack of a good animal model that closely resembles human IgAN. In this review, prevailing evidence for and against the use of immunosuppressive agents against IgAN will be discussed.

Corticosteroids

A relatively large quantity of data on corticosteroids was contributed by Japanese researchers in early years. Kobayashi et al. [4] reported that steroid treatment in 14 patients with proteinuria 1–2 g/day versus 29 control subjects was effective in lowering proteinuria, particularly in patients with baseline GFR >70 ml/min. After 10 years' follow-up, renal survival was 80 versus 34% [5]. These results were reproduced in 86 Italian patients in 1999 when Pozzi et al. [6] reported renoprotective effects of a 6-month course of steroid treatment. At 10 years, renal survival was better in the steroid group [7]. On the other hand, Lai et al. [8] found no therapeutic value of corticosteroids in Chinese patients. A recent meta-analysis [9] of 7 randomized control trials involving 386 subjects suggests that glucocorticoids have statistically significant effects on protecting renal function and reduction of proteinuria, but gastrointestinal tract reaction is a concern.

Cyclophosphamide in Combination with Corticosteroid

Evidence that pulse steroid plus intravenous or oral cyclophosphamide slow the rate of progression of advanced IgAN was provided by several groups worldwide.

In 2002, Ballardie et al. [10] showed in 38 patients with progressive loss of renal function that renal survival in cyclophosphamide-treated patients was considerably better at 5 years (72% compared with 6% in controls). Proteinuria and erythrocyturia reduced from 12 and 6 months of treatment, respectively. This study may be faulted, however, for suboptimal blood pressure control and insufficient use of medications that block the angiotensin system, the unusually poor survival rate of the placebo group, and the small number of patients. Tumlin et al. [11] conducted a prospective, uncontrolled, open-label trial of 12 patients with crescentic IgAN and clinically progressive disease. Treatment consisted of three doses of methylprednisolone at 15 mg/kg/day, followed by intravenous cyclophosphamide at 0.5 g/m^2/month for 6 months. Serum creatinine fell from 2.7 to 1.5 mg/dl, and proteinuria decreased from 4 to 1.3 g/day after treatment, suggesting a beneficial role of cyclophosphamide in crescentic glomerulonephritis. In another observational, uncontrolled study, Rasche et al. [12] obtained similar results in 21 patients with advanced IgAN treated with intravenous pulse cyclophosphamide (0.75 g/m^2/month) for 6 months together with low-dose oral prednisolone. More recently, Mitsuiki et al. [13] retrospectively examined the outcome of 35 patients with histologically advanced IgAN; 27 received prednisolone for 2 years and oral cyclophosphamide (50 mg/day) for 6 months, and the remaining 8 received supportive treatment. Renal prognosis was significantly better in the treatment group.

Overall, these studies suggest that combined cyclophosphamide/steroid therapy may benefit IgAN patients at very high risk of renal failure, namely those with a progressive decline in GFR and/or crescentic lesions. However, use of alkylating agents and long-term immunosuppression is not without side effects. More definitive evidence involving patients in sufficient numbers is required before this treatment can be widely accepted.

Cyclosporin

Cyclosporin is generally not used to treat IgAN. Lai et al. [14] conducted a randomized prospective single blind study of 19 patients with proteinuria >1.5 g/day. Patients who received cyclosporin had significant reduction of proteinuria, serum IgA, and increase of plasma albumin concentration compared with placebo. However, there was transient deterioration of renal function during treatment, despite within-range trough drug levels. The authors discourage indiscriminate use of cyclosporin in IgAN due to nephrotoxicity.

Azathioprine

Goumenos et al. [15] performed a retrospective analysis of 74 IgAN patients followed for 10 years, and found that long-term azathioprine combined with low-dose prednisone did not alter the clinical course compared to untreated controls.

The Japanese Pediatric IgA Nephropathy Treatment Study Group [16] reported significant reduction of proteinuria at 2 years with prednisolone/azathioprine treatment in children with newly diagnosed early IgAN. A recent prospective randomized study [17] of 207 subjects showed that the addition of azathioprine to corticosteroids did not provide additional benefits in terms of renal survival versus corticosteroids alone in the treatment of IgAN patients with proteinuria ≥1 g/24 h and plasma creatinine ≤2.0 mg/dl. Current data therefore suggest that the addition of azathioprine was ineffective and may even be potentially toxic.

Mycophenolate Mofetil

The first clinical report of MMF in IgAN was in the prevention of progression to allograft failure in recurrent IgAN of the transplant kidney [18]. To date, four randomized clinical trials have been published on the use of MMF in IgAN, which add more controversy than consensus.

The first randomized study, published in 2002 in the Chinese literature [19], was conducted in Beijing in which 62 Chinese patients with severe IgAN (urinary protein >2.0 g/day) received MMF or oral prednisone for at least 12 months. After 18 months' follow-up, the MMF group showed more significant improvement in proteinuria and serum lipids than the prednisone group.

In 2004, Maes et al. [20] treated 34 Belgian patients with impaired renal function, histologic unfavorable criteria and arterial hypertension, after instituting salt restriction and angiotensin-converting enzyme inhibitor therapy in all. After 3 years of follow-up evaluation, inulin clearances and proteinuria did not differ between the groups. In a similar study that recruited patients with even more advanced renal insufficiency using MMF as a 'salvage' therapy, Frisch et al. [21] reported a lack of efficacy and the study was terminated prematurely after observing a trend toward worse outcome in the MMF group.

In 2005, Tang et al. [22] treated 40 Chinese patients with mild tubulointerstitial lesions with persistent proteinuria >1 g/day despite full angiotensin blockade for 6 months. Twelve months after stopping MMF, the overall remission rate was significantly higher in MMF-treated patients whose proteinuria dropped to 62% of baseline, whereas urine protein in control patients increased to 120% of baseline. Serum interleukin 6 levels and, more intriguingly, in vitro binding of IgA to mesangial cells were elevated at baseline in both groups compared with normal healthy subjects; however, after MMF treatment these parameters were comparable to those of the healthy subjects. After 6 years' follow-up, the difference in proteinuria between the 2 groups was lost, but renal survival was significantly better in the MMF group [23].

Overall, MMF appears to be effective in reducing proteinuria in Chinese but not Caucasoid IgAN subjects. Therefore, ethnic differences may be one possible reason to account for the differences observed in these studies. Another possibility is the mild histologic grade in the study by Tang et al. [22] versus the moderate-to-severe grades in the studies by Maes et al. [20] and Frisch et al. [21]. Randomized clinical trials in North America [24] and Italy [25] are currently underway.

Conclusion on Choice of Immunomodulatory Therapy

This remains a controversial area. We advocate the use of immunomodulatory agents (cyclophosphamide for Caucasians and MMF for Orientals for 6 months) as an adjunctive therapy in patients with proteinuria >1 g/day despite achieving target blood pressure of 125/75 mm Hg with full renin-angiotensin blockade. More aggressive therapy should be reserved for patients with nephrotic-range proteinuria, crescentic lesions and/or rapidly progressive renal failure. On the other hand, patients with advanced renal failure (serum creatinine >300 µmol/l) and considerable tubulointerstitial fibrosis in the kidney will unlikely benefit from immunomodulation.

Acknowledgment

This study was supported by the S.K. Yee Medical Foundation (Project No. 210262).

References

1 Lai KN, To WY, Li PK, et al: Increased binding of polymeric lambda-IgA to cultured human mesangial cells in IgA nephropathy. Kidney Int 1996;49: 839–845.
2 Tang SC, Lai KN: The ubiquitin-proteasome pathway and IgA nephropathy: a novel link? Kidney Int 2009;75:457–459.
3 Samuels JA, Strippoli GF, Craig JC, et al: Immunosuppressive treatments for immunoglobulin A nephropathy: a meta-analysis of randomized controlled trials. Nephrology (Carlton) 2004;9: 177–185.
4 Kobayashi Y, Fujii K, Hiki Y, et al: Steroid therapy in IgA nephropathy: a prospective pilot study in moderate proteinuric cases. Q J Med 1986;61:935–943.
5 Kobayashi Y, Hiki Y, Kokubo T, et al: Steroid therapy during the early stage of progressive IgA nephropathy: a 10-year follow-up study. Nephron 1996;72: 237–242.
6 Pozzi C, Bolasco PG, Fogazzi GB, et al: Corticosteroids in IgA nephropathy: a randomised controlled trial. Lancet 1999;353:883–887.
7 Pozzi C, Andrulli S, Del Vecchio L, et al: Corticosteroid effectiveness in IgA nephropathy: long-term results of a randomized, controlled trial. J Am Soc Nephrol 2004;15:157–163.
8 Lai KN, Lai FM, Ho CP, et al: Corticosteroid therapy in IgA nephropathy with nephrotic syndrome: a long-term controlled trial. Clin Nephrol 1986;26: 174–180.
9 Cheng J, Zhang X, Zhang W, et al: Efficacy and safety of glucocorticoids therapy for IgA nephropathy: a meta-analysis of randomized controlled trials. Am J Nephrol 2009;30: 315–322.
10 Ballardie FW, Roberts IS: Controlled prospective trial of prednisolone and cytotoxics in progressive IgA nephropathy. J Am Soc Nephrol 2002;13: 142–148.
11 Tumlin JA, Lohavichan V, Hennigar R: Crescentic, proliferative IgA nephropathy: clinical and histological response to methylprednisolone and intravenous cyclophosphamide. Nephrol Dial Transplant 2003;18:1321–1329.
12 Rasche FM, Klotz CH, Czock D, et al: Cyclophosphamide pulse therapy in advanced progressive IgA nephropathy. Nephron Clin Pract 2003;93:c131-c136.
13 Mitsuiki K, Harada A, Okura T, et al: Histologically advanced IgA nephropathy treated successfully with prednisolone and cyclophosphamide. Clin Exp Nephrol 2007;11:297–303.
14 Lai KN, Lai FM, Li PK, et al: Cyclosporin treatment of IgA nephropathy: a short term controlled trial. Br Med J (Clin Res Ed) 1987;295:1165–1168.
15 Goumenos DS, Davlouros P, El Nahas AM, et al: Prednisolone and azathioprine in IgA nephropathy – a ten-year follow-up study. Nephron Clin Pract 2003;93:C58-C68.
16 Yoshikawa N, Ito H: Combined therapy with prednisolone, azathioprine, heparin-warfarin, and dipyridamole for paediatric patients with severe IgA nephropathy – is it relevant for adult patients? Nephrol Dial Transplant 1999;14:1097–1099.
17 Pozzi C, Andrulli S, Pani A, et al: Addition of azathioprine to corticosteroids does not benefit patients with IgA nephropathy. J Am Soc Nephrol 2010.
18 Nowack R, Birck R, van der Woude FJ: Mycophenolate mofetil for systemic vasculitis and IgA nephropathy. Lancet 1997;349:774.
19 Chen X, Chen P, Cai G, et al: A randomized control trial of mycophenolate mofeil treatment in severe IgA nephropathy. Zhonghua Yi Xue Za Zhi 2002;82:796–801.
20 Maes BD, Oyen R, Claes K, et al: Mycophenolate mofetil in IgA nephropathy: results of a 3-year prospective placebo-controlled randomized study. Kidney Int 2004;65:1842–1849.
21 Frisch G, Lin J, Rosenstock J, et al: Mycophenolate mofetil (MMF) vs. placebo in patients with moderately advanced IgA nephropathy: a double-blind randomized controlled trial. Nephrol Dial Transplant 2005;20: 2139–2145.
22 Tang S, Leung JC, Chan LY, et al: Mycophenolate mofetil alleviates persistent proteinuria in IgA nephropathy. Kidney Int 2005;68:802–812.

23 Tang SC, Tang AW, Wong SS, et al: Long-term study of mycophenolate mofetil treatment in IgA nephropathy. Kidney Int 2010;77:543–549.

24 Hogg RJ, Wyatt RJ: A randomized controlled trial of mycophenolate mofetil in patients with IgA nephropathy. BMC Nephrol 2004;5:3.

25 Dal CA, Amore A, Barbano G, et al: One-year angiotensin-converting enzyme inhibition plus mycophenolate mofetil immunosuppression in the course of early IgA nephropathy: a multicenter, randomised, controlled study. J Nephrol 2005;18:136–140.

Dr. Sydney C.W. Tang
Department of Medicine, Room 302, New Clinical Building
Queen Mary Hospital, University of Hong Kong
Hong Kong, SAR (China)
Tel. +852 22553879, E-Mail scwtang@hku.hk

Harabuchi Y (ed): Recent Advances in Tonsils and Mucosal Barriers of the Upper Airways.
Adv Otorhinolaryngol. Basel, Karger, 2011, vol 72, pp 50–52

Indication Criteria for Tonsillectomy in IgA Nephropathy Patients

Hirofumi Akagi[a] · Akira Doi[b] · Michiya Kosaka[c] · Kenshi Hattori[d] · Shin Kariya[e] · Kunihiro Fukushima[e] · Mitsuhiro Okano[e] · Kazunori Nishizaki[e] · Yu Masuda[e]

[a]Department of Otolaryngology, Incorporated Administrative Agency National Hospital Organization Minami-Okayama Medical Center, Okayama, [b]Division of Otolaryngology, Kochi Health Sciences Center, Kochi, [c]Kosaka ENT Clinic, [d]Hattori ENT Clinic, and [e]Department of Otolaryngology- Head and Neck Surgery, Okayama University Graduate School of Medicine, Dentistry and Pharmaceutical Sciences, Okayama, Japan

Abstract

We proposed the following indication criteria for tonsillectomy in patients with IgA nephropathy. (1) IgA nephropathy has been definitively diagnosed by an evaluation of the renal glomeruli during renal biopsy. (2) Tonsillectomy is indicated for patients who demonstrate grade I–III renal pathology and a serum creatinine level of 2.0 mg/dl or less during renal biopsy. However, even among patients who demonstrate grade IV disease or a serum creatinine level higher than 2.0 mg/dl during renal biopsy, surgery should be considered in the absence of contraindications for tonsillectomy, such as renal hypofunction, providing the patient wants to undergo surgery and informed consent is obtained. (3) The patient's medical history includes deterioration of urine findings during tonsillitis or acute upper respiratory inflammation. (4) Buried tonsils and the attachment of pus plugs to the tonsillar crypt are observed as local findings of the palatine tonsil. (5) Positive findings, especially positive urine findings (hematuria), are detected on the tonsillar provocation test. Items (1) and (2) are essential. Items (3) to (5) are indicative, as their inclusion has not been supported by previous studies.

We reported a retrospective case-control study of 71 patients with IgA nephropathy in order to assess the renal prognosis of this disease as a means of evaluating the long-term prognostic effect of tonsillectomy [1, 2]. Forty-one patients, including 19 males and 22 females, underwent tonsillectomy (group A), and 30 patients, including 13 males and 17 females, did not (group B). These patients were followed for more than 10 years after renal biopsy. In our reports, the clinical remission rate was 24.4% in group A and 13.3% in group B, the stable renal function rate was 82.9% in group A and 70.0% in group B, and the renal survival rate was 95.1% in group A and 73.3% in group B. The renal survival rate was significantly higher in group A than in group B. We investigated the indications for tonsillectomy in patients with IgA nephropathy based on these long-term treatment results and prognostic factors that are able to predict the effects of tonsillectomy. Based on our findings, we propose indication criteria for tonsillectomy in patients with IgA nephropathy.

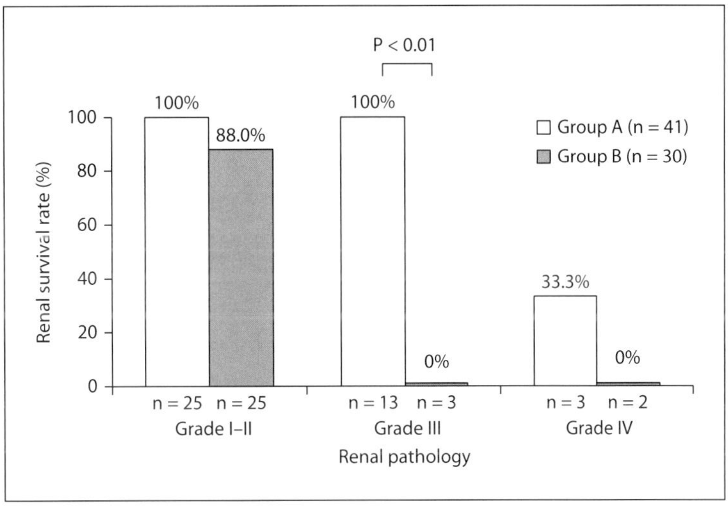

Fig. 1. Comparison of renal survival rates between groups A and B with respect to the difference in the grade of renal pathology.

Materials and Methods

The subjects were 71 patients, including 32 males and 39 females, who had a definite diagnosis of IgA nephropathy based on renal biopsy. They were divided into the 2 groups mentioned above (group A and B). The following 4 parameters were selected as prognostic factors [3]: (1) the presence or absence of a history of tonsillitis, (2) the presence or absence of pus plugs in the lacunae of the palatine tonsils, (3) the results of the tonsillar provocation test, and (4) renal pathology during renal biopsy.

Results and Discussion

A past history of tonsillitis, pus plugs in the lacunae of the palatine tonsils, and the results of the tonsillar provocation test were not useful for predicting the long-term effects of tonsillectomy in patients with IgA nephropathy.

A comparison of renal survival rates between groups A and B with respect to the difference in the grade of renal pathology [4] is shown in figure 1. Among the patients with grade I–II histopathological renal disorders (which show a good and a relatively good prognosis, respectively), the renal survival rates were 100 and 88.0% in groups A and B, respectively. Among the patients with grade III histopathological renal disorders (relatively poor prognosis group), the renal survival rates were 100 and 0% in groups A and B, respectively. Among the patients with grade IV histopathological renal disorders (poor prognosis group), the renal survival rates were 33.3 and 0% in groups A and B, respectively. Among the grade III patients, there was a significant difference between groups A and B.

Sato et al. [5] reported a comparison of renal survival rates between advanced IgA nephropathy groups treated by different methods with respect to the difference in serum creatinine levels at the time of renal biopsy. In this study, among the patients with a serum creatinine level of 2.0 mg/dl or less at the time of renal biopsy, the renal survival rate in the tonsillectomy group was 100% and was significantly higher than those in the other nontonsillectomy groups. Among the patients with a serum creatinine level higher than 2.0 mg/dl at the time of renal biopsy, the renal survival rate showed no significant difference between the groups.

Renal pathology and renal function were found to be useful prognostic factors for predicting the long-term effects of tonsillectomy in patients with IgA nephropathy.

Table 1. Indication criteria for tonsillectomy in patients with IgA nephropathy investigated by us

1	IgA nephropathy has been definitively diagnosed by an evaluation of the renal glomeruli during renal biopsy.
2	Tonsillectomy is indicated for patients who demonstrate grade I–III renal pathology and a serum creatinine level of 2.0 mg/dl or less during renal biopsy. However, even among patients who demonstrate grade IV disease or a serum creatinine level higher than 2.0 mg/dl during renal biopsy, surgery should be considered in the absence of contraindications for tonsillectomy, such as renal hypofunction, providing the patient wants to undergo surgery and informed consent is obtained.
3	The patient's medical history includes deterioration of urine findings during tonsillitis or acute upper respiratory inflammation.
4	Buried tonsils and the attachment of pus plugs to the tonsillar crypt are observed as local findings of the palatine tonsil.
5	Positive findings, especially positive urine findings (hematuria), are detected on the tonsillar provocation test.

Items (1) and (2) are essential.
Items (3) to (5) are indicative, as their inclusion has not been supported by previous studies.

Conclusions

Indication criteria for tonsillectomy in patients with IgA nephropathy, which were developed by us based on the findings we presented above, are shown in table 1. To date, no effective treatment for IgA nephropathy has been established. Even in patients with advanced histopathological renal disorders (grade III or lower), tonsillectomy should be aggressively considered when renal function is maintained to some degree.

References

1 Akagi H, Fukushima K, Kosaka M, Doi A, Okano M, Kariya S, Nishizaki K, Masuda Y: A 10-year retrospective case-control study for IgA nephropathy after tonsillectomy. ICS 2003;1257:147–150.

2 Akagi H, Kosaka M, Hattori K, Doi A, Fukushima K, Okano M, Kariya S, Nishizaki K, Sugiyama N, Shikata K, Makino H, Masuda Y: Long-term results of tonsillectomy as a treatment for IgA nephropathy. Acta Otolaryngol 2004;suppl 555:38–42.

3 Tomioka S, Miyoshi K, Tabata K, Hotta O, Taguma Y: Clinical study of chronic tonsillitis with IgA nephropathy treated by tonsillectomy. Acta Otolaryngol 1996;Suppl 523:175–177.

4 Sakai H, Abe K, Kobayashi Y, Koyama A, Shigematsu H, Harada T, Yoshikawa N, Arakawa M, Itoh H, Osawa G, Sakai O, Dohi K, Yamanaka N, Nagasawa T, Kurokawa K: Clinical guidelines of IgA nephropathy. Jpn J Nephrol 1995;37:417–421.

5 Sato M, Hotta O, Tomioka S, Horigome I, Chiba S, Miyazaki M, Noshiro H, Taguma Y: Cohort study of advanced IgA nephropathy: efficacy and limitations of corticosteroids with tonsillectomy. Nephron Clin Pract 2003;93:137–145.

Hirofumi Akagi
Department of Otolaryngology,
Incorporated Administrative Agency
National Hospital Organization Minami-Okayama Medical Center
4066 Hayashima, Hayashima-cho
Tsukubo-gun, Okayama 701-0304 (Japan)
Tel. +81 86 4821121, E-Mail akagih@s-okayama.hosp.go.jp

Harabuchi Y (ed): Recent Advances in Tonsils and Mucosal Barriers of the Upper Airways.
Adv Otorhinolaryngol. Basel, Karger, 2011, vol 72, pp 53–56

Periodontal and ENT Therapy in the Treatment of Pediatric Henoch-Schönlein Purpura and IgA Nephropathy

Chiyoko N. Inoue[a] · Sachiko Matsutani[b] · Masako Ishidoya[b] · Rikako Homma[b] · Yasushi Chiba[a] · Takako Nagasaka[c]

Department of [a]Pediatrics, [b]Otolaryngology and [c]Dentistry, Red Cross Sendai Hospital, Sendai, Japan

Abstract

Henoch-Schönlein purpura (HSP) and IgA nephropathy (IgAN) are both IgA1-related vasculitis caused by vascular deposition of IgA1-containing immune complexes. A pathological role of the tonsils in the development of HSP and IgAN has been suggested. Tonsils are a mucosa-associated lymphoid organ. Since oral and sinonasal cavities are anatomically directly connected to the tonsils, delivering exogenous antigens into the tonsils to induce local and systemic antibody responses, we examined the infectious status of these cavities when we treated HSP and IgAN. In 40 HSP children (6.7 ± 2.5 years), apical periodontitis, rhinosinusitis, and otitis media were identified in 21 (53%, 4.9 ± 2.8 affected teeth), 19 (48%), and 4 (10%) of them, whereas in 11 IgAN children (10.4 ± 2.5 years), these diseases were observed in 6 (55%, 5.8 ± 4.6 affected teeth), 2 (18%), and 0 (0%) of them, respectively. We first treated the patients with extensive eradiation of infectious foci, including antimicrobial treatment and root canal therapy. In 31 HSP patients, such dental and/or ENT therapy resulted in a complete cure without development of nephritis or recurrent attacks. For the remaining 9 HSP and 11 IgAN patients, we further performed tonsillectomy plus methylprednisolone (MP) pulse therapy to control their intractable symptoms, including aggravated purpura, recurrent HSP attacks or nephritis. Using this therapeutic strategy, all of the HSP patients attained clinical remission. All of the IgAN patients with various histological grades also achieved normalization of urinalysis by 7.2 ± 5.7 months after the start of steroid therapy. No relapses were observed in both diseases during follow-up for 2–10 years. In pediatric HSP and IgAN, apical periodontitis and rhinosinusitis may be involved in abnormal immune responses in both the tonsils and whole body. We conclude that extensive elimination of these infectious foci is beneficial to optimize the effect of tonsillectomy plus MP pulse therapy.

Henoch-Schönlein purpura (HSP) and IgA nephropathy (IgAN) are both IgA1-related vasculitides. Vascular deposition of the IgA1-containing immune complex plays a pathogenic role. HSP tends to affect children aged around 6 years with skin lesions, whereas IgAN lacks skin lesions and usually affects teenagers with a peak age of onset at around 12 years in Japan. Nephritis is associated with this vasculitis and is slowly progressive, resulting in end-stage renal failure in approximately 30% of the patients.

Children suffer from the common cold 3–8 times a year, and this is frequently complicated with rhinosinusitis. Rhinosinusitis usually resolves but occasionally persists for a few months without recognizable symptoms, becoming chronic rhinosinusitis. Children also tend to have dental caries. Dental caries in premature teeth easily invade through infected root canals into surrounding bony tissues, forming apical periodontitis. Apical periodontitis is a severe chronic infection containing billions of aerobic and anaerobic bacteria of more than 300 species in a single lesion [1]. Therefore, tonsils in children can be infected and inflamed, resulting in chronic tonsillitis. In addition, emerging evidence also suggest the role of periodontitis in inducing various types of vasculitis, including Berger's disease and necrotizing vasculitis by affecting vascular endothelial cell function [2].

'Tonsillectomy plus methylprednisolone (MP) pulse therapy' is a groundbreaking therapeutic strategy, which was begun in 1988 for adult IgAN [3]. In our institution, we have applied this therapeutic approach for pediatric IgAN as well as for intractable HSP since 1999 [4, 5]. In addition to performing this therapeutic procedure, we examined the infections of dental caries/apical periodontitis and rhinosinusitis, which could induce chronic tonsillitis, and thoroughly treated these infections. In this review, we summarize 10 years of our clinical experience.

Patients

The profile of 40 HSP patients was as follows. Mean age at onset was 6.7 years. Besides palpable purpura, more than 70% of the patients complained of abdominal pain and/or arthralgias, and 45% of them had both. There was a previous history of upper respiratory infection in 45% of the patients. In 5 patients, group A streptococcus was isolated from nasopharyngeal culture samples.

The profile of 11 patients was also as follows. The mean age at onset was 10.4 years. All patients exhibited hematuria and 82% of them excreted a significant amount of proteinuria, averaging 0.98 g/day. Seven patients were detected by annual urine screening for schoolchildren. Based on the renal pathology, all were suffering from diffuse proliferative glomerulonephritis, whereas 7 patients had active nephropathy with glomerular crescentic formation or capsular attachment.

Focal Infection in Patients of Henoch-Schönlein Purpura and IgA Nephropathy

Figure 1 shows the focal infections identified in the patients. In 40 HSP patients, the most commonly identified infection was dental caries (28/40, 70%) and apical periodontitis (21/40, 53%), followed by rhinosinusitis (19/40, 48%), and all were chronic. Forty-three percent of HSP patients had more than two simultaneous focal infections, for example, apical periodontitis and rhinosinusitis. On the other hand, chronic tonsillitis and otitis media were only found in a small amount of patients. In patients with IgAN, the prevalence of dental caries and apical periodontitis was also high (8/11, 73% and 6/11, 55%). In contrast to HSP, chronic rhinosinusitis in IgAN was much less common (2/11, 18%). Because rhinosinusitis is easy to resolve after the age of 7, the low prevalence of rhinosinusitis in IgAN may reflect a higher age at onset of IgAN. Otitis media was not identified in patients with IgAN.

Oral health status can be estimated by the DMFT score as a marker. DMFT is the total number of decayed, missing and filled teeth, representing a history of current and past dental health. The lower the score, the better the oral hygiene. In this study, the DMFT scores of our HSP patients was 5.0, which was slightly higher than that of the average Japanese (4.7 in 1999), but was significantly higher than that of American children (2.0 in 1987). On the other hand, the DMFT score in our IgAN patients was 5.9, which was much higher level than those reported from any other countries (e.g. USA, 1.3 in 1992) or average Japanese children (1.7 in 2007). This high DMFT score suggests a poor oral hygiene status in our HSP and IgAN patients.

Therapeutic Strategy and the Prognosis

Our therapeutic strategy for patients of HSP and IgAN is depicted in figure 2. On the day of diagnosis of HSP, dentists and otolaryngologists started exploration of the infectious foci. At the same time, intravenous antibiotic therapy was empirically started as a first-line therapy. In patients who had apical periodontitis in premature teeth, the affected teeth were extracted. When apical periodontitis was in the permanent teeth, extensive root-canal therapy was performed. For chronic rhinosinusitis, low-dose clarithromycin was prescribed until complete resolution was confirmed by sinus X-ray. Thirty-one patients reached clinical remission by conducting these therapies. However, 9 patients did not respond well to these therapies, exhibiting recurrent, prolonged, severe, or nephritic episodes. In these patients, we decided to suppress the disease activity

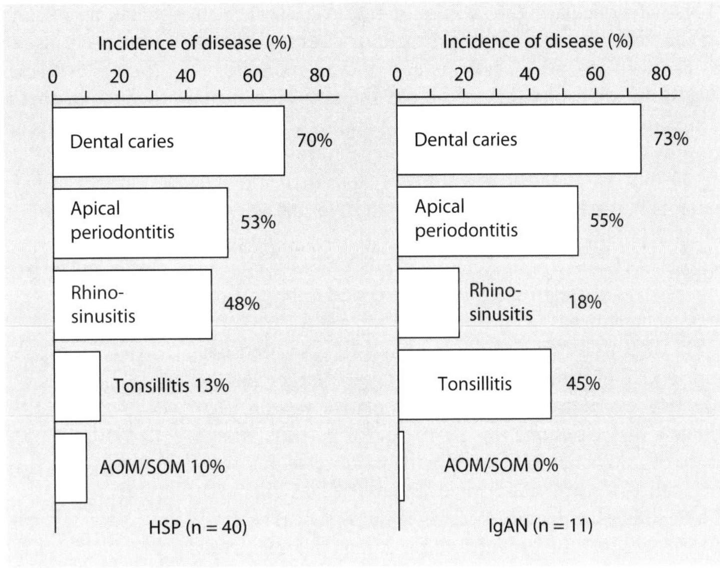

Fig. 1. Identified focal infection in patients with HSP and IgAN.

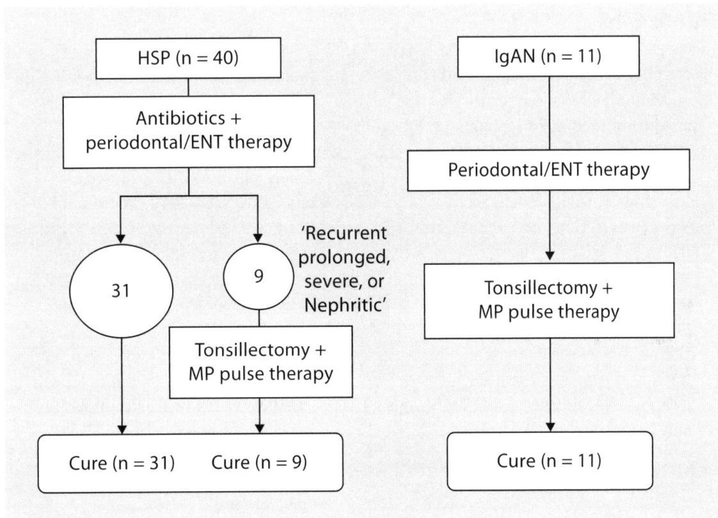

Fig. 2. Therapeutic strategy for HSP and IgAN.

by tonsillectomy plus MP pulse therapy. After these procedures, all the patients were cured. For IgAN, we also disinfected infectious foci. Tonsillectomy plus MP pulse therapy was then carried out followed by oral steroidal therapy for an average of 9.5 months, then all patients obtained clinical remission without any relapses.

In order to assess the effectiveness of our therapeutic regimen for HSP, we reviewed two eligible prospective studies and compared data on clinical outcomes, with renal complication as a marker. The occurrence of nephropathy in our study was only 3/40 (8%), which is significantly lower than those in other studies (e.g. 41% in the study by Ronkainen et al. [6]). This result demonstrates that our therapeutic approach greatly improves the long-term outcomes of pediatric HSP. We next estimated the effectiveness of our therapeutic approach for the prognosis of IgAN by calculating the remission rate every month after the start of steroid therapy. Proteinuria remission was observed in 10 and 11 patients at 6 and 12 months, respectively, after initiation of steroid therapy. Hematuria remission was observed in 7 and 9 patients at 6 and 12 months (respectively) after initiation of steroid therapy. By 20 months after the initiation of steroid therapy, all patients had achieved clinical remission. For all patients, hematuria remission was always preceded by proteinuria remission.

Two years' treatment with steroid and immunosuppressive agents has been a standard of care for pediatric IgAN. In a study by Yoshikawa et al. [7], who used disappearance of proteinuria as a surrogate marker for the effectiveness of treatment, the cumulative rate of proteinuria disappearance was 80.4% for 23 patients after 2 years of combination therapy with predonisolone, warfarin, dipyridamole, and mizoribine (PWDM therapy). On the other hand, a prospective study by Kawasaki et al. [8] showed that the prognosis after 2-year treatment was better for pediatric patients who underwent tonsillectomy plus MP pulse therapy than for those treated by PWDM therapy, with clinical remission rates of 75 vs. 56%, respectively. Our current study seems to show a better prognosis: all 11 patients achieved clinical remission by 20 months.

Conclusion

In pediatric HSP and IgAN, apical periodontitis, chronic rhinosinusitis and chronic tonsillitis may be involved in abnormal immune responses in both the tonsils and the whole body. Extensive elimination of these focal infections is beneficial to optimize the effect of tonsillectomy plus MP pulse therapy in curing the diseases.

References

1 Nair PN: Apical periodontitis: a dynamic encounter between root canal infection and host response. Periodontology 2000 1997;13:121–148.

2 Chen Y-W, Nagasawa T, Wara-Aswapati N, Ushida Y, Wang D, Takeuchi Y, Kobayashi H, Umeda M, InoueY, Iwai T, Ishikawa I, Izumi Y: Association between periodontitis and anti-cardiolipin antibodies in Buerger disease. J Clin Periodontol 2009;36:830–835.

3 Hotta O: Use of corticosteroids, other immunosuppressive therapies, and tonsillectomy in the treatment of IgA nephropathy. Semin Nephrol 2004;24:244–255.

4 Inoue CN, Chiba Y, Morimoto T, Nishio T, Kondo Y, Adachi M, Matsutani S: Tonsillectomy in the treatment of pediatric Henoch-Schoenlein nephritis. Clin Nephrol 2007;67:298–305.

5 Inoue CN, Nagasaka T, Matsutani S, Ishidoya M, Homma R, Chiba Y: Efficacy of early dental and ENT therapy in preventing nephropathy in pediatric Henoch-Schönlein purpura. Clin Rheumatol 2008;27:1489–1496.

6 Ronkainen J, Koskimies O, Ala-Houhala M, Antikainen M, Merenmies J, Rajantie J, Ormälä T, Turtinen J, Nuutinen M: Early prednisone therapy in Henoch-Schönlein purpura: a randomized, double-blind, placebo-controlled trial. J Pediatr 2006;149:241–247.

7 Yoshikawa N, Nakanishi K, Ishikura K, Hataya H, Iijima K, Honda M: Combination therapy with mizoribine for severe childhood IgA nephropathy. Pediatr Nephrol 2008;23:757–763.

8 Kawasaki Y, Takano K, Suyama K, Isome M, Suzuki H, Sakuma H, Fujiki T, Suzuki H, Hosoya M: Efficacy of tonsillectomy pulse therapy versus multiple-drug therapy for IgA nephropathy. Pediatr Nephrol 2006;21:1701–1706.

Chiyoko N. Inoue, MD, PhD
Department of Pediatrics, Red Cross Sendai Hospital
2–43–3, Taihaku-ku, Yagiyamahoncho
Sendai 982-8501 (Japan)
Tel. +81 22 243 1111, Fax +81 22 243 1101, E-Mail chnagano@sendai.jrc.or.jp

Harabuchi Y (ed): Recent Advances in Tonsils and Mucosal Barriers of the Upper Airways.
Adv Otorhinolaryngol. Basel, Karger, 2011, vol 72, pp 57–59

Tonsillectomy Combined with Steroid Pulse Therapy Induces Clinical Remission of IgA Nephropathy

Hiroyuki Komatsu · Shouichi Fujimoto

First Department of Internal Medicine, University of Miyazaki Hospital, Miyazaki, Japan

Abstract

Tonsillectomy combined with steroid pulse therapy has been a popular approach to treating IgA nephropathy (IgAN) in Japan for several years. However, little is understood about how such combined therapy affects the clinical course of IgAN. We therefore compared the effects of the combined therapy with those of steroid pulsing alone in a controlled study of patients with IgAN. The achievement ratio of clinical remission (CR), defined as the disappearance of urinary protein (UP) and occult blood (UOB), were compared between tonsillectomy combined with steroid pulse therapy (n = 35) and steroid pulse monotherapy (n = 20). The CR rate was higher in the group given combined therapy than that given monotherapy at the final observation 54.0 ± 21.2 months after the initial treatment (54.3 vs. 25.0%, p = 0.033). The Cox regression model showed that the combined therapy caused UP to disappear 6-fold more effectively than monotherapy. These findings suggest that tonsillectomy combined with steroid pulse therapy induces CR in patients with IgAN. Meanwhile, the indications for this therapy and verification of its positive long-term prognosis require urgent validation.

Tonsillectomy combined with steroid pulse therapy has received recent focus as a promising treatment for IgA nephropathy (IgAN) in Japan since Hotta et al. [1] reported that about 60% of patients with IgAN treated in this manner achieved clinical remission (CR) defined as the disappearance of proteinuria and hematuria. A nationwide survey of the combined therapy in Japan also showed that 45.6% of 2,746 patients who received the combined therapy between 2000 and 2006 achieved CR after 12 months, but that patient selection, injected quantities of steroids and CR rates vary among institutions [2].

We therefore conducted a nonrandomized controlled study to assess whether tonsillectomy combined with steroid pulse therapy causes CR more effectively than steroid pulse monotherapy among patients with IgAN [3]. Fifty-five patients were allocated to receive either combined therapy (n = 35) or monotherapy (n = 20), and repeated renal biopsies were obtained from 11 and 7 of the respective groups during the follow-up period. Both groups received intravenous methylprednisolone (0.5 g/day × 3 days), followed by

Table 1. Effect of tonsillectomy combined with steroid pulse therapy on IgA nephropathy

Authors	Year	Study design	Patient type	Number of patients	Follow-up months	Treatment	End-point	Results
Hotta et al. [1]	2001	cohort	adult	329	82	TSP vs. SP and/or OP	clinical remission rate	effect
Sato et al. [5]	2003	cohort	adult	70	70	TSP vs. OP±CPA	renal survival rate	no effect
Kawasaki et al. [6]	2006	RCT	child	32	37	TSP+WD vs. OP+WD+M	clinicopathological data	effect
Miyazaki et al. [7]	2007	NRCT	adult	101	60	TSP vs. SP vs. T	clinical remission rate	effect
Komatsu et al. [3]	2008	NRCT	adult	55	54	TSP vs. SP	clinical remission rate	effect
Kawaguchi et al. [8]	2010	cohort	adult	388	24 (median)	TSP vs. SP vs. T	clinical remission rate	effect

RCT = Randomized controlled trial; NRCT = nonrandomized controlled trial; TSP = tonsillectomy combined with steroid pulse therapy; SP = steroid pulse therapy; OP = oral prednisolone; CPA = cyclophosphamide; W = warfarin; D = dipyridamole; M = mizoribine; T = tonsillectomy.

oral prednisolone (initial dose, 0.5 mg/kg/day) for 12–18 months. The primary evaluation items were a 100% increase in serum creatinine (sCr) from baseline levels or the CR rate. Baseline clinicopathological data did not statistically differ between the groups given combined therapy or monotherapy (SBP, 122.0 ± 12.9 vs. 127.6 ± 16.6 mm Hg; UP, 1.06 ± 1.01 vs. 1.41 ± 1.05 g/day; sCr, 0.72 ± 0.29 vs. 0.84 ± 0.30 mg/dl). The CR rate was higher in the combined therapy than in the monotherapy group at 24 months after the initial treatment (61.8 vs. 17.6%; $p < 0.001$, χ^2 test), and the therapeutic effect persisted until the final observation at 54.0 ± 21.2 months (54.3 vs. 25.0%, $p = 0.033$, χ^2 test). None of combined therapy group achieved a 100% increase in sCr from the baseline level, whereas one patient in monotherapy group developed end-stage renal disease during the observation period. The histological findings of repeated biopsy specimens from 18 patients revealed significantly more reduced mesangial proliferation and IgA deposition in the group that received combined therapy. The Cox regression model adjusted for known risk factors (SBP, UP, sCr, and histological severity) showed that the combined therapy was about 6-fold more effective in causing the disappearance of UP than steroid pulse monotherapy. These findings suggest that tonsillectomy combined with steroid pulse treatment induces clinical remission more effectively than steroid pulse monotherapy in patients with IgAN.

A possible mechanism for IgAN onset and progression has been proposed [4]. The initial phase is chronic antigenic stimulation of the innate immune system by the tonsillar mucosa via the 'mucosa-bone marrow axis'. Thereafter, aberrantly glycosylated IgA1 derived from the bone marrow is deposited within the mesangial area. Tonsillectomy might act 'upstream' of the mechanism by eliminating antigenic stimuli from the tonsillar mucosa, whereas steroid pulse therapy acts 'downstream' by suppressing the abnormal immune response in the bone marrow, which leads to subsequent inflammation in renal glomeruli. Thus, intervention against both pathogenic mechanisms might have a better therapeutic effect on IgAN than steroid monotherapy.

Our study, however, has several limitations. We used the surrogate markers of proteinuria and/or hematuria remission to assess renal outcome. Patients with advanced IgAN accompanied by sCr levels of >2.0 mg/dl were excluded and the trial was not randomized. Other studies of the effectiveness of tonsillectomy combined with steroid pulse therapy have similar issues regarding study design, short follow-up periods, and lack of 'true' end-points such as renal survival rates (table 1). These Japanese studies also tended to select patients at the early phase of the disease, because Japan has an established annual health check-up system that monitors urinary parameters. In consequence, the effectiveness of the combined therapy for patients with advanced IgAN remains unclear at this stage. Long-term and larger observational studies should assess the effectiveness of the combined therapy on actual renal outcome. A randomized controlled trial is ideal to establish a high level of evidence in the field, although tonsillectomy is a surgical procedure. Furthermore, validation of the indication for combined therapy based on tonsillar and renal findings is an important and urgent concern for otolaryngologists and nephrologists.

References

1 Hotta O, Miyazaki M, Furuta T, Tomioka S, Chiba S, Horigome I, Abe K, Taguma Y: Tonsillectomy and steroid pulse therapy significantly impact on clinical remission in patients with IgA nephropathy. Am J Kidney Dis 2001;38:736–743.

2 Miura N, Imai H, Kikuchi S, et al: Tonsillectomy and steroid pulse (TSP) therapy for patients with IgA nephropathy: a nationwide survey of TSP therapy in Japan and an analysis of the predictive factors for resistance to TSP therapy. Clin Exp Nephrol 2009;13:460–466.

3 Komatsu H, Fujimoto S, Hara S, Sato Y, Yamada K, Kitamura K: Effect of tonsillectomy plus steroid pulse therapy on clinical remission of IgA nephropathy: a controlled study. Clin J Am Soc Nephrol 2008;3:1301–1307.

4 Hotta O: Use of corticosteroids, other immunosuppressive therapies, and tonsillectomy in the treatment of IgA nephropathy. Semin Nephrol 2004;24: 244–255.

5 Sato M, Hotta O, Tomioka S, Horigome I, Chiba S, Miyazaki M, Noshiro H, Taguma Y: Cohort study of advanced IgA nephropathy: efficacy and limitations of corticosteroids with tonsillectomy. Nephron Clin Pract 2003;93:c137–c145.

6 Kawasaki Y, Takano K, Suyama K, Isome M, Suzuki H, Sakuma H, Fujiki T, Suzuki H, Hosoya M: Efficacy of tonsillectomy pulse therapy versus multiple-drug therapy for IgA nephropathy. Pediatr Nephrol 2006;21: 1701–1706.

7 Miyazaki M, Hotta O, Komatsuda A, Nakai S, Shoji T, Yasunaga C, Taguma Y, Japanese Multicenter Study Group on Treatment of IgA Nephropathy (JST-IgAN): A multicenter prospective cohort study of tonsillectomy and steroid therapy in Japanese patients with IgA nephropathy: a 5-year report. Contrib Nephrol. Basel, Karger, 2007, vol 157, pp 94–98.

8 Kawaguchi T, Ieiri N, Yamazaki S, Hayashino Y, Gillespie B, Miyazaki M, Taguma Y, Fukuhara S, Hotta O: Clinical effectiveness of steroid pulse therapy combined with tonsillectomy in patients with immunoglobulin A nephropathy presenting glomerular haematuria and minimal proteinuria. Nephrology 2010;15:116–123.

Hiroyuki Komatsu
First Department of Internal Medicine, University of Miyazaki Hospital
5200 Kihara, Kiyotake
Miyazaki, 889-1692 (Japan)
Tel. +81 985 85 0872, E-Mail hkomatsu@fc.miyazaki-u.ac.jp

Harabuchi Y (ed): Recent Advances in Tonsils and Mucosal Barriers of the Upper Airways.
Adv Otorhinolaryngol. Basel, Karger, 2011, vol 72, pp 60–63

Aberrant Glycosylation of IgA1 and Anti-Glycan Antibodies in IgA Nephropathy: Role of Mucosal Immune System

Jan Novak[a] · Zina Moldoveanu[a] · Bruce A. Julian[a,b] · Milan Raska[a,e] · Robert J. Wyatt[c] · Yusuke Suzuki[f] · Yasuhiko Tomino[f] · Ali G. Gharavi[d] · Jiri Mestecky[a,b] · Hitoshi Suzuki[a,f]

Departments of [a]Microbiology and [b]Medicine, University of Alabama at Birmingham, Birmingham, Ala., [c]Children's Foundation Research Center at Le Bonheur Children's Medical Center, Memphis, Tenn., and [d]Department of Medicine, Division of Nephrology, College of Physicians and Surgeons, Columbia University, New York, N.Y., USA; [e]Department of Immunology, Palacky University in Olomouc, Olomouc, Czech Republic; [f]Department of Medicine, Division of Nephrology, Juntendo University Faculty of Medicine, Tokyo, Japan

Abstract

IgA nephropathy (IgAN), the most common glomerulonephritis, is characterized by mesangial IgA1-containing immunodeposits, proliferation of mesangial cells, and matrix expansion. Clinical onset is frequently heralded by synpharyngitic hematuria, macroscopic hematuria during an upper-respiratory tract infection. Clinical and laboratory data support a postulated extrarenal origin of the glomerular IgA1, likely derived from circulating immune complexes containing polymeric IgA1, deficient in galactose in the hinge-region *O*-glycans, bound by antiglycan antibodies. This aberrant IgA1 is produced by IgA1-secreting cells with abnormal activities of specific glycosyltransferases. The galactose deficiency affects IgA1 induced by mucosal antigens and elevated circulating levels of this abnormal IgA1 are hereditable, suggesting interactions of genetic and environmental factors. An abnormal mucosal immune response resulting in production of galactose-deficient IgA1 in IgAN patients is supported by several observations: the aberrant glycosylation affects mostly polymeric IgA1 produced by mucosal-associated IgA1-secreting cells (including those from tonsils), the synpharyngitic nature of the macroscopic hematuria, and the association of disease severity with polymorphisms of a pattern-recognition receptor, TLR9. Thus, IgAN is an auto-immune disease, induced by mesangial deposition of circulating complexes containing galactose-deficient IgA1. The aberrant glycosylation of IgA1 may reflect abnormal mucosal immune responses to infections of the upper respiratory tract in genetically predisposed individuals.

IgA nephropathy (IgAN), the most common type of glomerulonephritis in the world, is characterized by mesangial immunodeposits of IgA1, frequently accompanied by complement component 3, and IgG or IgM or both. Hematuria is typical and often includes episodes of macroscopic bleeding that coincide with mucosal infections, including those of the upper respiratory tract or digestive system. Proliferation of mesangial cells and expansion of extracellular matrix are found in patients with mild clinical disease, but progressive glomerular and interstitial sclerosis lead to end-stage renal failure within 20 years after diagnosis in 20–40% of patients. IgAN recurs in 50–60% of renal allografts; however, immune deposits in a kidney transplanted from a donor with subclinical IgAN into a patient with non-IgAN renal disease clear within several weeks. Moreover, idiotypic determinants are shared between the circulating complexes and the mesangial deposits, but a disease-specific idiotype has not been identified. These findings suggest that the cause of IgAN is extrarenal and is most likely due to deposition of circulating immune complexes containing IgA1 [1].

The apparent association between the immune complexes and upper-respiratory tract infections prompted an early search for antigens of environmental or microbial origin in the renal deposits. Although a variety of findings have been published, there is a current consensus that there is generally no IgAN-specific environmental or microbial antigen in renal immunodeposits.

Analysis of the glycosylation of IgA1 in patients with IgAN has provided new insights into the mechanisms underlying the formation of immune complexes and their deposition in the mesangium. Specifically, an aberrant glycosylation of IgA1 *O*-glycans, galactose deficiency, is a key pathogenetic factor contributing to the development of IgAN, as aberrantly glycosylated IgA1 is recognized by antiglycan antibodies (IgG and/or IgA1) [2, 3] and, consequently, immune complexes form. Circulating complexes in patients with IgAN contain IgA1 with galactose-deficient hinge-region *O*-glycans and this IgA1 is the predominant glycosylation variant of IgA1 in the mesangium. Collectively, these observations indicate that aberrant glycosylation of IgA1 plays a pivotal role in the pathogenesis of IgAN.

In humans, IgA1 represents one of the two structurally and functionally distinct subclasses of IgA. Unlike IgA2, IgM and IgG, IgA1 contains a structurally unique hinge-region segment between the first and second constant region domains of its heavy chains with up to six *O*-glycans consisting of *N*-acetylgalactosamine (GalNAc) with a β1,3-linked galactose; both residues may be sialylated. The carbohydrate composition of the *O*-glycans on normal human serum IgA1 is variable, with galactose-GalNAc disaccharide, and its mono- and di-sialylated variants as the prevailing forms. Galactose-deficient variants with terminal GalNAc or sialylated GalNAc are rarely found in the *O*-glycans of serum IgA1 of normal individuals, but are much more common in that of IgAN patients. The aberrant IgA1 predominates in the glomerular immunodeposits and in the circulating complexes and is produced though biosynthetic processes in IgA1-secreting cells [4].

O-glycans of IgA1 are synthesized in a stepwise manner, beginning with attachment of GalNAc to Ser or Thr catalyzed by a member of the UDP-GalNAc-transferase enzyme family. The *O*-glycan can be then extended by sequential attachment of galactose and/or sialic acid residues to the GalNAc. Addition of galactose is mediated by core 1 β1,3-galactosyltransferase (C1GalT1) that transfers galactose from UDP-galactose to the GalNAc. The stability of this enzyme during proteosynthesis depends on its interaction with the C1GalT1-specific molecular chaperone, Cosmc, that assists in the folding of the enzyme. In the absence of Cosmc, the C1GalT1 protein is degraded rapidly and the hinge region fails to receive its normal complement of galactose residues. The *O*-glycan structure is completed by a sialyltransferase that attaches sialic acid to the galactose. If sialic acid is linked to GalNAc prior to the attachment of galactose, this 'premature' sialylation by e.g., ST6GalNAcII precludes the subsequent attachment of galactose. Therefore, the relative activities of ST6GalNAcII and C1GalT1 directly influence the glycosylation of IgA1.

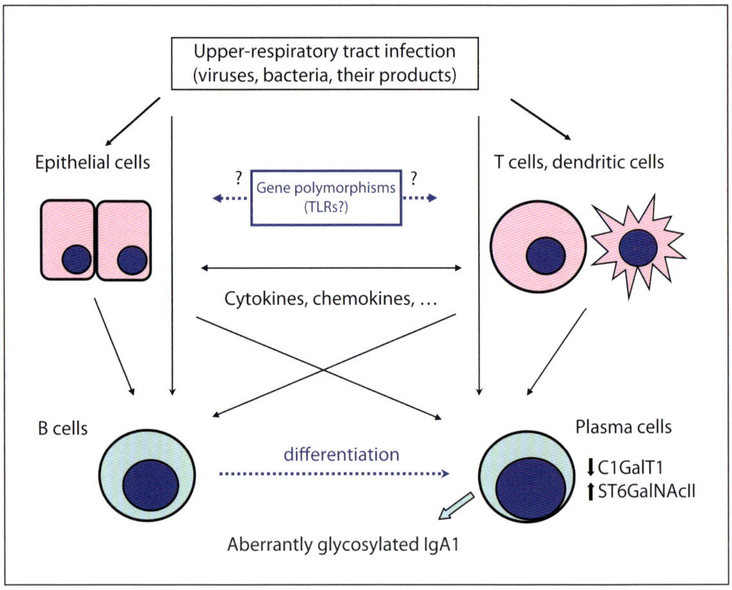

Fig. 1. Potential processes leading to the increased production of nephritogenic, aberrantly glycosylated, IgA1. We postulate that some of the events during an infection of the upper-respiratory tract, by viruses or bacteria, in a genetically predisposed individual send signals indirectly via cells in the mucosa (epithelial cells, T cells, dendritic cells) or directly to the B cells resulting in differentiation of IgA1-secreting plasma cells with altered expression and activity of the key glycosyltransferases and secretion of galactose-deficient IgA1.

Aberrant glycosylation in IgAN affects only IgA1, not other glycoproteins with *O*-glycans. This aberrancy of IgA1 is not due to variation in the coding sequence of the IgA1 hinge region, but rather to the abnormal regulation of particular enzymes in IgA1-producing cells. Specifically, the activity of C1GalT1 is reduced and that of ST6GalNAcII is elevated [4]. Consequently, these cells secrete IgA1 that contains terminal as well as sialylated GalNAc [4, 5]. The result is an increased fraction of IgA1 molecules in IgAN patients with *O*-glycans that are galactose-deficient and contain GalNAc that is frequently sialylated [4, 6].

It is of interest that the aberrant glycosylation affects the dimeric and polymeric but not the monomeric forms of the IgA1 secreted by the cells from patients with IgAN [4]. Similarly, it has been shown that a substantial portion of IgA1 in the mesangial deposits is polymeric [7]. These observations seem to imply mucosal origin of the pathogenic IgA1, as the polymeric J-chain-containing forms of IgA1 are mostly produced at mucosal sites. Moreover, it was shown that IgA1 synthesized in response to mucosally acquired antigens is galactose-deficient in the *O*-glycans [8]. However, the levels of aberrantly glycosylated IgA1 in the circulation of patients with IgAN are elevated and this phenotype is heritable. It is therefore possible that a combination of genetic and environmental factors is required for the overproduction of galactose-deficient IgA1 to cause IgAN. This conclusion is further supported by the observation that polymorphisms of one of the pattern-recognition receptors, TLR9, are associated with the clinical severity of IgAN [9]. One can thus envision a process wherein events during an infection of the upper-respiratory tract, by viruses or bacteria, in a genetically predisposed individual send signals indirectly via cells in the mucosa (epithelial cells, T cells, dendritic cells) or directly to the B cells resulting in differentiation of IgA1-secreting plasma cells with altered expression/activity of the key glycosyltransferases. The consequence would be increased production of nephritogenic, aberrantly glycosylated, IgA1 (fig. 1).

As outlined above, these issues of the interactions of IgA1-producing cells with microbiota of the upper-respiratory tract in IgAN patients are not well understood. Similarly, it is not clear where the cells secreting polymeric galactose-deficient IgA1 reside. Are tonsils an inductive site for these cells? To which tissues are then these cells directed and by what mechanisms? Do the cells that produce the polymeric galactose-deficient IgA1 home to peripheral lymphoid tissues, mucosal tissues or both [10]? Are the cells that synthesize the antiglycan antibodies also primed in tonsils, or in other sites of the upper-respiratory or digestive tract? These questions illustrate the important challenges that researchers and clinicians must answer to unravel the pathogenesis of IgAN. It can be hoped that new relevant information may be forthcoming from clinical trials involving tonsillectomy.

In summary, developments during the past decade have defined IgAN as an auto-immune disease, in which aberrantly glycosylated IgA1 is bound by antiglycan antibodies and the resultant immune complexes deposit in the renal mesangium and induce injury. Future studies are needed to define involvement of the mucosal immune system in the pathogenetic processes leading to the formation of the nephritogenetic IgA1-containing immune complexes.

Acknowledgements

The authors acknowledge grants from NIDDK supporting their research of IgAN, DK082753, DK078244, DK080301, DK075868, DK083663, DK071802, and DK077279, and by GAP302/10/1055 Czech Science Foundation and NT11081 Ministry of Health of the Czech Republic, and express their gratitude to the patients and their families for participation in various IgAN studies.

References

1 Julian BA, Novak J: IgA nephropathy: an update. Curr Opin Nephrol Hypertens 2004;13:171–179.
2 Suzuki H, Fun R, Zhang Z, Brown R, Hall S, Julian BA, Chatham WW, Suzuki Y, Wyatt RJ, Moldoveanu Z, Lee JY, Robinson J, Tomana M, Tomino Y, Mestecky J, Novak J: Aberrantly glycosylated IgA1 in IgA nephropathy patients is recognized by IgG antibodies with restricted heterogeneity. J Clin Invest 2009;119:1668–1677.
3 Tomana M, Novak J, Julian BA, Matousovic K, Konecny K, Mestecky J: Circulating immune complexes in IgA nephropathy consist of IgA1 with galactose-deficient hinge region and antiglycan antibodies. J Clin Invest 1999;104:73–81.
4 Suzuki H, Moldoveanu Z, Hall S, Brown R, Vu HL, Novak L, Julian BA, Tomana M, Wyatt RJ, Edberg JE, Alarcón GS, Kimberly RP, Tomino Y, Mestecky J, Novak J: IgA1-secreting cell lines from patients with IgA nephropathy produce aberrantly glycosylated IgA1. J Clin Invest 2008;118:629–639.
5 Leung JCK, Poon PYK, Lai KN: Increased sialylation of polymeric immunoglobulin A1: mechanism of selective glomerular deposition in immunoglobulin A nephropathy? J Lab Clin Med 1999;133:152–160.
6 Moldoveanu Z, Wyatt RJ, Lee J, Tomana M, Julian BA, Mestecky J, Huang W-Q, Anreddy S, Hall S, Hastings MC, Lau KK, Cook WJ, Novak J: Patients with IgA nephropathy have increased serum galactose-deficient IgA1 levels. Kidney Int 2007;71:1148–1154.
7 Monteiro RC, Halbwachs-Mecarelli L, Roque-Barreira MC, Noel LH, Berger J, Lesavre P: Charge and size of mesangial IgA in IgA nephropathy. Kidney Int 1985;28:666–671.
8 Smith AC, Molyneux K, Feehally J, Barratt J: *O*-Glycosylation of serum IgA1 antibodies against mucosal and systemic antigens in IgA nephropathy. J Am Soc Nephrol 2006;17:3520–3528.
9 Suzuki H, Suzuki Y, Narita I, Aizawa M, Kihara M, Yamanaka T, Kanou T, Tsukaguchi H, Novak J, Horikoshi S, Tomino Y: Toll-like receptor 9 affects severity of IgA nephropathy. J Am Soc Nephrol 2008;19:2384–2395.
10 Bene MC, Faure GC: Mesangial IgA in IgA nephropathy arises from the mucosa. Am J Kidney Dis 1988;12: 406–409.

Jan Novak
University of Alabama at Birmingham, Department of Microbiology
845 19th Street South, Room 734
Birmingham, AL 35294 (USA)
Tel. +1 205 934 4480, E-Mail jannovak@uab.edu

Harabuchi Y (ed): Recent Advances in Tonsils and Mucosal Barriers of the Upper Airways.
Adv Otorhinolaryngol. Basel, Karger, 2011, vol 72, pp 64–67

Reevaluation of the Mucosa-Bone Marrow Axis in IgA Nephropathy with Animal Models

Yusuke Suzuki[a] · Hitoshi Suzuki[a] · Daisuke Sato[a] · Tadahiro Kajiyama[a] · Keiko Okazaki[a] · Azusa Hashimoto[a] · Masao Kihara[a] · Kenji Yamaji[a] · Kenji Satake[a] · Junichiro Nakata[a] · Masashi Aizawa[a] · Jan Novak[b] · Yasuhiko Tomino[a]

[a]Division of Nephrology, Department of Internal Medicine, Juntendo University Faculty of Medicine, Tokyo, Japan; [b]Department of Microbiology, University of Alabama at Birmingham, Birmingham, Ala., USA

Abstract

Impaired immune regulation along the 'mucosa-bone marrow axis' has been postulated to play an important role in the pathogenesis of IgA nephropathy (IgAN). Animal models have allowed us to study such changes in detail. Recently, we established several useful animal models, including IgAN-prone mice. Using these animal models, our group is approaching the underlying mechanisms by which bone marrow and mucosal cell interrelate and finally induce this disease. Accumulating evidence from these approaches suggests that there is dysregulation of innate and cellular immunity in IgAN resulting in changes in the mucosal immune system. These changes appear to be closely linked to disruption of mucosal tolerance, resulting in abnormal priming and dissemination of cells to sites such as the bone marrow where they are responsible for synthesis of nephritogenic IgA. Our clinical studies further support these ideas and indicate that the tonsils may be a major mucosal priming site in human IgAN. In addition, our findings also suggest clinical application of nephritogenic IgA (IgA1) as a biological marker and possible future treatment strategies that focus on manipulating the priming and dissemination of these memory cells in order to prevent the appearance of nephritogenic IgA (IgA1) in the systemic compartment.

There is no clear disease-specific treatment strategy for IgA nephropathy (IgAN) principally due to the lack of a comprehensive understanding of this multifactorial disease. Clinical evidence from kidney transplantation indicate that pathogenesis of IgAN mainly links to abnormality of mucosal immune system, rather than abnormality of renal intrinsic cell [1]. On the other hand, studies of bone marrow (BM) or BM transplantation (BMT) in human patients with IgAN [1] suggest that nephritogenic IgA seems to be overproduced in systemic immune sites, such as BM. In the 1980s, based on elegant series of studies, van Es and coworkers hypothesized that there is 'mucosa-BM axis' in which there is continual trafficking of responsible cells in IgA immune system between mucosal sites and BM in IgAN [reviewed in 2]. It is widely accepted that a pathological role of aberrantly glycosylated IgA1 in IgAN [reviewed in 2, 3]. Recent studies showed that IgAN patients have increased serum levels of galactose-deficient IgA1 (GdIgA1) [4]. However, the origin of the responsible cells producing the GdIgA1 and their localization are still obscure. How can we study the production of nephritogenic IgA in the mucosa-BM axis of IgAN? Since it is practically very difficult to approach this axis in a human system, a number of investigators have therefore used experimental animal models [1]. Recent studies demonstrated that the aberrantly glycosylated IgA is also involved in the pathogenesis of murine IgAN [1, 5]. We have recently established IgAN-prone mouse model which is genetically and clinically very close to human IgAN [6]. Here, we describe how experimental animal models have provided a better understanding of the mucosa-BM axis and how this data may be applicable to human IgAN.

Major Sites and Responsible Cells for Production of the Nephritogenic IgA

The ddY mouse is a well-known model of spontaneous IgAN [1]. These mice develop mesangial proliferative glomerulonephritis with striking deposition of IgA in the mesangium, resembling human IgAN [1, 6]. We found that ddY mice can be classified into three groups, early-onset (~20 weeks; 35%), late-onset (~40 weeks; 35%) and quiescent groups (30%) by histological grading in serial biopsies [6]. A genomewide association analysis indicated that the susceptibility to murine IgAN is partly regulated by specific loci syntenic to the gene of human familial IgAN [6]. These results support this prone mice model for examining the pathogenesis of IgAN [6].

Using this model, we have confirmed that transplantation of BM from these early-onset mice to control mice results in the development of IgAN, resembling human IgAN [7]. In contrast, BMT from quiescent or control mice to onset ddY mice abrogates glomerular injury and the mesangial deposition. These findings suggest that the BM may be a reservoir of memory cells capable of synthesizing IgA with a propensity for mesangial deposition and triggering glomerulonephritis.

To test the possibility that these responsible cells are disseminated to other lymphoid tissues, we transferred whole-spleen cells from the IgAN-prone mice into SCID mice. Not only BMT but also the cell transfer could reconstitute the murine IgAN in SCID mice [unpubl. data], suggesting that the responsible cells may be disseminated to systemic lymphoid tissues. BMT from IgAN-prone mice into alymphoplasia mice further indicated that germinal center and peripheral lymphoid tissues including lamina propria are not requisite for maturation of B cells producing nephritogenic IgA [8]. Tonsillectomy has a favorable effect on long-term renal survival in IgAN patients. In addition, tonsillectomy with steroid pulse therapy can be more effective therapy for IgAN than tonsillectomy alone, indicating that certain cases of IgAN require not only tonsillectomy but also additional steroid pulse therapy. Since the additional steroid therapy may principally attenuate the activity of the responsible leukocytes rather than local inflammation, these findings also suggest that the responsible cells may be disseminated to other tissues than tonsils. We evaluated responses of IgAN patients to treatments combining tonsillectomy with steroid pulse therapy [unpubl. data]. There were two types of patients, those who required tonsillectomy alone for reduction of serum GdIgA1 serum levels and those who needed additional steroid pulse therapy. These observations seem to suggest that the responsible cells producing GdIgA1 are predominantly in tonsils in a fraction of patients, whereas they may be disseminated from tonsils to other tissues in the other subset of IgAN patients [unpubl. data]. Therefore, tonsillectomy may remove the major mucosal tissue serving as a site for new priming and as a reservoir of the pathogenic IgA-producing cells and, thus, reduce the subsequent dissemination of these cells into other tissues, such as BM and spleen. Furthermore, the additional steroid pulse therapy may target not only renal inflammation but also already disseminated pathogenic cells into the systemic lymphoid tissues.

Mucosal Immune Priming in the Generation of Nephritogenic IgA

Since mucosal infections including tonsillitis exacerbate IgAN, it has been discussed that mucosal encounter of exogenous antigens could play a key role in the development of IgAN. Toll-like receptors (TLRs) are a family of pathogen-recognition molecules for suitable defense mechanisms in innate immunity [9]. Innate immune system of vertebrates is able to distinguish bacterial/viral DNA from self-DNA by detecting unmethylated CpG oligonucleotides (ODN) in particular base contexts ('CpG motifs') via pattern recognition receptors, such as TLR9 [9]. We recently found overexpression of TLR9 mainly on tonsillar plasmacytoid dendritic cells (pDC) in some patients with IgAN [unpubl. data]. These patients with high TLR9 expression exhibited a rapid and successful therapeutic response to combined tonsillectomy and steroid pulse therapy [unpubl. data], suggesting that tonsillar TLR9 activation may be involved in the pathogenesis of IgAN. To further investigate, we nasally administered CpG ODN to the IgAN-prone mice and found that glomerular damage was worsened in association with greater mesangial IgA deposition and higher serum IgA levels [10], suggesting that TLR9 binding and activation may represent a final common pathway for immune activation by the above-mentioned exogenous antigens in IgAN. Importantly, CpG DNA alone may enhance the serum levels of IgA and IgA/IgG immune complexes and thereby promote mesangial IgA and glomerular injury.

Conclusion

Insights from experimental models in the mucosa-BM axis discussed here suggest that patients with IgAN have an impaired mucosal immune system with dysregulation of innate immunity.

References

1 Suzuki Y, Tomino Y: Potential immunopathogenic role of the mucosa-bone marrow axis in IgA nephropathy: insights from animal model. Semin Nephrol 2008;28:66–77.
2 van den Wall Bake AW, Daha MR, van Es LA: Immunopathogenetic aspects of IgA nephropathy. Nephrologie 1989;10:141–145.
3 Novak J, Julian BA, Tomana M, Mestecky J: IgA glycosylation and IgA immune complexes in the pathogenesis of IgA nephropathy. Semin Nephrol 2008;28:78–87.
4 Moldoveanu Z, Wyatt RJ, Lee JY, Tomana M, Julian BA, Mestecky J, Huang WQ, Anreddy SR, Hall S, Hastings MC, Lau KK, Cook WJ, Novak J: Patients with IgA nephropathy have increased serum galactose-deficient IgA1 levels. Kidney Int 2007;71:1148–1154.
5 Nishie T, Miyaishi O, Azuma H, Kameyama A, Naruse C, Hashimoto N, Yokoyama H, Narimatsu H, Wada T, Asano M: Development of immunoglobulin A nephropathy-like disease in β-1,4-galactosyltransferase-I-deficient mice. Am J Pathol 2007;170:447–456.
6 Suzuki H, Suzuki Y, Yamanaka T, Hirose S, Nishimura H, Toei J, Horikoshi S, Tomino Y: Genome-wide scan in a novel IgA nephropathy model identifies a susceptibility locus on murine chromosome 10, in a region syntenic to human IGAN1 on chromosome 6q22–23. J Am Soc Nephrol 2005;16:1289–1299.
7 Suzuki H, Suzuki Y, Aizawa M, Yamanaka T, Kihara M, Pang H, Horikoshi S, Tomino Y: Th1 polarization in murine IgA nephropathy directed by bone marrow-derived cells. Kidney Int 2007;72:319–327.

8 Aizawa M, Suzuki Y, Suzuki H, Pang H, Kihara M, Yamaji K, Horikoshi S, Tomino Y: Roles of bone marrow, mucosa and lymphoid tissues in pathogenesis of murine IgA nephropathy. Contrib Nephrol. Basel, Karger, 2007, vol 157, pp 164–168.

9 Akira S, Takeda K: Toll-like receptor signaling. Nat Rev Immunol 2004;4:499–511.

10 Suzuki H, Suzuki Y, Narita I, Aizawa M, Kihara M, Yamanaka T, Kanou T, Tsukaguchi H, Novak J, Horikoshi S, Tomino Y: Toll-like receptor 9 affects severity of IgA nephropathy. J Am Soc Nephrol 2008;19:2384–2395.

Yusuke Suzuki
Division of Nephrology, Department of Internal Medicine, Juntendo University Faculty of Medicine
Hongo 2–1–1, Bunkyo-ku
Tokyo 113-8421 (Japan)
Tel. +81 3 5802 1065, E-Mail yusuke@juntendo.ac.jp

Harabuchi Y (ed): Recent Advances in Tonsils and Mucosal Barriers of the Upper Airways.
Adv Otorhinolaryngol. Basel, Karger, 2011, vol 72, pp 68–70

IgA Nephropathy and Aberrant Glycosylation of Tonsillar, Serum and Glomerular IgA1

Yoshiyuki Hiki[a] · Akihiko Ito[b] · Yoshihiro Yamamoto[a] · Koichiro Yamamoto[a] · Hitoo Iwase[b]

[a]School of Health Sciences and Medicine, Fujita Health University, Aichi, and [b]Department of Otorhinolaryngology and Biochemistry Kitasato University, Kanagawa, Japan

Abstract

Human IgA1, which is the predominant subtype deposited in the glomeruli in IgA nephropathy (IgAN), has a unique mucin-like structure in its hinge region. Several studies suggested that the IgA1 molecules in IgAN patients had an aberrant structure of O-glycans. The paper summarizes the analyses of O-glycan structure in the IgA1 molecules taken from tonsils, sera and glomeruli of patients with IgAN. Hypoglycosylation, especially hypogalactosylation of O-glycans has been observed not only in serum and glomerular IgA1 but also in tonsillar IgA1.

Tonsillar IgA

Amelio et al. [1] indicated that serum IgA levels were significantly lower in tonsillectomized cases compared to nontonsillectomized individuals. The results are of interest for nephrologists, because IgAN patients have significantly high levels of serum IgA. This would be expected that tonsillectomy was effective in IgAN patients from the aspect of the quantity of IgA. The long-term effectiveness of tonsillectomy was subsequently observed by Xie et al. [2].

Tonsillar extracts were obtained using sucrose density gradient ultracentrifugation. The production of IgA/g tonsil was significantly higher in tonsillar tissue taken from IgAN patients than in those of controls ($p = 0.04$). The IgA1/IgA2 ratio in IgAN patients was significantly increased compared to that of patients with chronic tonsillitis ($p < 0.01$). It was suggested that there was a disordered production of IgA in the tonsils of some IgAN patients [3]. Hypoglycosylated IgA was also evaluated using antisynthetic IgA1 hinge peptide (sHP) antibody, which would strongly recognize hypoglycosylated IgA1. The binding of the antibody to IgA was significantly higher in tonsillar extracts of IgAN patients than in controls ($p = 0.015$), suggesting that IgA1 produced from tonsils is significantly hypoglycosylated in IgAN [4].

Glomerular and Serum IgA1

Mass Spectrometry Analyses

In our previous study [5], the mass spectrometry peak distribution of hinge glycopeptides of IgA1 taken from glomeruli, and from pooled sera

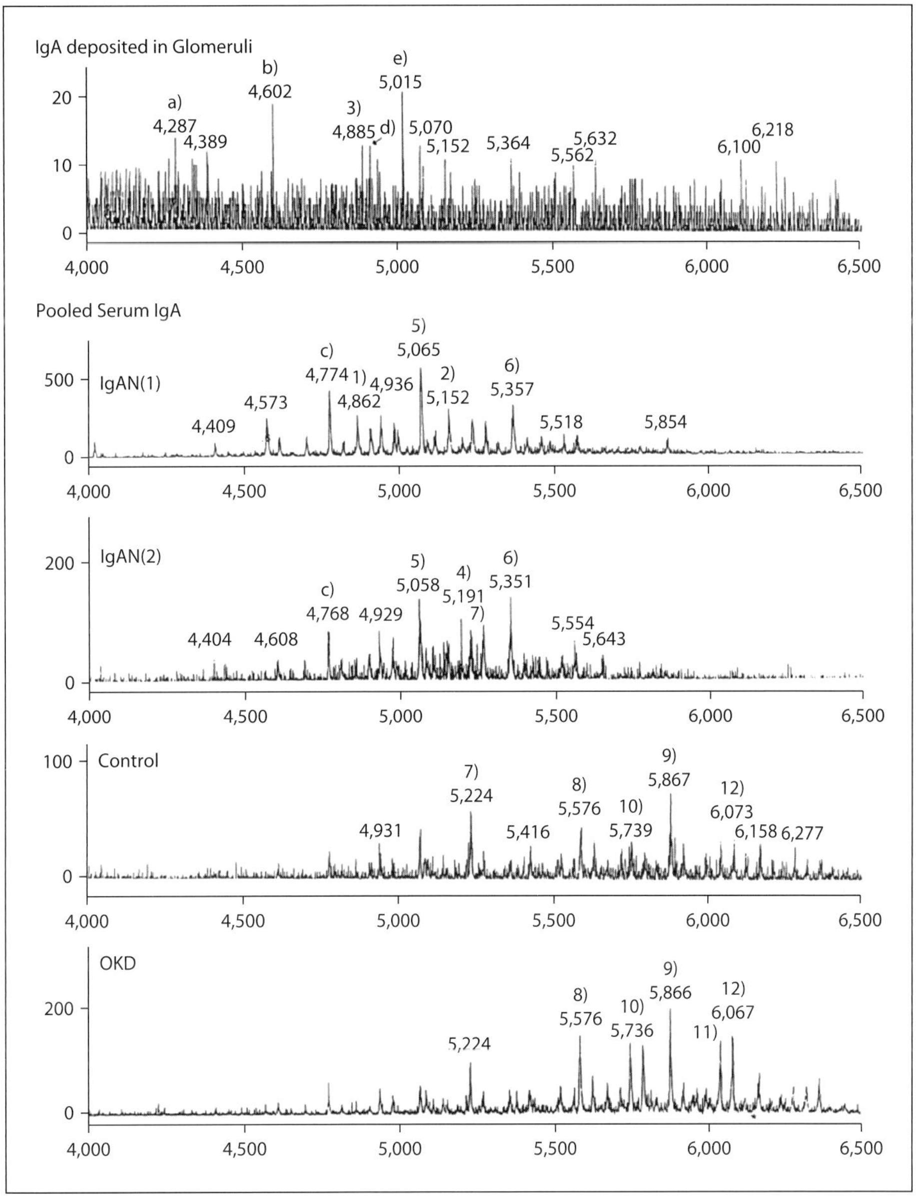

Fig. 1. Molecular weight peak distributions of hinge glycopeptides from glomerular and serum IgA1. Those of IgAN patients shifted to the left compared to those of the two control samples, suggesting that the molecular weights of hinge glycopeptides tend to be smaller in glomerular and serum IgA1 in IgAN.

of IgAN patients shifted to the left, compared to those of two control samples (fig. 1). As the molecular weight of the peptide core is constant, the results suggested that the hinge glycopetide of IgA1 was hypoglycosylated in IgAN. Recently, Odani et al. [6] analyzed the O-glycan structure of IgA1 hinges in 30 IgAN patients and 30 controls, and found some glycoforms, which were frequently detected in IgAN patients. The IgA1 hinge region of IgAN patients frequently had more GalNAc exposed residues lacking galactose (Tn antigens).

Helix aspersa Lectin ELISA [7]

Binding assay between *Helix aspersa* (HAA) and serum IgA pretreated with sialidase was performed by ELISA. As the HAA lectin recognizes exposed GalNAc residues (Tn), the assay could evaluate GalNAc and sialylated GalNAc residues. HAA-IgA-binding levels were significantly higher in IgAN patients compared to the other two control groups (vs. control or other kidney diseases, $p < 0.02$). The clinical features of IgAN patients in the high binding group and in the normal binding group were quite similar.

These results suggested that aberrancy of O-glycans plays a role in IgA deposition but did not associate with the severity of IgAN. Further studies are required to examine the induction of tissue damage and progression of IgAN.

Acknowledgements

The authors dedicate this paper to the late Dr. Yukio Shibayama, a practicing physician, who cured Hiki Yoshiyuki of IgAN by tonsillectomy 40 years ago.

References

1 Amelio RD, Palmisano L, Moli SL, Seminara R, Aiuti F: Serum and salivary IgA levels in normal subjects: comparison between tonsillectomized and non-tonsillectomized subject. Int Archs Allergy Appl Immun 1982;68: 256–259.

2 Xie Y, Nishi S, Ueno M, Imai N, Sakatsume M, Narita I, Suzuki Y, Akazawa K, Shimada H, Arakawa M, Gejyo F: The efficacy of tonsillectomy on long-term renal survival in patients with IgA nephropathy. Kidney Int 2003;63: 1861–1867.

3 Itoh A, Iwase H, Takatani T, Nakamura I, Hayashi M, Kobayashi Y, Hiki Y, Okamoto M: Disordered balance of IgA subclass production in the tonsils of some IgA nephropathy patients. J Nephrol 2005;18:575–581.

4 Itoh A, Iwase H, Takatani T, Nakamura I, Hayashi M, Oba K, Hiki Y, Kobayashi Y, Okamoto M: Tonsillar IgA1 as a possible source of hypoglycosylated IgA1 in the serum of IgA nephropathy patients. Nephrol Dial Transplant 2003;18:1108–1114.

5 Hiki Y, Odani H, Takahashi M, Yasuda Y, Nishimoto A, Iwase H, Shinzato T, Kobayashi Y, Maeda K: Mass spectrometry proves under-O-glycosylation of glomerular IgA1 in IgA nephropathy. Kidney Int 2001;59:1077–1085.

6 Odani H, Yamamoto K, Iwayama S, Iwase H, Takasaki A, Takahashi K, Fujita Y, Sugiyama S, Hiki Y: Evaluation of the specific structures of IgA1 hinge glycopeptide in 30 IgA nephropathy patients by mass spectrometry. J Nephrol. 2010; 23:70–76.

7 Shimozato S, Hiki Y, Odani H, Takahashi K, Yamamoto K, Sugiyama S: Serum under-galactosylated IgA1 is increased in Japanese patients with IgA nephropathy. Nephrol Dial Transplant 2008;23: 1931–1939.

Dr. Yoshiyuki Hiki
Fujita Health University, Shcool of Health Sciences
1–98 Dengakugakubo
Kutsukake-cho, Toyoake, Aichi 470-1192 (Japan)
Tel. +81 562 93 2510, E-Mail yyhiki@fujita-hu.ac.jp

Harabuchi Y (ed): Recent Advances in Tonsils and Mucosal Barriers of the Upper Airways.
Adv Otorhinolaryngol. Basel, Karger, 2011, vol 72, pp 71–74

Abnormalities of Glycogenes in Tonsillar Lymphocytes in IgA Nephropathy

Tatsuyuki Inoue[a] · Hitoshi Sugiyama[a,b] · Masashi Kitagawa[a] · Keiichi Takiue[a] · Hiroshi Morinaga[a] · Yoko Kikumoto[a] · Yohei Maeshima[a] · Kunihiro Fukushima[c] · Kazunori Nishizaki[c] · Hirofumi Akagi[d] · Yoshiyuki Hiki[e] · Hirofumi Makino[a]

[a]Department of Medicine and Clinical Science, [b]Center for CKD and Peritoneal Dialysis, [c]Otolaryngology, Okayama University Graduate School of Medicine, Dentistry, and Pharmaceutical Sciences, and [d]Department of Otolaryngology, National Hospital Organization Minami-Okayama Medical Center, Okayama, and [e]Department of Nephrology, Fujita Health University, Toyoake, Japan

Abstract

Glycosylation, which represents the most complex post-translational modification, plays a pivotal role during protein maturation, and is orchestrated by numerous glycosyltransferases. Aberrant O-glycosylation of serum and tonsillar IgA1 is presumed to be one of the pathogeneses of IgA nephropathy (IgAN). However, the synthesis of underglycosylated IgA1 in tonsils has not yet been characterized. This study investigated tonsillar B lymphocytes of IgAN using tonsils from patients with chronic tonsillitis and sleep apnea syndrome. Gene expression of β1,3-galactosyltransferase (β3GalT), Cosmc, UDP-N-acetyl-α-D-galactosamine: polypeptide N-acetylgalactosaminyl-transferase 2, were significantly downregulated in tonsillar CD19-positive B lymphocytes from IgAN patients compared to control as determined by real-time RT-PCR. In contrast, the level of sialyltransferase was not significantly different among the three groups. Tonsillar B cell β3GalT gene expression significantly correlated with estimated GFR and negatively correlated with proteinuria and glomerular or interstitial injury score. Double immunofluorescent staining showed that some IgA-positive cells in the intrafollicular area were also positive for β3GalT staining. Western blotting showed the protein expression of β3GalT in the tonsils to significantly decrease in IgAN in comparison to the controls. These data suggest the downregulation of β3GalT in tonsillar B lymphocytes to be closely associated with the clinical characteristics of IgAN.

IgA nephropathy (IgAN) is the most common glomerulonephritis worldwide [1]. The structure of O-glycans in the hinge region of IgA1 has been well studied, and considerable evidence has revealed the involvement of aberrantly glycosylated IgA1 in the pathogenesis of IgAN [2, 3]. Multiple O-glycans of IgA1 are assembled by the stepwise addition of monosaccharides. Glycogenes encode proteins involved in glycan synthesis, such as glycosyltransferases [4]. The analysis of human glycogenes has indicated that the Cosmc mRNA expression level in the peripheral B cells of IgAN is significantly decreased [5].

In IgAN patients, an upper respiratory tract infection is often related to relapse and it manifests as macroscopic hematuria and renal dysfunction. The mechanism of underglycosylated IgA production in tonsils has not yet been fully elucidated. Because O-glycans in IgA molecules are produced by glycosyltransferases, we hypothesize that dysregulation of glycosyltransferases is associated with aberrant O-glycosylation in tonsillar IgA1 and with the clinical characteristics of IgAN.

β3GalT, Cosmc, and pp-GalNAc-T2 Genes Are Downregulated in Tonsillar CD19-Positive B Lymphocytes in IgA Nephropathy

The differential regulation of glycogenes related to O-glycosylation was analyzed in the IgA1 hinge region [6]. The gene expression of β3GalT, the enzyme responsible for O-galactosylation, decreased significantly in patients with IgAN in comparison to those of CT ($p < 0.01$) or SAS ($p < 0.01$) in tonsillar CD19-positive cells. The level of Cosmc decreased significantly in IgAN in comparison to CT ($p < 0.05$) and SAS ($p < 0.01$) controls. Similarly, pp-GalNAc-T2, an essential enzyme for the initiation of O-glycosylation of the IgA1 hinge region, decreased significantly in IgAN in comparison to CT ($p < 0.05$) and SAS ($p < 0.01$). The gene expression of ST3Gal and ST6GalNAc II and III increased in patients with IgAN compared with SAS; however, the difference was not statistically significant.

Qin et al. [5] reported that peripheral B lymphocytes exhibited a significantly lower level of Cosmc gene expression in IgAN than in normal control, while no apparent difference was observed in β3GalT expression. It is likely that β3GalT gene expression is differentially regulated in peripheral and tonsillar B lymphocytes in IgAN. The core 1 structure is an intermediate in the synthesis of most extended O-glycan structures and may be further modified by the addition of sialic acid. There are some controversies about ST6GalNAc II gene expression between peripheral CD19-positive B cells [7] and IgA1-producing cell lines derived from IgA and CD19 double-positive B cells [8] of IgAN patients. Tonsillar CD19-positive B lymphocytes ST6GalNAc II gene expression increased in IgAN patients compared with that in SAS, although the increase was not statistically significant increase ($p = 0.27$). The regulation and expression of glycosyltransferases in tonsils may have complex changes in biosynthetic pathways of O-glycans in IgAN.

Relationship between the Expression of Tonsillar β3GalT and Clinical or Renal Pathological Parameters in IgA Nephropathy

The relationship between the gene expression of β3GalT in tonsillar B lymphocytes and the clinical manifestations were analyzed in IgAN patients [6]. The level of β3GalT gene expression significantly positively correlated with renal function as expressed by eGFR ($r = 0.586$, $p = 0.0003$), and also significantly negatively correlate with daily proteinuria ($r = -0.404$, $p = 0.018$), IGL score ($r = -0.539$, $p = 0.002$), and tubulointerstitial injury ($r = -0.532$, $p = 0.002$). There were no significant differences of the levels of eGFR in the lower β3GalT expression group in either CT or SAS. Neither Cosmc nor pp-GalNAc-T2 gene in tonsillar CD19-positive B lymphocytes showed any association with the clinical or pathological parameters in IgAN.

Considering that renal dysfunction, proteinuria, and tubulointerstitial injury are prognosis marker at presentation in IgAN [1], a downregulated β3GalT gene expression may also be a prognostic marker for these states.

Expression of β3GalT Protein in Tonsillar B Cells

The majority of CD19-positive B lymphocytes (86.1%) expressed surface IgA as assessed by flow cytometry. In morphometric analysis of tonsils in IgAN, the intrafollicular area was expanded as compared to CT and SAS. Immunohistochemical analysis revealed the presence of numerous CD19-positive cells both in the follicle and intrafollicular areas. Both IgA-positive cells and some β3GalT-positive cells were observed in the intrafollicular area of patient tonsils. Double immunofluorescent staining showed that some IgA-positive cells in the intrafollicular area were also positive for β3GalT staining. In Western blot analysis, the expression level of tonsillar β3GalT in IgAN was observed to significantly decrease in comparison to the tonsillar extracts from CT ($p < 0.01$) and SAS ($p < 0.01$).

Because the expression of β3GalT in the tonsillar tissue was previously uncharacterized, we demonstrated for the first time that β3GalT-positive cells were localized to the intrafollicular area and crypt epithelium of tonsil tissues derived from IgAN patients used by specific antibody [9]. We also observed a decrease in β3GalT expression in the tonsillar tissues of IgAN, as revealed by a western blotting. β3GalT gene inducers include 5-azacytidine and sodium n-butyrate, both of which may suppress the degradation of β3GalT [10].

Conclusions

We herein demonstrated the downregulation of β3GalT gene in the tonsillar B lymphocytes from patients with IgAN. Previously, only two reports have described underglycosylated IgA1 in tonsillar tissue specimens from patients with IgAN [3, 11]. Because galactosylation of IgA1 is regulated by galactosyltransferases including β3GalT, our findings may partly explain the agalacto type O-glycans in tonsils described in the previous reports. The regulation and expression of glycosyltransferases in tonsils may have complex changes in biosynthetic pathways of O-glycans in IgAN.

In conclusion, a downregulation of β3GalT gene expression may be a prognostic marker for IgAN. Moreover, normalization of β3GalT gene and protein expression in tonsils using pharmacological manipulation may be novel therapeutic approaches to combat the progression of renal dysfunction in patients with IgAN.

References

1 Barratt J, Feehally J: IgA nephropathy. J Am Soc Nephrol 2005;16:2088–2097.

2 Hiki Y, Kokubo T, Iwase H, Masaki Y, Sano T, Tanaka A, Toma K, Hotta K, Kobayashi Y: Underglycosylation of IgA1 hinge plays a certain role for its glomerular deposition in IgA nephropathy. J Am Soc Nephrol 1999;10:760–769.

3 Horie A, Hiki Y, Odani H, Yasuda Y, Takahashi M, Kato M, Iwase H, Kobayashi Y, Nakashima I, Maeda K: IgA1 molecules produced by tonsillar lymphocytes are under-O-glycosylated in IgA nephropathy. Am J Kidney Dis 2003;42:486–496.

4 Narimatsu H: Human glycogene cloning: focus on beta 3-glycosyltransferase and beta 4-glycosyltransferase families. Curr Opin Struct Biol 2006;16:567–575.

5 Qin W, Zhou Q, Yang LC, Li Z, Su BH, Luo H, Fan JM: Peripheral B lymphocyte beta1,3-galactosyltransferase and chaperone expression in immunoglobulin A nephropathy. J Intern Med 2005;258: 467–477.

6 Inoue T, Sugiyama H, Hiki Y, Takiue K, Morinaga H, Kitagawa M, Maeshima Y, Fukushima K, Nishizaki K, Akagi H, Narimatsu Y, Narimatsu H, Makino H: Differential expression of glycogenes in tonsillar B lymphocytes in association with proteinuria and renal dysfunction in IgA nephropathy. Clin Immunol 2010;136:447–455.

7 Ding JX, Xu LX, Zhu L, Lv JC, Zhao MH, Zhang H, Wang HY: Activity of alpha2,6 sialyltransferase and its gene expression in peripheral B lymphocytes in patients with IgA nephropathy. Scand J Immunol 2009;69:174–180.

8 Suzuki H, Moldoveanu Z, Hall S, Brown R, Vu HL, Novak L, Julian BA, Tomana M, Wyatt RJ, Edberg JC, Alarcon GS, Kimberly RP, Tomino Y, Mestecky J, Novak J: IgA1-secreting cell lines from patients with IgA nephropathy produce aberrantly glycosylated IgA1. J Clin Invest 2008;118:629–639.

9 Narimatsu Y, Ikehara Y, Iwasaki H, Nonomura C, Sato T, Nakanishi H, Narimatsu H: Immunocytochemical analysis for intracellular dynamics of C1GalT associated with molecular chaperone, Cosmc. Biochem Biophys Res Commun 2008;366:199–205.

10 Ju T, Cummings RD: Protein glycosylation: chaperone mutation in Tn syndrome. Nature 2005;437:1252.

11 Itoh A, Iwase H, Takatani T, Nakamura I, Hayashi M, Oba K, Hiki Y, Kobayashi Y, Okamoto M: Tonsillar IgA1 as a possible source of hypoglycosylated IgA1 in the serum of IgA nephropathy patients. Nephrol Dial Transplant 2003;18: 1108–1114.

Dr. Hitoshi Sugiyama
Department of Medicine and Clinical Science
Center for Chronic Kidney Disease and Peritoneal Dialysis
Okayama University Graduate School of Medicine
Dentistry, and Pharmaceutical Sciences
2-5-1 Shikata-cho Kita-ku
Okayama 700-8558 (Japan)
Tel. +81 86 235 7235, E-Mail hitoshis@md.okayama-u.ac.jp

Harabuchi Y (ed): Recent Advances in Tonsils and Mucosal Barriers of the Upper Airways.
Adv Otorhinolaryngol. Basel, Karger, 2011, vol 72, pp 75–78

Microarray Analysis of Tonsils of IgA Nephropathy Patients

Hirotsugu Iwatani[a] · Kenichiro Iio[a] · Yasuyuki Nagasawa[a] · Ryohei Yamamoto[a] · Arata Horii[b] · Daisuke Okuzaki[c] · Hidenori Inohara[b] · Hiroshi Nojima[c] · Enyu Imai[a] · Hiromi Rakugi[a] · Yoshitaka Isaka[a]

[a]Geriatric Medicine and Nephrology and [b]Otolaryngology, Osaka University Graduate School of Medicine, and [c]Molecular Genetics, Research Institute for Microbial Diseases, Osaka University, Suita, Osaka, Japan

Abstract

IgA nephropathy (IgAN) is the most common primary glomerulonephritis. Its close relation with the tonsils is well known because tonsillitis sometimes causes aggravation of urinary findings or macrohematuria. However, the genes specific to the tonsils of IgAN patients are not clarified. To clarify the specific gene expression in the tonsils of IgAN patients, we performed tonsillectomy and corticosteroid IV therapy as a treatment of IgAN, analyzed the gene expression in the tonsils by microarray and compared it with that in tonsils from chronic tonsillitis patients. The upregulated genes seem to be categorized into two groups: muscle-related genes and immune-related genes. The downregulated genes include the polymeric Ig receptor (pIgR) which was reportedly involved in single nucleotide polymorphism (SNP) of Japanese IgAN patients.

A close relationship between IgAN and the tonsil is well known; however, gene expression specific to the tonsils of IgAN has not been clarified.

Of 73 consecutive biopsy-proven adult IgAN patients who underwent tonsillectomy combined with steroid pulse as a treatment in Osaka University Hospital from 2004 to 2007, we enrolled 23 patients whose proteinuria and hematuria were completely ameliorated within 2 years after tonsillectomy. We analyzed the gene expression in the tonsils using microarray [1], and compared it with that of patients with chronic tonsillitis undergoing tonsillectomy (n = 22). One case in the IgAN group was eliminated because of the small amounts of RNA. The patients characteristics are shown in table 1 [1]. Up- and down-regulated genes are summarized in table 2 [1]. Upregulated genes appear to be categorized into two groups. One group belongs to the muscle-related genes such as myosin heavy polypeptide 1, nebulin, sarcolipin, and small muscle protein. Tonsils in chronic tonsillitis patients were obviously larger than those in IgAN patients and the structural difference has already been reported [2]. The upregulation of these muscle-related genes might reflect the structural differences. The other group includes immune-related genes such as CALB2, DUSP27 and CXCL11. In downregulated genes, pIgR was also an immune-related gene.

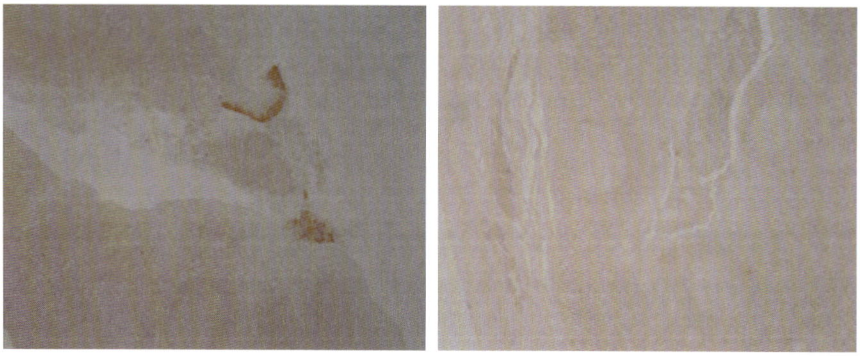

Fig. 1. Immunohistochemical analysis of pIgR in tonsils of control and IgAN.

Table 1. Patient characteristics

	IgAN group (n=23)	Control group (n=22)
Age, years	32 (24–46)	31 (20–40)
Sex (female/total)	11/23	12/22
Cr, mg/dl	0.85 (0.7–1.0)*	0.7 (0.5–0.8)
Proteinuria, g/day	0.38 (0.10–0.51)	0
CRP, mg/dl	0 (0–0)	0 (0–0.2)
IgA, mg/dl	320 (225–392)	261 (211–394)
ASO, IU/ml	80 (60–320)**	320 (160–2,560)
ASK	53 (34.5–100.5)*	119.9 (49.5–234.4)
C3, mg/dl	92 (85–100)	104 (86–122.5)
C4, mg/dl	19 (18–23.3)	22 (20–25.5)
CH50, U/ml	40.5 (36.5–47.1)	45.8 (38.2–49.4)
History of macrohematuria	10/23	0/22
Period to remission of proteinuria, months	3.9 (0.6–6.5)	
Period to remission of hematuria, months	6.5 (5.1–10.7)	

* $p < 0.05$, ** $p < 0.01$ median (interquartile range).

We also confirmed the fold changes of some genes in table 2 using real-time PCR [1]. The results were as follows: fold change in IgAN compared to control for CALB2 is 2.419, DUSP27 1.834, APOBEC2 1.452, CXCL11 1.936 and pIgR –2.193, which were consistent with microarray analysis. We made further analysis for pIgR clinically because it was reported to be associated with the SNP of Japanese patients with IgAN [3] and basically because its intestinal

Table 2. List of up- and down-regulated top 10 genes in tonsils of IgAN compared to control

Gene no.	Fold change	Primary sequence name	Sequence description
Up regulated			
1	3.44597	AF319957	FKSG22 (FKSG22) mRNA, complete cds
2	3.3604	MYH1	myosin, heavy polypeptide 1, skeletal muscle, adult (MYH1), mRNA
3	3.2843	CALB2	calbindin 2, 29kDa (calretinin) (CALB2), transcript variant CALB2, mRNA [NM_001740]
4	2.48523	DUSP27	DUSP27
5	2.19025	HBG1	hemoglobin, gamma A (HBG1), mRNA [NM_000559]
6	2.12117	APOBEC2	apolipoprotein B mRNA editing enzyme, catalytic polypeptide-like 2 (APOBEC2), mRNA
7	2.10019	CXCL11	chemokine (C-X-C motif) ligand 11 (CXCL11), mRNA
8	2.08785	NEB	nebulin (NEB), mRNA
9	2.07118	SLN	sarcolipin (SLN), mRNA
10	2.04012	SMPX	small muscle protein, X-linked (SMPX), mRNA
Down regulated			
1	–5.70085	NM_152399	hypothetical protein FLJ30834 (FLJ30834), mRNA
2	–3.8934	ALB	albumin (ALB), mRNA
3	–2.89827	C20orf114	chromosome 20 open reading frame 114 (C20orf114), mRNA
4	–2.48895	CGREF1	cell growth regulator with EF hand domain 1 (CGREF1), mRNA
5	–2.35137	PIGR	polymeric immunoglobulin receptor (PIGR), mRNA
6	–2.31104	CHGB	chromogranin B (secretogranin 1) (CHGB), mRNA
7	–2.26152	AI916628	AI916628 wa28h04.xl NCI_CGAP_Kid11 Homo sapiens cDNA clone IMAGE:2299447 3', mRNA sequence [AI916628]
8	–2.24077	PLUNC	palate, lung and nasal epithelium carcinoma associated (PLUNC), transcript variant 1, mRNA
9	–2.23702	THC2439430	ALU8_HUMAN (P39195) Alu subfamily SX sequence contamination warning entry, partial (14%) [THC2439430]
10	–2.19688	SCGB3A1	secretoglobin, family 3A, member 1 (SCGB3A1), mRNA

RNA of the high IgA ddY mouse, an IgAN model mouse, was reported to be decreased [4]. One of the mechanisms of high serum IgA in the ddY mouse may be explained by the decreased excretion of IgA into the mucosal surface from the intestine due to the decreased expression of pIgR that is engaged in the trans-epithelial transport of IgA. We stained 10% formalin/PBS-fixed paraffin-embedded section of tonsil with antihuman secretory component antibody (Santa Cruz Biotechnology, Inc., Calif., USA) as described previously [1]. Based on our preliminary analysis, the expression of pIgR tends to be lower in tonsils of IgAN than in those of control. Further analysis is necessary.

In conclusion, we confirmed that some muscular genes related with tonsil structure were elevated and some immune-related genes were up- or down-regulated in tonsils of IgAN patients. The pIgR was downregulated in the tonsils of IgAN patients.

References

1 Iio K, Nagasawa Y, Iwatani H, et al: Microarray analysis of tonsils in immunoglobulin A nephropathy patients. Biochem Biophys Res Commun 2010;393: 565–570.

2 Xie Y, Nishi S, Ueno M, et al: The efficacy of tonsillectomy on long-term renal survival in patients with IgA nephropathy. Kidney Int 2003;63:1861–1867.

3 Obara W, Iida A, Suzuki Y, et al: Association of single-nucleotide polymorphisms in the polymeric immunoglobulin receptor gene with immunoglobulin A nephropathy (IgAN) in Japanese patients. J Hum Genet 2003;48:293–299.

4 Yanagihara T, Kumagai Y, Norose Y, et al: Age-dependent decrease of polymeric Ig receptor expression and IgA elevation in ddY mice: a possible cause of IgA nephropathy. Lab Invest 2004;84:63–70.

Hirotsugu Iwatani
Geriatric Medicine and Nephrology, Osaka University, Graduate School of Medicine
2–2 Yamadaoka
Suita, Osaka 565-0871 (Japan)
Tel. +81 6 6879 3857, E-Mail hiro@kid.med.osaka-u.ac.jp

Harabuchi Y (ed): Recent Advances in Tonsils and Mucosal Barriers of the Upper Airways.
Adv Otorhinolaryngol. Basel, Karger, 2011, vol 72, pp 79–82

Reactive Arthritis Induced by Tonsillitis: A Type of 'Focal Infection'

Shigeto Kobayashi[a] · Ginichiro Ichikawa[b]

[a]Department of Rheumatology, Juntendo University Koshigaya Hospital, Fukuroyama Koshigaya-shi, Saitama, and
[b]Department of Otolaryngology Juntendo University School of Medicine, Bunkyo-ku, Tokyo, Japan

Abstract

Objective: The clinical manifestation of reactive arthritis (ReA) induced by tonsillitis is demonstrated. **Methods:** Medical records of 21 patients with ReA induced by tonsillitis were analyzed. **Results:** Nine male and 12 female patients were recorded. The mean age was 31.7 years ranging from 20 to 51 years. The mean duration of arthritis was 29.8 months (2 weeks to 10 years). Acute or recurrent origoarthritis involved in ankle, knee and sternoclavicular joints associated with Achilles tendon enthesitis were demonstrated. Thirteen of 21 (62%) patients were demonstrated positive for ASO and/or ASK. Group A streptococcus was demonstrated in 12 of 21 (57.1%) patients and other bacteria were demonstrated by culture of tonsillar swab or from resected tonsillar microabscess. No bacteria was demonstrated in synovial fluid from 3 patients. Rheumatoid factor was demonstrated only in 2 of 21 patients. HLA-B39 and BW61 (B40) were significantly demonstrated in 5 and 7 patients ($p = 0.0004$, 0.0006, respectively) compared with those of healthy controls. All patients were treated with antibiotics and nonsteroidal anti-inflammatory drugs (NSAIDs). Eight of 21 patients underwent tonsillectomy. Arthritis ceased after the treatments and no recurrence was found. **Discussion:** Sterile inflammatory arthritis induced by tonsillitis was cured by resection of the microabscess in the tonsils. Therefore, ReA induced by tonsillitis is one form of 'focal infection'.

Reactive arthritis (ReA) has been defined as an acute sterile arthritis developing soon after or during an infection elsewhere in the body and with the live micro-organism not entering the joint [1]. Conventionally, ReA induced by certain species of bacteria is confined to HLA-B27-related arthritis or, as formerly called, 'Reiter's syndrome'. However, ReA induced by other species of bacteria is completely unrelated to HLA-B27: a non-HLA-B27-related ReA is for instance group A α-hemolytic streptococcus-induced arthritis. 'Poststreptococcal reactive arthritis (PSRA)', a new clinical manifestation of streptococcal infection, has been introduced [2].

Previously, we described ReA induced by tonsillitis. We demonstrated that ReA was cured by tonsillectomy in several patients [3]. We here describe 21 adult cases of ReA-induced tonsillitis.

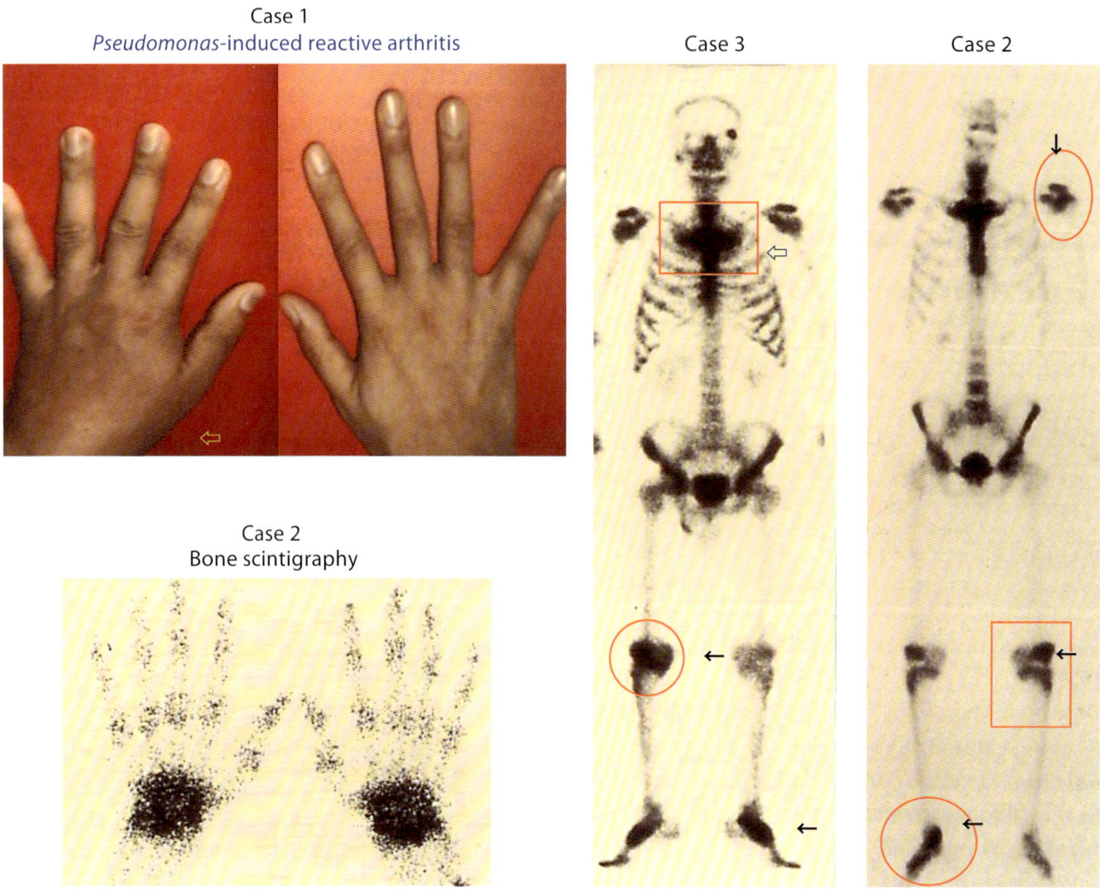

Fig. 1. Acute or recurrent origoarthritis with ankle, knee and sernoclavicular joints associated with the Achilles tendon enthesitis. Case 1 from Kobayashi, Clin Rheumatol 1996;15:516–520.

Patients and Methods

The medical records of 21 patients with ReA induced by tonsillitis and diagnosed and treated at Juntendo Hospital were analyzed [3].

Results

Nine male and 12 female patients were recorded. The mean age (± SD) was 31.7 ± 8.6 years, ranging from 20 to 51 years (median 30 years). The mean duration of arthritis was 29.8 ± 35.8 months (median 24 months, ranging from 2 weeks to 10 years). Acute or recurrent origoarthritis with ankle, knee and sternoclavicular joints associated with Achilles tendon enthesitis were demonstrated (fig. 1). Two patients had anterior uveitis [4], 3 had erythema marginatum and 3 had nonspecific abdominal pain [3]. Thirteen of 21 (62%) patients were demonstrated positive for ASO and/or ASK. Group A streptococcus was demonstrated in 12 of 21 (57.1%) patients and *Staphylococcus, Pseudomonas aeruginosa,* group B streptococcus and *Chlamydia trachomatis*

Table 1. Clinical manifestation of 'subacute rheumatoid arthritis'

1	Gender (male:female) and age of onset: 1:2, 20–30 decades
2	Arthritis begins during and/or after infection especially tonsillitis ameliorated
3	Polyarthritis continues from several weeks to 2 years
4	Oligoarthritis prone to affect knees and feet; elbow and wrist joints not frequent
5	Negative tests of Waalar-rose test and rheumatoid factors; increased finding of ASLO is sometimes found but the titers turned negative during the course
6	No radiographic bone destruction is found

Shichikawa et al: Jpn Clin Orthoped 1967;2:907–914

were demonstrated by culture of tonsillar swab or from resected tonsillar microabscess. Synovial fluid from 3 patients was cultured and no bacteria were demonstrated. Rheumatoid factor (RF) was demonstrated in 2 of 21 (9.5%), antinuclear antibody in 7 of 21 (33.3%), and anticardiolipin antibody in 6 of 18 (33.3%) patients [5]. Proteinuria (>100 mg/dl) was demonstrated in 8 of 21 (38.1%) patients. HLA-B typing was determined in 15 patients. HLA-B39 and BW61 (B40) were significantly demonstrated 5 and 7 patients ($p = 0.0004, 0.0006$, OR 11.4 and 7.26, respectively) compared with those of healthy controls [3]. All patients were treated with antibiotics and NSAIDs. Eight of 21 patients underwent tonsillectomy. Arthritis ceased after the treatments and no recurrence was found. Carditis was not demonstrated in any of the patients even though no prophylactic antibiotic treatment was given.

Discussion

Most of our patients have PSRA, even though other bacteria in tonsillar microabscesses can induce ReA [6, 7]. Therefore, PSRA is not an adequate name for this disease. 'Tonsillitis-induced ReA' or 'ReA induced by tonsillitis' seems suitable. There has been much discussion on the difference between PSRA and ARF. Recently, PSRA and acute rheumatic fever (ARF) are thought to be different presentations of the same disease [8]. The increased number of our patients having HLA-B39 and/or BW61(B40) has a special implication since HLA-B39 was significantly demonstrated among HLA-B27-negative ankylosing spondylitis patients in Japan; furthermore, an amino acid homology was demonstrated between HLA-B39 and HLA-B27 [9]. From 1950, the concept of PSRA had been reported among French rheumatologists called 'rhrumatisme articular subaigu de l'adulte, rheumatisme post-angineux, and/or subacute rheumatism' (table 1). The clinical and laboratory manifestation is very similar to that of PSRA.

Sterile inflammatory arthritis was cured by resection of microabscess in tonsils. Therefore, tonsillitis-induced ReA is one form of 'focal infection' although the name of this diagnosis was discarded [10]. The term 'focal infection' should be reinstated since many patients with palmoplanter pustulosis (PPP), chronic psoriasis, IgA nehropathy and tonsillitis-induced ReA were cured or their diseases were ameliorated by tonsillectomy, as reported in this International symposium.

References

1 Aho K, Leirisalo-Repo H: Reactive arthritis. Clin Rheum Dis 1985;11:25–40.

2 Fink CW: The role of the streptococcus in poststreptococcal reactive arthritis and childhood polyarteritis nodosa. J Rheumatol 1991;(suppl 29):14–20.

3 Kobayashi S, Tanaka M, Tamura N, et al: Reactive arthritis induced by tonsillitis. Arthritis Rheum 1992;(suppl 25): D182:S244.

4 Kobayashi S, Tamura N, Ikeda M, Sakuraba K, Matsumoto T, Hashimoto H: Uveitis in adult patients with post-streptococcal reactive arthritis: the first two cases reported associated with uveitis. Clin Rheumatol 2002;21:533–535.

5 Tamura N, Kobayashi S, Hashimoto H: Anticardiolipin antibodies in patients with post-streptococcal reactive arthritis. Ann Rheum Dis 2002;61:374.

6 Tamura N, Kobayashi S, Hashimoto H, Hoirose S: Reactive arthritis induced by *Vibrio parahaemolyticus*. J Rheumatol 1993;20:1062–1063.

7 Kobayashi S, Tamura N, Ichikawa G, Takasaki Y, Hashimoto H: Reactive arthritis induced by *Pseudomonas aeruginosa*. Clin Rheumatol 1996;15:516–517.

8 Tutar E, Atalay S, Yilmaz E, Ucar T, Kocak G, Imamoglu A: Poststreptococcal reactive arthritis in children: is it really a different entity from rheumatic fever? Rheumatol Int 2002;22:80–83.

9 Yamaguchi A, Tsuchiya N, Mitsui H, et al: Association of HLA-B39 with HLA-B27-negative ankylosing spondylitis and pauciarticular juvenile rheumatoid arthritis in Japanese patients: evidence for a role of the peptide-anchoring B pocket. Arthritis Rheum 1995;38: 1672–1677.

10 Phillips I: Discarded diagnoses, focal infection. Lancet 2002;360:1795–1796.

Shigeto Kobayashi, MD, PhD
Department of Rheumatology, Juntendo University Koshigaya Hospital
560 Fukuroyama Koshigaya-shi
Saitama 343-0032 (Japan)
Tel. +81 48 975 0321, E-Mail shigeto@juntendo.ac.jp

Harabuchi Y (ed): Recent Advances in Tonsils and Mucosal Barriers of the Upper Airways.
Adv Otorhinolaryngol. Basel, Karger, 2011, vol 72, pp 83–85

Tonsil-Related Skin Diseases and Possible Involvement of T Cell Co-Stimulation in Chronic Focal Infection

Satomi Kobayashi

Division of Dermatology, Seibo International Catholic Hospital, Tokyo, Japan

Abstract

Some inflammatory skin diseases are known to be related to tonsil focal infection at their onset. Administration of antibiotics is adequate treatment in most acute or subacute cases. However, chronic focal infections in the tonsils could cause chronic skin diseases like pustulosis palmaris et plantaris (PPP), and it is our frequent experience that tonsillectomy leads to a dramatic and persistent improvement of PPP skin lesions. The expression of inducible co-stimulator (ICOS), a co-stimulatory receptor on activated T cells, was significantly higher in tonsil tissues from PPP patients than in tonsil tissues from non-PPP patients. Moreover, ICOS expression in tonsil tissues from 3 patients with psoriasis vulgaris that was strongly suspected to be related to tonsil focal infection was also high, suggesting that the activation of T cells via ICOS costimulation in focal infections likely triggers inflammation associated with tonsil-related skin diseases. PPP is notable today for paradoxically induced skin lesions in patients treated with TNF-α antagonists for rheumatoid arthritis, Crohn's disease, psoriasis and psoriatic arthritis. It is important to clarify the immunological milieu in PPP not only for the treatment approach but also for understanding these unexpected reactions.

Tonsil-Related Skin Diseases and Pustulosis palmaris et plantaris

Some inflammatory skin diseases are known to be related to tonsil focal infection at their onset (fig. 1). Among them, most acute or subacute skin diseases are supposedly attributable to allergic hypersensitivity to streptococcal antigens, and administration of antibiotics is enough for their treatment. However, silent and chronic focal infections in the tonsils could cause chronic skin diseases, and tonsillectomy is often efficient in those cases. Pustulosis palmaris et plantaris (PPP) is a chronic dermatitis characterized by sterile intra-epidermal pustules associated with erythematous scaling on the palms and soles. Although an average of 5–7 years of symptomatic therapy is required for any improvement, tonsillar and oral chronic infections such as apical periodontation are well known to be largely involved in the onset of PPP, and a tonsillectomy and dental treatment rapidly improve the skin lesions. A tonsillectomy leads to the reduction of serum levels of IL-8 and IL-6 in PPP patients [1]. In addition, an in vitro stimulation of tonsillar T cells with α-streptococcal antigens from patients with PPP-enhanced production of IL-6,

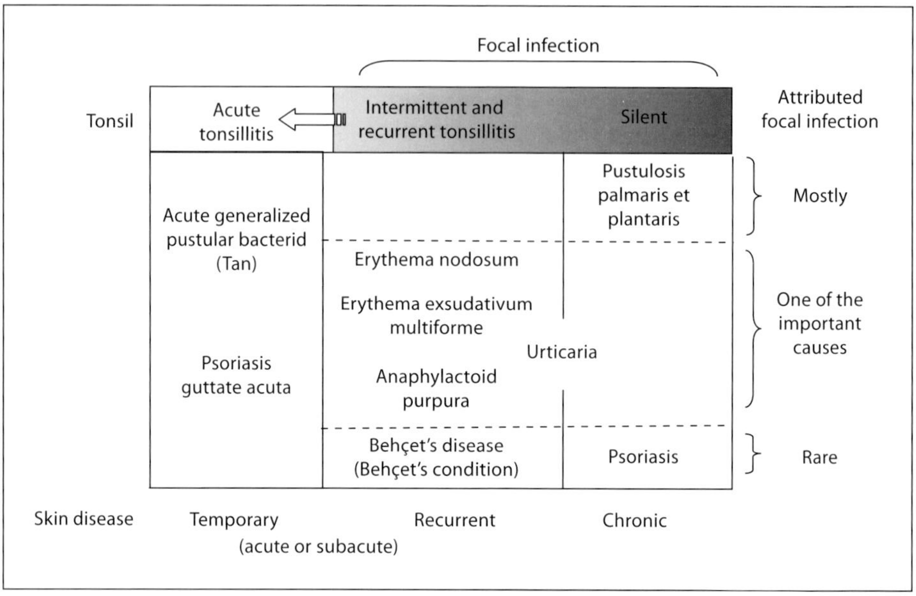

Fig. 1. Tonsil-related skin diseases.

interferon (IFN)-γ, tumor necrosis factor (TNF)-α [2], and the expression of cutaneous lymphocyte-associated antigen (CLA), a homing receptor related to migration into the skin, and transforming growth factor (TGF)-β production [3].

Inducible Co-Stimulator Expression at the Site of Chronic Focal Infection

Inducible co-stimulator (ICOS) [4] is a member of CD28 family that binds to its ligand, B7h, on antigen-presenting cells and provides costimulatory signals to augment T cell proliferation and the production of various cytokines [4]. The expression of ICOS was higher in tonsil tissues from PPP patients than in tonsil tissues from non-PPP patients. ICOS expression in tonsil tissues from 3 patients with psoriasis vulgaris that was strongly suspected to be related to tonsil focal infection was also high. The expression levels of ICOS on T cells in the peripheral blood were similar to those on cells from non-PPP patients (fig. 2). On tonsillar antigen-presenting cells, the expression of B7h was clearly induced on infiltrated cells in the epithelium of the tonsillar crypt in PPP patients as seen on immunohistochemical staining, and appeared to enhance co-stimulation at the tonsils in PPP resulting in the production in T cells of various cytokines like IL-4, IL-5, IL-10, IFN-γ and TNF-α. However, even though numerous ICOS+ T cells were detected in psoriatic skin, only a few were detected in PPP skin, suggesting that ICOS-B7h interactions probably did not occur in PPP skin lesions.

Silent and Chronic Tonsillar Infection Sites

The mechanisms of these results suggest that the activation of T cells via ICOS co-stimulation in focal infections likely triggers the skin inflammation associated with PPP by supplying proinflammatory cytokines, thus resulting in tissue damage. However, the role of ICOS in the silent and chronic tonsillar infection sites of the tonsil has not yet been elucidated. There are some ICOS gene haplotypes

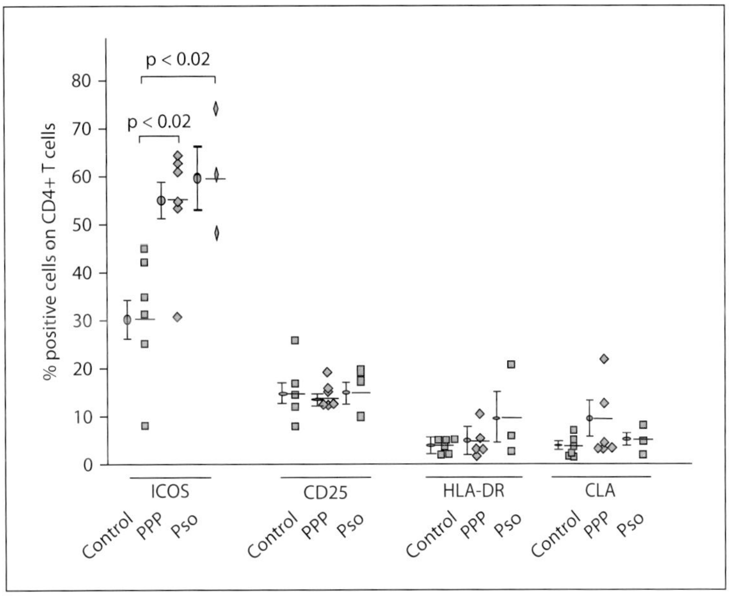

Fig. 2. ICOS and other T cell activation markers on tonsillar T cells.

that correlate with IL-10 secretion from ICOS+ T cells, and the question of a relation between ICOS+ T cells and regulatory T cells comes up. PPP is notable today for paradoxically induced skin lesions in patients treated with TNF-α antagonists, and an imbalance between TNF-α and IFN-α could be supposed to promote the paradox. It is important to clarify the immunological milieu in PPP not only for the treatment approach but also for understanding these unexpected reactions.

References

1 Yamamoto T, Katayama I, Nishioka K: Restricted usage of the T-cell receptor Vβ repertoire in tonsillitis in association with palmoplantar pustulosis. Acta Derm Venereol (Stockh) 1998;78: 161–163.

2 Murakata H, Harabuchi Y, Kataura A: Increased interleukin-6, interferon-γ and tumour necrosis factor-α production by tonsillar mononuclear cells stimulated with alpha-streptococci in patients with pustulosis palmaris et plantaris. Acta Otolaryngol (Stockh) 1999;119:384–391.

3 Nozawa H, Kishibe K, Takahara M, Harabuchi Y: Expression of cutaneous lymphocyte-associated antigen (CLA) in tonsillar T-cells and its induction by in vitro stimulation with alpha-streptococci in patients with pustulosis palmaris et plantaris (PPP). Clin Immunol 2005;116: 42–53.

4 Hutloff A, Dittrich AM, Beier KC, Eljaschewitsch B, Kraft R, Anagnostopoulos I, Kroczek RA: ICOS is an inducible T-cell co-stimulator structurally and functionally related to CD28. Nature1999;397:263–266.

Satomi Kobayashi
Division of Dermatology, Seibo International Catholic Hospital
2-5-1 Nakaochiai, Shinjuku-ku
Tokyo 161-8521 (Japan)
Tel. +81 3 3951 1111, E-Mail satomik@derm.twmu.ac.jp

Harabuchi Y (ed): Recent Advances in Tonsils and Mucosal Barriers of the Upper Airways.
Adv Otorhinolaryngol. Basel, Karger, 2011, vol 72, pp 86–88

Clinical Outcome of Tonsillectomy for Palmoplantar Pustulosis and Etiological Relationship between Palmoplantar Pustulosis and Tonsils

Miki Takahara

Department of Otolaryngology- Head and Neck Surgery, Asahikawa Medical College, Asahikawa, Hokkaido, Japan

Abstract

Palmoplantar pustulosis (PPP) is famous for causing typical tonsillar focal diseases. Clinical improvement of PPP rash after tonsillectomy was seen in 109 (94%) of 116 patients by subjective self-assessment, and 52 (88%) of 59 patients by objective Palmoplantar Pustulosis Area and Severity Index (PPPASI) scoring. Flow-cytometric analyses revealed that expression of activation markers (CD25 and HLA) class II increased on tonsillar T cells from PPP and IgAN patients. Moreover, expressions of skin-homing receptors (CLA and CCR6) increased on tonsillar T cells from PPP patients. In addition, the expressions were enhanced by stimulation of indigenous bacteria. Moreover, those expressions also increased in peripheral T cells, and decreased after tonsillectomy. Immunohistchemical analyses revealed that the ligands of those receptors (E-selectin and chemokine ligand 20) were expressed in lesions of skin. On the basis of our findings, migration of tonsillar T cells on which several homing receptors express by hyperimmune response against indigenous bacteria have a critical role in the pathogenesis of tonsillar focal diseases.

Clinical Evaluation of Tonsillectomy for Palmoplantar Pustulosis Patients

Clinical improvement of palmoplantar pustulosis (PPP) rash after tonsillectomy was evaluated in 116 patients with PPP by subjective self-assessment on a scale of 1 to 10, and in 59 PPP patients by the objective Palmoplantar Pustulosis Area and Severity Index (PPPASI) score. As a result, improvement at the last visit was seen in 109 (94%) of 116 patients by subjective evaluation, and 52 (88%) of 59 patients by PPPASI scoring (fig. 1). These findings suggest that tonsillectomy is a very effective treatment for PPP.

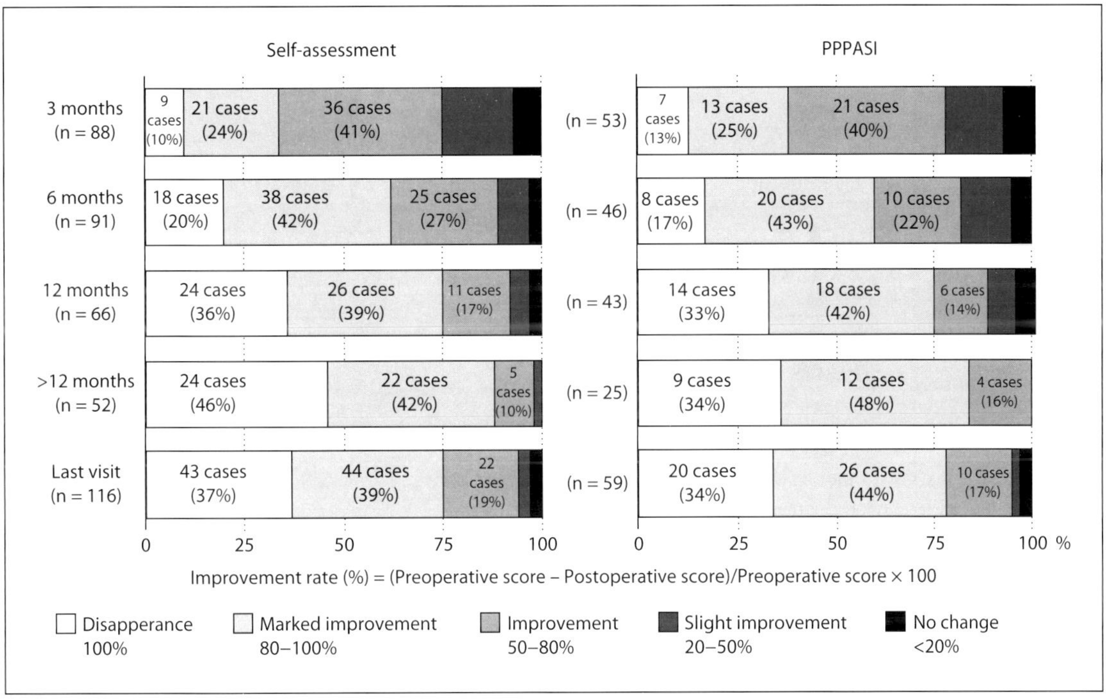

Fig. 1. Improvement factor of PPP rash after tonsillectomy in evaluation of the subjective self-assessment or the objective PPPASI score.

Research Progress for the Pathogenesis of Tonsillar Focal Disease

Normally, the palatine tonsil does not have a serious immune response against indigenous bacteria by immunologic tolerance; however, hyperresponses against α-streptococci was seen in tonsils from PPP patients. In tolerance, activation of T cells is strictly controlled by several factors including cytotoxic T lymphocyte antigen-4 (CTLA4) and TGF-β. On tonsillar T cells from PPP, expression of activation markers such as CD25 and HLA class II increased [1]. Moreover, CTLA4 mRNA increased, and Smad7 mRNA, the inhibitory molecule of TGF-β intracellular signaling, decreased in tonsillar T cells from PPP patients [1]. Therefore, CTLA4 and Smad7 are related to the hyperactivation of tonsillar T cells from the patients.

In the next step, we focused on cutaneous lymphocyte antigen (CLA), CC chemokine receptor 6 (CCR6), because it is reportedly related to migration of T cells to skin. Expressions of CLA and CCR6 increased on tonsillar and peripheral blood T cells from PPP patients [2, 3]. In addition, the expressions on peripheral blood T cells decreased after tonsillectomy [2, 3]. Moreover, stimulation of α-streptococci enhanced the expressions (fig. 2) [2, 3]. In the PPP skin lesions, E-selectin (ligand of CLA)/CC and chemokine ligand 20 (CCL20; ligand of CCR6) was expressed [2, 3].

On the basis of our findings, migration of tonsillar T cells on which several homing receptors express by a hyperimmune response against indigenous bacterium into the lesions have a critical role in the pathogenesis of tonsillar focal diseases.

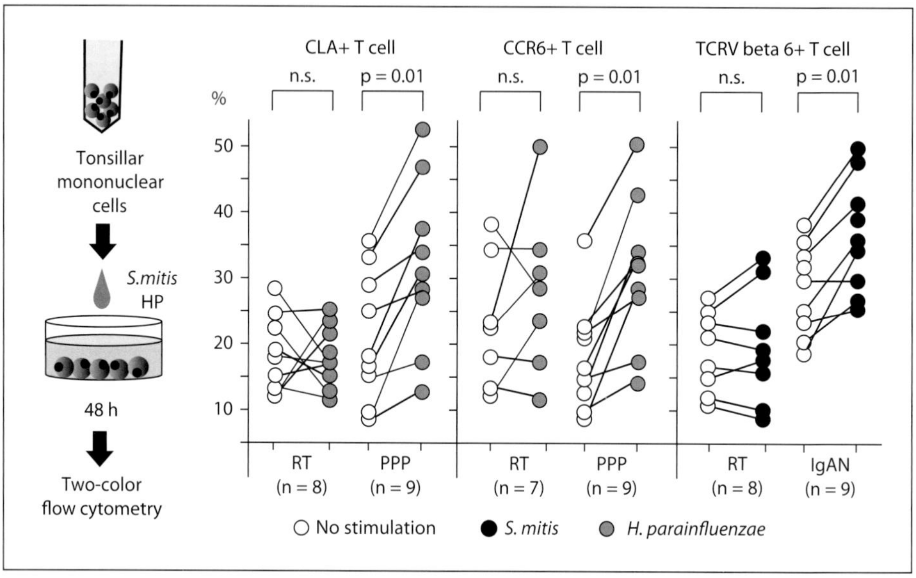

Fig. 2. Alternation of CLA, or CCR6 expression on tonsillar T-cell by stimulation of α-streptococci.

References

1 Takahara M, Kishibe K, Nozawa H, Harabuchi Y: Increase of activated T-cells and up-regulation of Smad7 without elevation of TGF-beta expression in tonsils from patients with pustulosis palmaris et plantaris. Clin Immunol 2005; 115:192–199.

2 Nozawa H, Kishibe K, Takahara M, Harabuchi Y: Expression of cutaneous lymphocyte-associated antigen (CLA) in tonsillar T-cells and its induction by in vitro stimulation with alpha-streptococci in patients with pustulosis palmaris et plantaris (PPP). Clin Immunol 2005;116: 42–53.

3 Yoshizaki T, Bandoh N, Ueda S, Nozawa H, Goto T, Kishibe K, Takahara M, Harabuchi Y: Up-regulation of CC chemokine receptor 6 on tonsillar T cells and its induction by in vitro stimulation with α-streptococci in patients with pustulosis palmaris et plantaris. Clin Exp Immunol 2009;157 :71–82.

Miki Takahara
Department of Otolaryngology- Head and Neck Surgery, Asahikawa Medical College
Midorigaoka E2–1–1–1
Asahikawa, Hokkaido, 078-8510 (Japan)
Tel. +81 166 68 2554, Fax +81 166 68 2559, E-Mail miki@asahikawa-med.ac.jp

Harabuchi Y (ed): Recent Advances in Tonsils and Mucosal Barriers of the Upper Airways.
Adv Otorhinolaryngol. Basel, Karger, 2011, vol 72, pp 89–92

Triggering Role of Focal Infection in the Induction of Extra-Palmoplantar Lesions and Pustulotic Arthro-Osteitis Associated with Palmoplantar Pustulosis

Toshiyuki Yamamoto

Department of Dermatology, Fukushima Medical University, Fukushima, Japan

Abstract

Palmoplantar pustulosis (PPP) is a chronic inflammatory disorder characterized by sterile pustules predominantly involving the palms and soles of middle-aged women. Whether PPP is the acral type of pustular psoriasis or a distinct entity has long been discussed; however, the clinical features of PPP are really heterogeneous and different between Asians and Caucasians, which may depend on the race with backgrounds of different HLAs. PPP is closely related with psoriasis, but considered to be a distinct entity in Japan. Although the pathogenesis of PPP is still poorly understood, PPP is a representative skin disorder showing a close relationship with focal infections such as tonsillitis, chronic sinusitis, and dental infection. In particular, tonsillitis often triggers or deteriorates PPP. In Japanese patients, regions other than the palms and soles are occasionally affected manifesting scaly erythemas which resemble psoriasis, and solitary pustules are also seen. Some of these extra-palmoplantar lesions are induced by the Koebner phenomenon or occur after focal infections. Further, arthralgia is also induced on the sternum, clavics, sacroiliac joints, and upper ribs following focal infections. This paper makes a focus on the triggering role of focal infection in the induction of extra-palmoplantar lesions as well as arthralgia (putulotic arthro-osteitis).

Palmoplantar pustulosis (PPP) is a chronic disease characterized by sterile pustules intermingled with scaly erythemas, vesicles and hyperkeratosis occurring at distinct sites on the palms and soles, precipitated with several factors, i.e. focal infection, smoking, and dental metal allergy. In this paper, triggering role of focal infection in PPP is discussed.

Extra-Palmoplantar Lesions

Although PPP lesions are typically confined to the palms and soles, clinical manifestations resembling psoriasis, namely, thin, scaly erythemas, occasionally appear on extra-palmoplantar areas such as the forearms, elbows, dorsa of the feet, lower legs, knees, and buttocks (fig. 1a) [1]. Compared with psoriasis, infiltration of the erythema is mild and the lesions are not well

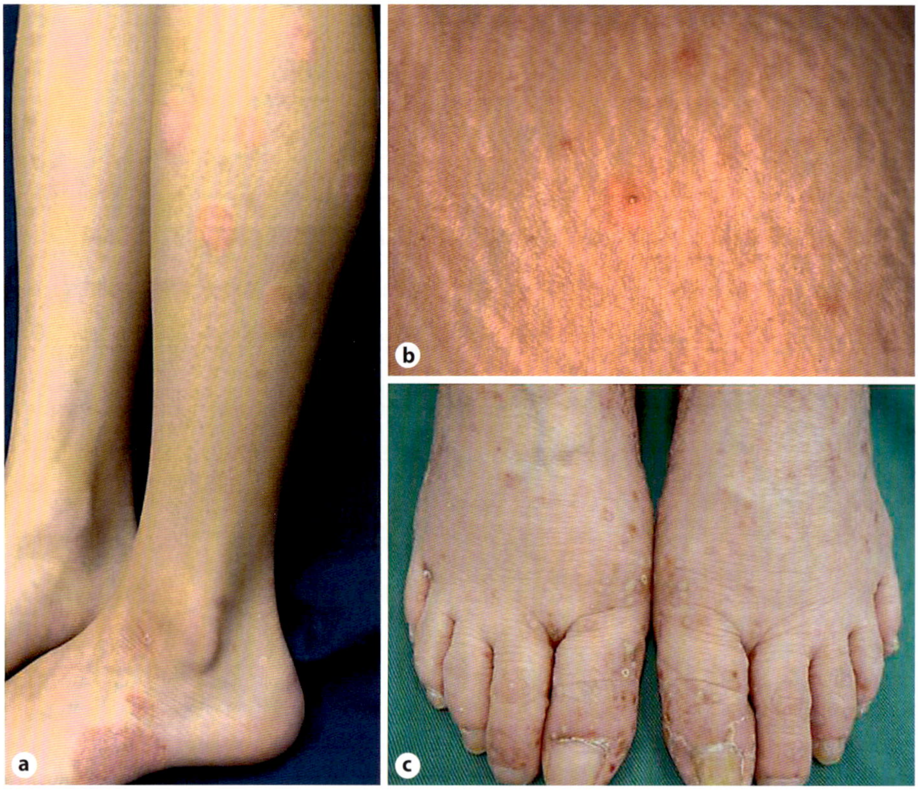

Fig. 1. **a** Scaly erythemas on the lower legs. **b** Extra-palmoplantar lesions are sometimes presented as scattered pustules on the body. **c** Prominent pustule formation on the dorsa of the foot following tonsilar infection.

demarcated; however, these have sometimes been misdiagnosed as a complication of psoriasis. Those extra-palmoplantar lesions develop both acutely and chronically. In the chronic type, cutaneous lesions are apt to develop on the mechanically stimulated areas [2] and are called the Koebner phenomenon. Histological features show mild acanthosis with focal parakeratosis and exocytosis. Infiltration of lymphocytes into the epidermis is mainly composed of T cells, which also express cutaneous lymphocyte-associated antigen (CLA), a homing receptor which binds to E-selectin on endothelial cells and facilitates T cell migration into the inflamed skin. However, the accumulation of neutrophils under the corneal layer, known as Munro's microabscess, is not seen, and dilation of the capillaries in the papillary dermis is absent. Perivascular infiltration of mononuclear cells in the upper dermis is seen. Therefore, there are no specific findings and many features overlap with those of eczematous reaction. Multiple parakeratotic foci alternating with orthohyperkeratosis are useful [3]. Also, solitary pustules suddenly occur, although less frequently, following focal infection (fig. 1b). In rare cases, a number of erythematous lesions with scaling may suddenly appear on the trunk accompanied by joint pain, following focal infections such as tonsillitis, dental infections, and sinusitis. A biopsy specimen taken from a pustular lesion may reveal spongiform abscesses.

Pustulotic Arthro-Osteitis

Although there are no definite data analyzing large samples, patients presenting with extra-palmoplantar lesions show severe cutaneous as well as joint manifestations. Sternocostoclavicular hyperostosis is frequently associated with PPP, and characterized by periosteal and endosteal hyperossification of the sternum, clavics, sacroiliac joint, and upper ribs. Patients complain of severe pain and swelling in these areas. This condition is worsened by focal infections, e.g. streptococcal throat infection, and the pain associated with sternocostoclavicular hyperostosis is mitigated by systemic administration of antibiotics or the surgical removal of focal infections, as with a tonsillectomy. In rare cases, severe pain persists even after surgery, and pain management sometimes requires oral cyclosporine [4]. The clinical symptoms of sternocostoclavicular hyperostosis and the cutaneous manifestations parallel each other, and biopsy specimens of the joint reveal nonspecific inflammation. Migration of streptococcal specific T cells from the tonsil into skin and joints may occur.

Role of Focal Infection

It is well known that focal infection, i.e. tonsillitis, chronic sinusitis, dental infection, tympanitis or cholecystitis, triggers or deteriorates PPP. Tonsillar infection occasionally triggers sudden onset of cutaneous eruption not only on the palms/soles, but on the extra-palmoplantar areas, with or without arthralgias (fig. 1c). Further, tonsillectomy frequently improves and even completely releases cutaneous as well as skeletal involvement associated with PPP. Of interest, serum levels of interleukin-6 (IL-6) and IL-8 were both dramatically reduced to normal levels in relation to clinical improvement [5]. IL-8 is a potent chemoattractant and activator for neutrophils, and has been suggested to play an important role in pustular formation. In addition to the marked clearance of palmoplantar lesions, extra-palmoplantar lesions also disappear following tonsillectomy, and, further, severe sternocostoclavicular pain is immediately improved. Other than tonsillitis, odontogenic infection also triggers the exacerbation of PPP. These facts strongly suggest a key triggering role of focal infection leading to a sequential event inducing PPP.

Pathophysiology

The characteristic histopathological features of PPP exhibit intraepidermal infiltration of polymorphonuclear neutrophils forming pustules. Although the mechanisms of neutrophil chemotaxis towards the epidermis are unknown, selective accumulation of neutrophils could be supposed to be caused by the local generation of neutrophil-specific chemoattractants, i.e. IL-8, C5a, platelet-activating factor, and leukotriene B_4, and lesional keratinocytes may play an important role in eliciting neutrophilic inflammatory response mechanisms. Additionally, more or less numbers of CD4-positive T cells are infiltrated below and around the pustules in the skin, which are suggested to play an important role by releasing inflammatory cytokines. Tonsillar T cells express CLA in patients with PPP, which may migrate into the skin. CLA-positive T cells identify a population of memory effector T cells. In vitro, bacterial infection such as α-streptococci activates tonsillar T cells to enhance CLA expression [6] and cytokine production such as IL-6, TNF-α, and interferon-γ (IFN-γ) [7]. Tonsillar crypt epithelial cells of PPP tonsils secrete high amounts of IL-6 [8]. Inducible co-stimulator (ICOS) is induced on T cells, and its ligand B7h is expressed in lymphoid and nonlymphoid tissues. The interaction between ICOS and B7h is supposed to be one of the important pathways in the inflammatory and immunological process. Recent studies show that ICOS expression is higher in the tonsil tissues as well as in skin lesions in PPP [9]. Heat shock proteins (HSPs) are recognized by γδ T cell receptors and Toll-like receptors 2 and 4, and are suggested to develop autoimmunity after bacterial infection. Antibodies that react with HSP65 can be found in the sera of patients with PPP, suggesting that HSP-producing chronic infectious bacteria might trigger PPP. These data suggest that activated tonsillar T cells by infection migrate into the skin forming cutaneous lesions in PPP via a number of inflammatory cytokines. C-C chemokine receptor, CCR6, expression on both tonsilar and peripheral blood T cells was upregulated in patients with PPP [10]. In vitro stimulation with α-streptococcal antigen significantly enhanced CCR6 expression on tonsillar T cells in patients with PPP [10]. Further, bacterial products stimulate the enhanced production of IL-23, which triggers T cells to produce IL-17. IL-17 promotes neutrophil migration via the release of CXC chemokines. The IL-23/IL-17 inflammatory pathway is recently suggested to be central to the inflammatory and pustular types of psoriasis, and may also be important in PPP.

References

1 Yamamoto T: Extra-palmoplantar pustulosis associated with palmoplantar pustulosis. J Eur Acad Dermatol Venereol 2009;23:1227–1232.

2 Yamamoto T, Yokozeki H, Tsuboi R: Koebner phenomenon associated with palmoplantar pustulosis. J Eur Acad Dermatol Venereol 2007;21:990–992.

3 Aydin O, Engin B, Oguz O, Ilvan S, Demirkesen C: Non-pustular palmoplantar psoriasis: is histologic differentiation from eczematous dermatitis possible? J Cutan Pathol 2008;35: 169–173.

4 Yamamoto T, Kimura K, Katayama I, Nishioka K: Successful treatment of severe arthralgia associated with palmoplantar pustulosis with low-dose oral cycloporin A. J Dermatol 1995;22: 512–514.

5 Yamamoto T, Katayama I, Nishioka K: Restricted usage of the T-cell receptor Vβ repertoire in tonsillitis in association with palmoplantar pustulosis. Acta Derm Venereol (Stockh) 1998;78: 161–163.

6 Nozawa H, Kishibe K, Takahara M, Harabuchi Y: Expression of cutaneous lymphocyte-associated antigen (CLA) in tonsillar T-cells and its induction by in vitro stimulation with alpha-streptococci in patients with pustulosis palmaris et plantaris (PPP). Clin Immunol 2005;116:42–53.

7 Murakata H, Harabuchi Y, Kataura A: Increased interleukin-6, interferon-gamma and tumor necrosis factor-alpha production by tonsillar mononuclear cells stimulated with alpha-streptococci in patients with pustulosis palmaris et plantaris. Acta Otolaryngol 1999;119:384–391.

8 Koshiba S, Ichimiya S, Nagashima T, Tonooka A, Kubo T, Kikuchi T, Hmi T, Sato N: Tonsillar crypt epithelium of palmoplantar pustulosis secretes interleukin-6 to support B-cell development via p63/p73 transcription factors. J Pathol 2008;214:75–84.

9 Sakiyama H, Kobayashi S, Dianzani U, Ogiuchi H, Kawashima M, Uchiyama T, Yagi J: Possible involvement of T cell co-stimulation in pustulosis palmaris et plantaris via the induction of inducible co-stimulator in chronic focal infections. J Dermatol Sci 2008;50:197–207.

10 Yoshizaki T, Bandoh N, Ueda S, Nozawa H, Goto T, Kishibe K, Takahara M, Harabuchi Y: Up-regulation of CC chemokine receptor 6 on tonsilar T cells and its induction by in vitro stimulation with α-streptococci in patients with pustulosis palmaris et plantaris. Clin Exp Immunol 2009;157:71–82.

Toshiyuki Yamamoto
Department of Dermatology, Fukushima Medical University
Hikarigaoka 1
Fukushima 960-1295 (Japan)
Tel. +81 24 547 1307, E-Mail toyamade@fmu.ac.jp

Harabuchi Y (ed): Recent Advances in Tonsils and Mucosal Barriers of the Upper Airways.
Adv Otorhinolaryngol. Basel, Karger, 2011, vol 72, pp 93–96

Role of Biofilms in Chronic Inflammatory Diseases of the Upper Airways

L. Calò[a] · G.C. Passàli[a] · J. Galli[a] · G. Fadda[b] · G. Paludetti[a]

Institutes of [a]Otorhinolaringology and [b] Microbiology, Catholic University of the Sacred Heart, Rome, Italy

Abstract

The objective of our studies was to document the presence of bacterial biofilms in recurrent and chronic infectious diseases of the upper airways (UA) (adenoiditis, tonsillitis, chronic rhinosinusitis) and to assess the association between the presence of biofilm and the maintenance of a chronic inflammation. **Methods:** 16 surgical samples of tonsils and adenoids from patients with UA infections and 24 samples of ethmoid mucosa from patients who underwent endoscopic sinus surgery for chronic rhinosinusitis (CRS) were cultured using conventional methods and subjected to scanning electron microscopy (SEM) to detect evidence of biofilm. **Results:** Bacterial biofilms were observed in 57.5% of chronically infected UA mucosa; in 41.7% of ethmoid mucosa of CRS patients they were significantly ($p < 0.001$) associated with a marked destruction of ciliated epithelium. **Discussion:** Our studies confirm that biofilm formation plays a role in UA infections, it not only explains the resistance of these infections to antibiotic therapy, but also represents an important element that contributes to the maintenance of a chronic inflammatory reaction.

Bacterial biofilms are communities of microbial cells enclosed in a self-produced polymeric matrix (EPS), a three-dimensional structure composed of water, exopolysaccharides, proteins and DNA. Bacterial organisms within the biofilm use an intercellular communication system based on the secretion of small signaling molecules (quorum sensing). The protected organization of the biofilm guarantees bacterial survival in hostile environments, the exchange of genetic material and the resistance to host's defense system, both innate and specific immunity [1]. Bacteria within biofilms can tolerate levels of antimicrobial agents 1,000 times higher then when they present in a planktonic form. In the EPS, subpopulations of microbial cells, known as 'persisters', can survive to drug therapy. 'Persisters' demonstrate tolerance to antibiotics. In fact when the concentration of antibiotics reduces, these cells repopulate the biofilm and, as a nidus of infection, periodically release bacteria in planktonic form. Biofilms have been identified also in various medical devices used in otorhinolaryngology, including tympanostomy tubes, voice prostheses, endotracheal tubes and cochlear implant removed because of recurrent infections. Moreover, it is nowadays well known that biofilms can directly colonize mucosal tissues, producing chronic and recurrent infections resistant to antibiotic. The upper airways seem to

Table 1. Results obtained by sample's culture and biofilms identification

Samples	n (%) of samples with biofilms	n (%) of samples with positive cultures	Micro-organisms isolated (n)
Adenoid tissue (n = 8)	8 (100)	7 (86.5)	*H. influenzae* (6) *S. pyogenes* (1) α-hemolytic streptococcus (1)
Tonsil (n = 8)	5 (62.5)	5 (62.5)	*S. aureus* (3) α-hemolytic streptococcus (5)
Ethmoid sinus mucosa (n = 24)	10 (41.7)	24 (100)	*M. catarrhalis* (6) *H. influenzae* (12) *S. pyogenes* (4) *S. aureus* (2) *S.epidermidis* (1) *S. pneumoniae* (3)
Total (n = 40)	23/40 (57.5)	36/40 (90)	

be at high risk for this type of colonization [2]. The objective of our studies was to document the presence of bacterial biofilms in recurrent and chronic infectious diseases of the upper airways (adenoiditis, tonsillitis, chronic rhinosinusitis) and to assess the association between the presence of biofilm and the maintenance of a chronic inflammation.

Materials and Methods

We examined 40 samples of upper respiratory tract tissues obtained from 36 patients: 28 adults (mean 45 years), 8 children (mean 6 years) consecutively admitted to the ENT clinic and affected by recurrent upper airways (UA) infections, as documented by clinical history, hematochemical findings, and computed tomography scans. For all patients, surgical treatment was planned after repeated cycles of specific antibiotic therapy.

Surgical samples included tonsillar tissue (n = 8) and adenoid tissue (n = 8) from patients who underwent adenotonsillectomy, and ethmoid mucosa (n = 24) from patients who underwent endoscopic sinus surgery for chronic rhinosinusitis (CRS). All specimens were cultured using conventional methods and subjected to scanning electron microscopy (SEM) to detect evidence of biofilm.

Results

The results are summarized in table 1.

90% (36, n: 40) of the tissue specimens were culture-positive. Bacterial biofilms (associated in most cases with coccoid bacteria) were observed in 57.5% of the adenoid and tonsil tissue samples and in 41.7% of ethmoid mucosa of CRS. *Haemophilus influenzae* was the most commonly isolated bacterium, especially in adenoid tissue and pathologic ethmoid mucosa (fig. 1). Focusing our attention on mucosal alterations in 10 ethmoid samples in which bacterial biofilm were present, we found a marked destruction of the epithelium with a complete absence of cilia, while in ethmoid samples without biofilms, the epithelium was well represented in 5 cases (n = 24) despite a positive culture result, and partially damaged with a consistent inflammatory cells representation in 9 cases (n = 24). Moreover, the presence of biofilm was significantly associated with an abnormal ciliary state and with the presence of *H. influenzae* ($p = 0.001$). χ^2 test Yates correction for qualitative variables and the Kruskal-Wallis test for quantitative

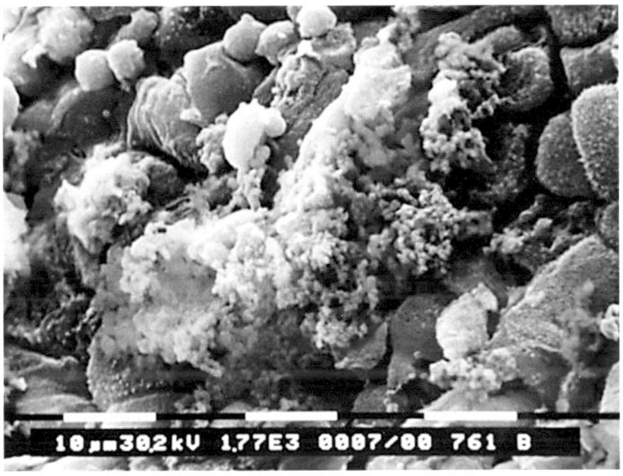

Fig 1. Biofilm in CRS.

ones. The statistically significant level was set at p = 0.05.

Conclusions

A recent paper describes biofilms as 'the most successful forms of life in earth' [3], and many studies have been published from the first description by Antonie van Leeuwenhoek in the 16th century about micro-organisms bound to a surface in the form of dental plaque. The introduction of scanning electron microscopy and, more recently, of confocal laser scanning microscopy has offered the possibility to perform direct and accurate observation of bacteria and their complex organization. It has been demonstrated that about 99% of all bacteria exist in biofilms and the Centers for Disease Control and Prevention estimate that at least 65% of all human bacterial infectious processes involve biofilms [4]. Biofilm formation is a dynamic process that begins with the casual attachment of one or more bacteria to an inorganic or organic surface. The attachment of bacteria is facilitated, on inorganic materials (prosthesis or medical devices), by the presence of an irregular surface, and, on organic surfaces, by cilia or flagella, or organic polymeric liquids such as blood, saliva or respiratory secretions. Biofilm development is characterized by consecutive stages mediated by molecular messengers and by acetylated lactones, also called autoinducers, which interact with the surface receptors and regulate gene expression. This mechanism is known as 'quorum sensing'. These adaptations determine increased resistance to antibiotics and host-defense mechanisms correlated to the EPS capacity to absorb or limit antibiotic distribution, the particular biofilm organization, characterized by the transport system of proteic material and the rich net of water channels in the glycocalyx (particularly elaborate in its peripheral area but limited in the biofilm core), and, finally, the environmental heterogeneity within the biofilm, with different pH gradients and oxygen concentrations. These differences in metabolic and environmental conditions allow bacteria to survive within the biofilm core, without reproducing for a long period of time, as spores. In our experience, all tissue samples were culture positive and the most frequently isolated bacteria *(H. influenzae, Streptococcus* alpha hemolytic [commensal], *Streptococcus pyogenes* and *Staphylococcus aureus)* were isolates usually identified in pediatric recurrent UA infections [5].

The high incidence of bacterial biofilms in adenoid and tonsil tissue and ethmoid samples may help explain the difficult eradication of bacterial species involved in these chronic infective processes. However, no certain conclusion can be drawn on the role of the above-mentioned bacterial species in biofilm formation in our samples.

Only recently, did some authors introduce the use of fluorescent in situ hybridization (FISH), and immunostaining combined with confocal laser scanning microscopy, to prove that the bacterial species isolated in mucosal biofilms are the same pathogens commonly associated with chronic infections [6], and show that chronic ad enotonsillitis is probably a result of multiple overlapping infections caused by different pathogens, and the spectrum of micro-organisms changes in parallel with the displacement in the lymphoid tissue and the age of the patient. Also, the high percentage of bacterial biofilms in our specimens (41.7%) confirms, as described by others [7], the association between biofilm evidence and chronic rhinosinusitis. Nevertheless, although biofilms represent an important factor in the resistance to medical therapy and in the persistence of sinusal infections, their role in the physiopathological process still remains unclear. The significant correlation in our study between the presence of biofilm and the damage of the nasosinusal epithelium could justify the CRS recurrence after endoscopic surgery, as stated by Bendouah et al. [8], even if it is difficult establish whether colonization of the nasal mucosa by biofilms is the consequence or the cause of complete ciliated epithelium destruction and alterations in clearance [9, 10]. With the availability of new techniques, such as scanning electron and confocal laser microscopy, semiquantitative methods to quantify biofilm production in vitro, and, finally, FISH, should be possible to observe the presence of mucosal biofilms in almost all cases, explain the resistance to antibiotics and host immune response, and, finally, clarify the effective etiopathogenic role of biofilms in sustaining chronic inflammatory mucosal reactions.

Our research, which is consistent with data in the literature, would be an early contribution to other studies in order to define a standardized diagnostic method and discover new therapeutic approaches to prevent biofilm formation.

References

1 Costerton JW, Stewart PS, Greenberg EP: Bacterial biofilm: a common cause of persistent infections. Science 1999;284:1318–1322.
2 Hall-Stoodley L, Hu FZ, Gieseke A, et al: Direct detection of bacterial biofilms on the middle-ear mucosa of children with chronic otitis media. JAMA 2006;296: 202–211.
3 Flemming HC, Wingender J: The biofilm matrix. Nat Rev Microbiol 2010;8: 623–633.
4 Galli J, Calò L, Ardito F, Imperiali M, Bassotti E, Fadda G, Paludetti G: Biofilm formation by *Haemophilus influenzae* isolated from adeno-tonsil tissue samples, and its role in recurrent adenotonsillitis. Acta Otorhinolaryngol Ital 2007;27:134–138.
5 Saylam G, Tatar EC, Tatar I, Ozdek A, Korkmaz H: Association of adenoid surface biofilm formation and chronic otitis media with effusion. Arch Otolaryngol Head Neck Surg 2010;136: 550–555.
6 Winther B, Gross BC, Hendley JO, Early SV: Location of bacterial biofilm in the mucus overlying the adenoid by light microscopy. Arch Otolaryngol Head Neck Surg 2009;135:1239–1245
7 Palmer J: Bacterial biofilms in chronic rhinosinusitis. Ann Otol Rhinol Laryngol suppl 2006;196:35–39.
8 Bendouah Z, Barbeau J, Hamad WA, Desrosiers M: Biofilm formation by *Staphylococcus aureus* and *Pseudomonas aeruginosa* is associated with an unfavorable evolution after surgery for chronic sinusitis and nasal polyposis. Otolaryngol Head Neck Surg 2006;134:991–994.
9 Galli J, Calò L, Ardito F, Imperiali M, Bassotti E, Passàli GC, La Torre G, Paludetti G, Fadda G: Damage to ciliated epithelium in chronic rhinosinusitis: what is the role of bacterial biofilms? Ann Otol Rhinol Laryngol 2008;117:902–908.
10 Galli J, Ardito F, Calò L, Mancinelli L, Imperiali M, Parrilla C, Picciotti PM, Fadda G: Recurrent upper airway infections and bacterial biofilms. J Laryngol Otol 2007;121:341–344.

Giulio Cesare Passàli
Institute of Otorhinolaringology, Catholic University of the Sacred Heart
p.le A. Gemelli 1
IT–00168 Rome (Italy)
Tel. +39 3331727194, E-Mail giulio.passali@rm.unicatt.it

Harabuchi Y (ed): Recent Advances in Tonsils and Mucosal Barriers of the Upper Airways.
Adv Otorhinolaryngol. Basel, Karger, 2011, vol 72, pp 97–99

Regulation of Microbiota by Antimicrobial Peptides in the Gut

Koji Masuda[a] · Kiminori Nakamura[a,b] · Sawako Yoshioka[a] · Rie Fukaya[a] · Naoki Sakai[a,b] · Tokiyoshi Ayabe[a,b]

Innate Immunity Laboratory, [a]Graduate School of Life Science, and [b]Department of Cell Biological Science, Faculty of Advanced Life Science, Hokkaido University, Sapporo, Hokkaido, Japan

Abstract

The antimicrobial peptide is one of major effectors of the innate immunity, and is common in the entire multicellular organisms. In mammals, one family of antibacterial peptide named defensins plays a central role in host defense, especially in the epithelial surface such as oral cavity, skin and the intestine. Recently, the importance of the antimicrobial peptides has been widely recognized. The epithelium of the gut is a largest surface that is exposed to various pathogens in the environment. It is the Paneth cells that produce antimicrobial peptides, α-defensins in the small intestine. Paneth cells contribute to mucosal innate immunity by sensing bacteria and releasing microbicidal activities mostly from activated α-defensins. In mice, α-defensins, named cryptdins, consisted of six major isoforms (cryptdin-1 to cryptdin-6), and among those cryptdin-4 is the most microbicidal, suggesting that cryptdin-4 has a pivotal role in innate immunity. Paneth cell α-defensins have selective activities against commensal bacteria which may be associated with compositions of intestinal microbiota in vivo and homeostasis of the entire intestine. In addition, Paneth cell α-defensins appeared to be regulated topographically to control intestinal integrity.

Antimicrobial peptides are gene-encoded effectors in the innate immunity from plant to human, and microbicidal, cationic small peptides. Antimicrobial peptides have a broad spectrum, active against bacteria, fungi, protozoa and certain viruses, and have a low occurrence of resistance [1]. In mammals, many epithelial cells express antimicrobial peptides. In the airway including nasopharynx and lung, the skin, and many other tissues, epithelial cells express β-defensins and chathelicidins. One of the small intestinal epithelial cell lineages, the Paneth cell, produces antimicrobial peptides, named α-defensins [2].

Antimicrobial Peptides in the Gut

Paneth cell α-defensins are the only antimicrobial peptides produced and released by the small intestinal epithelium. Mammalian α-defensins are 3–4 kDa cationic peptides with six cysteines which form invariantly placed 3 disulfide bonds [2]. Paneth cells are normally specific to the base of the small intestinal crypts, where they are recognized by their large, apically oriented granules

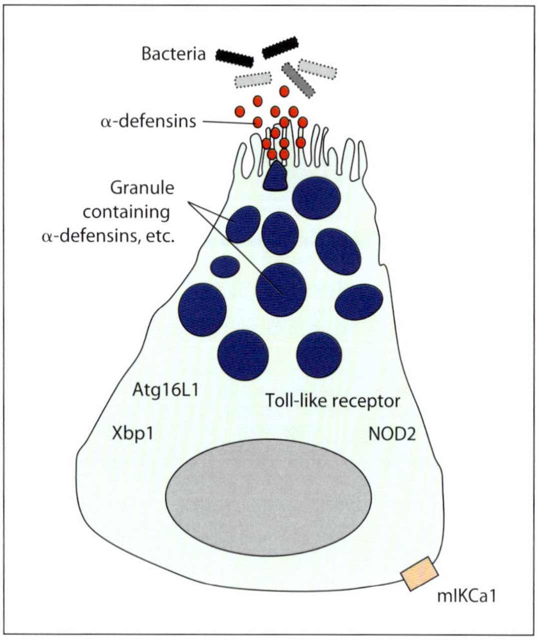

Fig. 1. Paneth cells in the innate immunity. Paneth cell α-defensins are secreted into the lumen of the small intestine. Molecules expressing in Paneth cells and involved in the innate immunity may have a key role to understand certain diseases such as Crohn disease.

containing α-defensins. Paneth cell α-defensins, cryptdins, cryptdin-1 to cryptdin-6 (Crp1-Crp6) in mouse, HD5 and HD6 in human, have potent in vitro microbicidal activities. Among the cryptdins, cryptdin-4 (Crp4) is known to have the most potent bactericidal activities [3]. It has been shown that Paneth cells contribute to the mucosal immunity by sensing bacteria and releasing granules containing α-defensins at effective concentrations [4–7].

Paneth Cell α-Defensins and the Gut Microbiota

Cryptdins elicit potent bactericidal activities against noncommensal bacteria, and Crp4 has the most potent activities. Bactericidal activities are known to correlate with permeabilization of live *Escherichia coli*, with equilibrium binding to *E. coli* membrane phospholipids. It has been reported that disulfide bonds of Crp4 have no effect on the bactericidal activities against noncommensal bacteria demonstrated by Cys-to-Ala mutagenesis [8]. Recently, Salzman et al. [9] showed that significant HD5-dependent changes in microbiota composition, but not in total bacterial numbers were detected in the small intestine of the HD5 transgenic mice. It suggests a new homeostatic role of α-defensins. It has been known that MMP-7 null mice which lack activated cryptdins in Paneth cells only accumulate inactive precursors and no active, processed cryptdins. Mastroianni et al. [10] reported that abundant active cryptdins are recovered from the colonic lumen of the MMP-7 null mice. It suggests that cryptdins may play a role not only in the small intestine but also in the colonic lumen. Masuda et al. [11] revealed that a Paneth cell α-defensin, native cryptdin-4 showed only small or no bactericidal activities against intestinal commensal microbiota such as *Bifidobacterium bifidum*, *Lactobacillus casei* and *Bacteroides thetaiotaomicron*, whereas it showed potent bactericidal activities against intestinal noncommensal microbiota such as *Salmonella typhimurium* and *Staphylococcus aureus*. In this study, we showed that cryptdins have selective bactericidal activity against commensal bacteria. Taken together, these findings suggest a new role for antimicrobial peptides in the intestinal homeostasis, and also provide an insight into the mechanisms of innate intestinal immunity (fig. 1) [12]. In relation to inflammatory bowel disease, it was reported that the proform of a human Paneth cell α-defensin, HD5, was reduced in some patients with Crohn disease [13]. The reduced pro-HD5 was degraded by trypsin, a processing enzyme of HD5 in vivo and the bactericidal activity was diminished. Those recent advances further inspire us to understand the role of antimicrobial peptides in health and diseases.

Acknowledgments

This work was partially supported by a Grant-in-Aid for Knowledge Cluster Phase II, Sapporo Bio-S, a Grant-in-Aid for Scientific Research on Priority Areas, and a Grant-in-Aid for Scientific Research from The Ministry of Education, Culture, Sports, Science and Technology of Japan.

References

1 Zasloff M: Antimicrobial peptides of multicellular organisms. Nature 2002;415:389–395.
2 Selsted ME, Ouellette AJ: Mammalian defensins in the antimicrobial immune response. Nat Immunol 2005;6:551–557.
3 Ouellette AJ, Hsieh MM, Nosek MT, Cano-Gauci DF, Huttner KM, Buick RN, Selsted ME: Mouse Paneth cell defensins: primary structures and antibacterial activities of numerous cryptdin isoforms. Infect Immun 1994;62:5040–5047.
4 Wilson CL, Ouellette AJ, Satchell DP, Ayabe T, López-Boado YS, Stratman JL, Hultgren SJ, Matrisian LM, Parks WC: Regulation of intestinal α-defensin activation by the metalloproteinase matrilysin in innate host defense. Science 1999;286:113–117.
5 Ayabe T, Satchell DP, Wilson CL, Parks WC, Selsted ME, Ouellette AJ: Secretion of microbicidal α-defensins by intestinal Paneth cells in response to bacteria. Nat Immunol 2000;1:113–118.
6 Ayabe T, Satchell DP, Pesendorfer P, Tanabe H, Wilson CL, Hagen SJ, Ouellette AJ: Activation of Paneth cell α-defensins in mouse small intestine. J Biol Chem 2002;277:5219–5228.
7 Ayabe T, Ashida T, Kohgo Y, Kono T: The role of Paneth cells and their antimicrobial peptides in innate host defense. Trends Microbiol 2004;12:394–398.
8 Maemoto A, Qu X, Rosengren KJ, Tanabe H, Henschen-Edman A, Craik DJ, Ouellette AJ: Functional analysis of the α-defensin disulfide array in mouse cryptdin-4. J Biol Chem 2004;279:44188–44196.
9 Salzman NH, Hung K, Haribhai D, Chu H, Karlsson-Sjoberg J, Amir E, Teggatz P, Barman M, Hayward M, Eastwood D, Stoel M, Zhou Y, Sodergren E, Weinstock GM, Bevins CL, Williams CB, Bos NA: Enteric defensins are essential regulators of intestinal microbial ecology. Nat Immunol 2010;11:76–83.
10 Mastroianni JR, Ouellette AJ: α-defensins in enteric innate immunity: functional Paneth cell α-defensins in mouse colonic lumen. J Biol Chem 2009; 284:27848–27856.
11 Masuda K, Sakai N, Nakamura K, Yoshioka S, Ayabe T: Bactericidal activity of mouse α-defensin, cryptdin-4 predominantly affects non-commensal bacteria. J Innate Immun 2011;in press, DOI: 10.1159/000322037.
12 Ouellette AJ: Paneth cells and innate mucosal immunity. Curr Opin Gastroenterol 2010;6:547–553.
13 Tanabe H, Ayabe T, Maemoto A, Ishikawa C, Inaba Y, Sato R, Moriichi K, Okamoto K, Watari J, Kono T, Ashida T, Kohgo Y: Denatured human α-defensin attenuates the bactericidal activity and the stability against enzymatic digestion. Biochem Biophys Res Commun 2007; 358:349–355.

Tokiyoshi Ayabe, MD, PhD
Department of Cell Biological Science, Faculty of Advanced Life Science, Hokkaido University
Kita-21, Nishi-11, Kita-ku
Sapporo, Hokkaido 001-0021 (Japan)
Tel. +81 11 706 9049, E-Mail ayabe@sci.hokudai.ac.jp

Harabuchi Y (ed): Recent Advances in Tonsils and Mucosal Barriers of the Upper Airways.
Adv Otorhinolaryngol. Basel, Karger, 2011, vol 72, pp 100–102

Evidence of the Local Immune Status in the Human Larynx

Tadashi Nakashima · Hideichiro Tomita · Shun-ichi Chitose

Department of Otolaryngology, Head and Neck Surgery, Kurume University School of Medicine, Kurume, Japan

Abstract

We have studied the presence of local immunity in the larynx and its role and development of laryngeal glands in the human larynx. The local immune status in laryngeal secretion or related tissue specimens from the laryngeal ventricle was examined and the results were analyzed between individuals with or without head and neck cancer. Laryngeal secretions or mucosal tissue specimens were obtained during the microscopic laryngeal surgery or at the time of the surgery of the larynx. The laryngeal secretion contained immunological factors such as IgG, IgM, IgA or secretory IgA (SIgA). The mean level of SIgA of the mucosal tissue was low in patients with the benign laryngeal disease and considerably decreased in patients with previous radiation therapy. The level of SIgA in the laryngeal secretion closely correlated to the level of SIgA in the mucosal tissue. From the present study, we confirmed the actual presence of local immune function in the human larynx. Furthermore, the local immune status is affected by either the presence of malignancy or the treatment to the larynx such as radiation.

The larynx is endowed with a rich supply of glandular tissues and the laryngeal mucosa is covered with mucous materials. We have been studying the role of laryngeal mucus fluid and reported that such secretions, produced in the laryngeal glands, are not only necessary as a lubricant for vocal fold vibration but also important for local defense status of the laryngeal mucosa [1, 2].

The laryngeal glands are mainly contained in the laryngeal ventricle and the concentration of glandular tissue increases as they grow. However, there have been few reports regarding the actual status of local immunity based on immunological factors in the laryngeal secretion. Knowledge of the mucosal immune status in the larynx should provide a valuable baseline for understanding the immunological status of laryngeal disorders.

Materials and Methods

Approval for this study was obtained from the Institutional Review Board of the Kurume University School of Medicine.

Mucus fluid in the laryngeal ventricle was locally collected during microscopic laryngeal surgery or at the time of surgical removal of the larynx from 72 human adults (66 males, 6 females; age ranging from 52 to 84 years). Sixty-two of 72 were patients with head and neck cancer and the other 10 patients has other benign disease such as aspiration. There were 11 patients who had a history of radiotherapy to the neck. In patients whose false vocal cord was free from tumor invasion, a mucosal tissue specimen was also extracted. For comparison, the serum and sputa of the same individual were also examined in some patients.

The levels of immunoglobulins (IgG, IgA and IgM) were measured quantitatively using turbidimetric immunoassay (TIA) or electro-chemiluminescence immunoassay (ECLIA) (SRL Laboratories, Tokyo, Japan). The level of secretory IgA was measured using the enzyme immunoassay (ELISA; Medical & Biological Laboratories, Nagoya, Japan).

Statistical Analysis

Statistically significant correlations between the mean levels of each patient group were determined by Cochran-Cox, using the 'Stat View' software package (Abacus Concepts, Calif., USA). $p < 0.05$ was considered to indicate statistical significance.

Results

Measurement of Immunoglobulins

The mean concentration of each immunoglobulin in the serum was 11.95 mg/ml (IgG), 2.53 mg/ml (IgA) and 0.84 mg/ml (IgM). SIgA was not determined. The mean concentration of each immunoglobulin in the sputa was 0.26 mg/ml (IgG), 0.20 mg/ml (IgA), 0.01 mg/ml (IgM) and 199.2 μg/ml (SIgA). The mean concentration of each immunoglobulin in the laryngeal fluid was 0.53 mg/ml (IgG), 0.13 mg/ml (IgA), 0.02 mg/ml (IgM) and 69.6 μg/ml (SIgA). Although the mean concentration of each immunoglobulin was rather low as compared to the serum, the laryngeal fluid was found to contain immunoglobulins. The mean level of IgA or SIgA in laryngeal secretion was lower than those in sputa.

The mean level of immunoglobulins of the laryngeal secretion and tissue was compared according to the patients' characteristics. In patients with benign laryngeal disease, the mean concentration was of 0.16 mg/ml (IgG), 0.07 mg/ml (IgA), 0.01 mg/ml (IgM) and 90.1 μg/ml (SIgA). In the cancer group, the mean concentration was 0.53 mg/ml (IgG), 0.14 mg/ml (IgA), 0.02 mg/ml (IgM) and 74.6 μg/ml (SIgA), but was 0.67 mg/ml (IgG), 0.15 mg/ml (IgA), 0.03 mg/ml (IgM) and 42.5 μg/ml (SIgA) in patients who had previously received radiotherapy. Because of the limited number of patients examined, however, no significant difference was observed between each group.

In the tissue specimens obtained from false cords, the mean level was 3.14 mg/wg for IgG, 0.99 mg/ml for IgA, 0.17 mg/ml for IgM and 129.1 μg/ml for SIgA. The mean level of IgM (0.07 mg/ml) and SIgA (70.60 μg/ml) in the benign group was significantly lower than in the cancer group ($p < 0.05$). The SIgA of the radiotherapy group was also lower than in the cancer group. However, no absolute difference was detected.

In patients whose samples of the laryngeal secretion and the mucosal tissue were obtained simultaneously, the correlation of the level of immunoglobulins in each individual was examined. IgG or IgM did not show any correlation between each value. A slight correlation was found in the case of IgA. In contrast, a statistically significant correlation was found between the level of SIgA of laryngeal secretion and the mucosal tissue.

Discussion

It is well established that mucosal immunity by external secretions is present in either respiratory or gastrointestinal passages. In particular, locally produced secretory IgA is the predominant immunoglobulin in mucosal immunity [3, 4]. Using an immunofluorescent method, we have previously demonstrated that IgA-producing plasma cells are numerous in the submucosal or periglandular area of the human larynx, thus suggesting that the local immune system is active in the human larynx [1].

In a previous report of local immunity of the human larynx, Mogi et al. [5] first observed that laryngeal secretions have much the same amount of IgG and other immunoglobulins as those obtained from nasal secretion and tracheobronchial washings. According to their observations, they determined the mean level of IgA and secretory component (SC) of the laryngeal secretion to be 0.62 mg/ml and 61 μg/ml whereas that of nasal secretions was 0.54 mg/ml and 97 μg/ml. The level of IgA in the laryngeal secretion in our observation is lower than their results.

The examined mucosa obtained from the false cord is thought to include epithelial or subepithelial tissues which include glandular tissue and stroma. It was interesting to note that the mean levels of IgM and SIgA in the benign group are lower than in the cancer group ($p < 0.05$).

It should also be emphasized that the level of secretory immunoglobulin in laryngeal secretions or tissue specimens was found to have decreased in the group that had previously undergone radiotherapy to the neck. In our recent study of the larynx in patients who received radiotherapy to the neck, the laryngeal glands were often found to have been replaced with fibrous connective tissue [6]. As the ratio of serous-type glandular acini also decreased, not only the voice function but also the local defense function of the larynx might thus be impaired. Further studies on the importance of local immune acuity and the expression of tumor markers are now underway.

References

1 Nakashima T, Komiyama S, Makishima K, Takeda K, Hiroto I: Immunopathological study of the larynx: IgA distribution and secretory activity. Ann Otol Rhinol Laryngol 1980;89:359–365.

2 Nakashima T, Makishima K, Komiyama S, Takeda K, Hiroto I: Local immune system in the developing fetal larynx. Laryngoscope 1980;91:398–407.

3 Tomasi TB Jr, Jan EM, Solomon A, Prendergast RA: Characteristics of an immune system common to certain external secretions. J Exp Med 1965;121:101–124.

4 Brandtzaeg P: Mucosal and glandular distribution of immunoglobulin components: differential localization of free and bound SC in secretory epithelial cells. J Immunol 1974;112:1553–1559.

5 Mogi G, Watanabe N, Maeda S, Umehara T: Laryngeal secretions: an immunological and immunohistological study. Acta Otolaryngol (Stockh) 1979;87:129–141.

6 Nakashima T, Tomita H, Tsuda S, Chitose S: Radiotherapy of the neck influences the distribution of laryngeal secretory glands. J Laryngol Otol 2005;119: 976–980.

Tadashi Nakashima
Department of Otolaryngology, Head and Neck Surgery, Kurume University School of Medicine
67 Asahi-machi
Kurume 830-0011 (Japan)
Tel, +81942317575, E-Mail orlkaku@med.kurume-u.ac.jp

Harabuchi Y (ed): Recent Advances in Tonsils and Mucosal Barriers of the Upper Airways.
Adv Otorhinolaryngol. Basel, Karger, 2011, vol 72, pp 103–106

Short Review on Sublingual Immunotherapy for Patients with Allergic Rhinitis: from Bench to Bedside

Hideyuki Kawauchi · Kaoru Goda · Miki Tongu · Takaya Yamada · Noriaki Aoi · Ichiro Morikura · Takashi Fuchiwaki

Department of Otorhinolaryngology, Shimane University, Faculty of Medicine, Izumo, Japan

Abstract

Sublingual immunotherapy has been considered to be a painless and effective therapeutic treatment for allergic rhinitis, and is known as type 1 allergy of the nasal mucosa. So far, its mechanism of action has been elucidated employing peripheral blood serum and lymphocytes in an antigen-specific fashion. Because of the limitations in sampling human materials, there is still controversy among many reports between clinical efficacy and laboratory data. Therefore, its mechanism of action needs to be investigated further by using promising animal models such as rodents and monkeys. Bearing this in mind, in our present study, we successfully constructed an effective murine model for sublingual immunotherapy in allergic rhinitis in which mice were administered ovalbumin (OVA) sublingually followed by intraperitoneal sensitization and nasal challenge.

Allergic Rhinitis and Regulatory Mechanism for Allergic Inflammation

Allergic rhinitis is one of the commonest types of allergic inflammation affecting 10–25% of the world's population, and its prevalence has increased over the last decade. Allergic rhinitis is characterized by a predominant Th2 response, antigen-specific IgE synthesis and infiltration of eosinophils into the nasal mucosa [1]. The type 1 allergic response is largely divided into two phases, namely systemic response at the induction phase and allergic inflammation in the eliciting phase. The eliciting phase is further divided into two phases, namely immediate phase and late phase. To consider the pathologies of type 1 allergic inflammation, we should now distinguish between the induction phase and the eliciting phase, even though there is always a mixture of these two phases in normal human nasal mucosa. The hygiene hypothesis in line with helper T cell dichotomy has been proposed by a large number of investigators and many plausible hypotheses are available to understand allergic inflammation in comparison with infective inflammation.

More recently, regulatory T cells, defined as CD4+CD25+ FoxP3+ T cell subpopulations, have been focused on as key players to downregulate excessive Th1 or Th2 pathologies such as autoimmune disease or allergy. These regulatory T cell subpopulations are considered to be efficiently developed in a circumstance of low hygiene and high pathogen/adjuvant burden. Regulatory T cells producing IL-10 and/or TGF-β are induced not only in atopic patients by successful immunotherapy, but also during natural allergen exposure in healthy people.

Regulatory T cells can control and regulate all the effector mechanisms activated during allergy and the Th2 responses through the production of IL-10/TGF-β and/or cell-cell contact. IL-10 is a potent suppressor of total and allergen-specific IgEs, whereas it induces an antibody isotype switch towards IgG4. TGF-β also decreases IgE production and induces an immunoglobulin isotype switch towards IgA. IL-10 and TGF-β act directly or indirectly on the human airways to decrease both mucus production and airway hyperreactivity.

Antigen-Specific Subcutaneous – and Sublingual – Immunotherapy

In the 5th edition of Japanese guidelines of allergic rhinitis, specific immunotherapy is recommended and introduced. So we need a more elegant and safe immunotherapy rather than the conventional one, and now sublingual immunotherapy has been in trials with T cell epitopes of cedar pollen in patients suffering from cedar pollenosis. Peptide immunotherapy with the T cell epitope of allergens (percutaneously or sublingually) is now in the process of clinical trials in Japan.

For the better understanding of sublingual immunotherapy, we need information such as standardization of antigens for immunotherapy, clinical efficacy, safety, mechanism of action, and aim for early intervention. Allergen-specific immunotherapy is associated with an improved tolerance to allergen challenge, with a decrease in immediate- and late-phase allergic inflammation [2]. Allergen-specific immunotherapy also modifies cellular and humoral responses to the allergen. The ratio of Th1 cytokines to Th2 cytokines is increased following allergen-specific immunotherapy, and functional regulatory T cells are induced. Production of blocking antibodies, IgG1, IgG4 and IgA, is induced and these immunoglobulins compete with IgE for allergen binding, thereby decreasing the allergen capture and presentation that is facilitated by the IgE in complex with FcεRI or FcεRII.

Sublingual immunotherapy has previously been shown in many clinical studies to modulate allergen-specific Th2 responses with a decrease in the IgE to IgG4 ratio, and its mechanism has been considered similar to that of subcutaneous immunotherapy [3–7]. Here, we address some new findings of the immunological mechanisms of sublingual immunotherapy such as decrease in the IgE/IgG4 ratio, induction of IL-10-producing Tregs and allergen-specific T cell tolerance, etc. Cosmi's group have performed a clinical long-term study for sublingual immunotherapy in patients with perennial rhinitis with *Dermatophagoides* and came to the conclusion that the effects of SLIT is downregulation of Dp-specific IgE , enhancement of IFN-γ with Th cells, downregulation of Dp-specific proliferation, and enhancement of IL-10 production. On the other hand, in their clinical study of patients with birch pollenosis, Bohler et al. [8] found that transient induction of regulatory T cells immediately after SLIT is followed by long-term allergen-specific peripheral tolerance (anergy) and immune deviation (from Th2 to Th1 milieu). Then, why do we choose sublingual immunotherapy as a new therapeutic method rather than subcutaneous immunotherapy?

Sublingual immunotherapy requires much more amounts of allergen than subcutaneous immunotherapy, but it has several benefits in comparison with subcutaneous immunotherapy [9]. Sublingual immunotherapy is pain-free and safer than subcutaneous immunotherapy, because the amount of mast cells is least in the sublingual mucosal tissue. Another benefit is that patients can carry out the immunotherapy procedure by

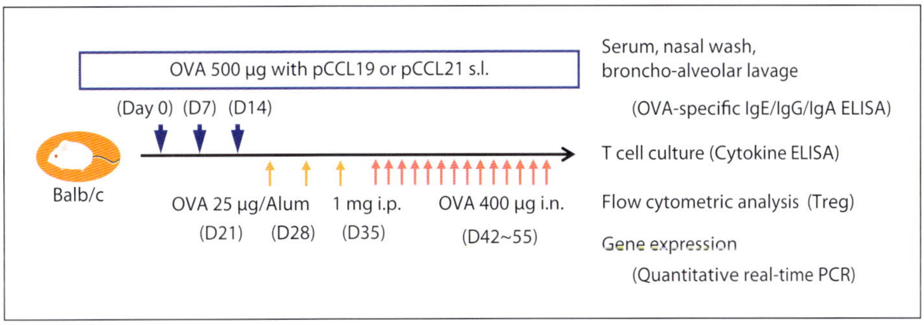

Fig. 1. Induction of allergic rhinitis and sublingual immunotherapy: Mice were sensitized by intraperitoneal injections (i.p.) of 25 μg of OVA with 1 mg of alum every week for three times and were nasally challenged (i.n.) with 400 μg of OVA for 14 consecutive days. For sublingual treatment (s.l.), 4 μl of PBS alone or PBS containing 500 μg of OVA was applied on the sublingual mucosa of anesthetized mice before sensitization. Mice and specimens: 6- to 8-week-old Balb/c mice were used. After the final nasal challenge, serum, nasal wash and broncho-alveolar lavage (BAL) were collected. Single cells of spleen, cervical lymph node (CLN), nasopharynx-associated lymphoid tissue (NALT), and nasal passage were harvested from the mice.

themselves at home after reaching the allergen maintenance dose, thus necessitating fewer visits to the outpatient clinic. To solve the problem of sublingual immunotherapy requiring a high dose of allergen, improvement of the allergen delivery system is necessary. One possible way is to modify immunocompetent cells such as dendritic cells for the efficient induction of regulatory T cells and the production of allergen-specific IgGs.

Experimental Data in Our Murine Allergic Rhinitis Model and Future Goal

Sublingual immunotherapy has been considered to be a painless and effective therapeutic treatment for allergic rhinitis, which is a known as type 1 allergy of the nasal mucosa. So far, its mechanism of action has been elucidated by employing peripheral blood serum and lymphocytes in an antigen-specific fashion. Controversy still exists between many reports regarding the clinical efficacy and laboratory data of this method because of the limitations in sampling human material. Therefore, its mechanism of action needs to be further investigated using promising animal models such as rodents and monkeys. Bearing this in mind, in our present study, we successfully constructed an effective murine model for sublingual immunotherapy in allergic rhinitis in which mice were administered ovalbumin (OVA) sublingually followed by intraperitoneal sensitization and nasal challenge. The materials and methods are shown in detail in figure 1. To summarize our experimental data, sublingually treated mice showed significantly decreased allergic responses as well as suppressed Th2 immune responses and sublingual administration of OVA did not alter the frequency of CD4+CD25+ regulatory T cells (Tregs), but led to upregulation of Foxp3- and IL-10-specific mRNAs in the Tregs of cervical lymph nodes (CLN). These results suggest that IL-10 expressing CD4+CD25+Foxp3+ Tregs in CLN are involved in the suppression of allergic responses [10].

Conclusion

The future goal, from the research and clinical aspects, is that antigen dosing via the sublingual route should be precisely examined with T cell epitopes to increase clinical efficacy and avoid adverse events. Different types of antigen delivery systems should be developed to replace the conventional methods.

Acknowledgement

This study was supported by Grant-in-Aids from the Japanese Ministry of Education, and Agriculture.

References

1 Gelfand EW: Inflammatory mediators in allergic rhinitis. J Allergy Clin Immunol 2004;114:S135–S138.

2 Larche M, Akdis CA, Valenta R: Immunological mechanisms of allergen-specific immunotherapy. Nat Rev Immunol 2006;6:761–771.

3 Wilson DR, Torres Lima M, Durham SR: Sublingual immunotherapy for allergic rhinitis: systematic review and meta-analysis. Allergy 2005;60:4–12.

4 Song JH, Kim JI, Kwon HJ, et al: CCR7-CCL19/CCL21-regulated dendritic cells are responsible for effectiveness of sublingual vaccination. J Immunol 2009;182:6851–6860.

5 Ciprandi G, Fenoglio D, Cirillo I, et al: Sublingual immunotherapy: an update on immunologic and functional effect. Allergy Asthma Proc 2007;28:40–43.

6 Okubo K, Gotoh M, Fujieda S, et al: A randomized double-blind comparative study of sublingual immunotherapy for cedar pollinosis. Allergol Int 2008;57:265–227.

7 Moingeon P, Batard T, Fadel R, et al: Immune mechanisms of allergen-specific sublingual immunotherapy. Allergy 2006;61:151–165.

8 Bohler B, et al: SLIT induces IL-10-producing Tregs and allergen-specific T cell tolerance. J Allergy Clin Immunol 2007;120:707–713.

9 Yamanaka K, Yuta A, Kakeda M, et al: Induction of IL-10-producing regulatory T cells with TCR diversity by epitope-specific immunotherapy in pollinosis. J Allergy Clin Immunol 2009;124:842–845, e7.

10 Goda K, Kawauchi H, et al: An investigation of the mechanism of sublingual immunotherapy: an experimental data in murine allergic rhinitis model. Jpn J Stomatopharyngol 2009;22:31–33.

Dr. Hideyuki Kawauchi
Department of Otorhinolaryngology, Shimane University, Faculty of Medicine
89–1 Enya-cho
Izumo City, Shimane 693-8501 (Japan)
Tel. +81 853 20 2273, E-Mail kawauchi@med.shimane-u.ac.jp

Harabuchi Y (ed): Recent Advances in Tonsils and Mucosal Barriers of the Upper Airways.
Adv Otorhinolaryngol. Basel, Karger, 2011, vol 72, pp 107–109

Differential Properties of Mucous Glycoproteins Produced by Allergic Inflammation and Lipopolysaccharide Stimulation in Rat Nasal Epithelium

Takeshi Shimizu · Shino Shimizu

Department of Otorhinolaryngology, Shiga University of Medical Science, Otsu, Shiga, Japan

Abstract

To examine the differential properties of mucous glycoproteins, we produced hyperplastic and metaplastic changes in goblet cells of rat nasal epithelium by intranasal instillation of ovalbumin (OVA) in OVA-sensitized rats, and by intranasal lipopolysaccharides (LPS) instillation. The epithelial mucosubstance was quantitatively examined by AB-PAS and lectin histochemistry. The newly produced mucin after OVA challenge or LPS instillation contained a high amount of sulfomucin and a low amount of neutral glycoprotein: LPS-induced mucin contained more sulfomucin (70.1% of total) and less neutral glycoprotein (8.6%) than OVA-induced mucin (sulfomucin 33.6%, neutral glycoprotein 41.8%). Four of the lectins, PNA, MAL II, SNA, UEA I, stained some of the mucosubstance, indicating the presence of galactose-N-acetylgalactosamine, α2,3-linked and α2,6-linked sialic acid-galactose, and fucose residues. After LPS instillation, the reactivity was higher for galactose-N-acetylgalactosamine (64.8% of total) and α2,3-linked sialic acid-galactose (75.8%) than after saline instillation (3.5 and 19.1%, respectively) or OVA challenge (5.8 and 32.3%). A 2-fold increase in mucin mRNA (rat Muc5ac) expression was induced after LPS instillation or OVA challenge. These results indicate that mucin mRNA expression increases similarly after LPS instillation or OVA challenge, however, carbohydrate compositions of newly produced mucin are different between the two groups.

Mucous glycoproteins (mucin) are large heterogeneous macromolecules, containing oligosaccharide chains attached to peptide backbones encoded by several MUC genes. Hypersecretion of mucus is a common characteristic of airway inflammation. Mucin differs in the sugar groups and the extent of sialylation and sulfation of the oligosaccharide structure in different hypersecretory conditions. The alteration of these oligosaccharide structures or peptide backbones may affect the physicochemical properties of mucus in disease. However, little is known about the disease-related changes of mucin character and mucin gene expression in airway inflammation and biological roles of these changes are still unclear. We hypothesized that the extent of sialylation and sulfation of the terminal sugar residues, and mucin gene expression, are different between mucins produced by allergic inflammation and by lipopolysaccharide (LPS) stimulation.

In the present study, we evaluated (1) the amount of sialomucin and sulfomucin by alcian blue-periodic acid-Schiff (AB-PAS) histochemistry, (2) the terminal sugar residues by lectin histochemistry, and (3) mRNA expression of the rat Muc5ac gene in rat nasal epithelium, produced by allergic inflammation or LPS stimulation.

Materials and Methods

We produced allergic inflammation and LPS-induced inflammation in rat nasal epithelium. Hypertrophic and metaplastic changes of goblet cells were induced by intranasal instillation of ovalbumin (OVA) in OVA-sensitized rats, and by intranasal LPS instillation. Rats were killed at 24 h after the last intranasal instillation. The nasal cavity was transversely sectioned at the level of incisive papilla, and histopathological changes of nasal septal epithelium were examined. The percent area of intraepithelial mucosubstance was quantitatively measured by the image analyzer.

Tissue sections were stained with AB-PAS and lectin histochemistry. Some of the mucosubstance in rat nasal epithelium reacted with four of the lectins: *Arachis hypogaea* (PNA), *Maackia amurensis II* (MAL-II), *Sambucus nigra* (SNA), and *Ulex europaeus I* (UEA-I). The expression of rat Muc5ac mRNA in rat nasal epithelium is also examined. The instillation methods, tissue preparations, AB-PAS and lectin staining, and methods for RT-PCR were described previously [1–3].

Results and Conclusions

Rat Muc5ac mRNA Expression

LPS stimulation and OVA challenge induces goblet cell metaplasia and mucus production in nasal epithelium of sensitized rats, whereas only a few goblet cells were observed in control rats. Quantitative examination revealed significant increase of epithelial mucosubstance after LPS stimulation and OVA challenge in OVA-sensitized rats. Both LPS stimulation and OVA challenge significantly increased rat Muc5ac mRNA expression compared with animals treated with saline instillation. However, there was no difference between LPS stimulation and OVA challenge.

AB-PAS Histochemistry

Four types of mucosubstance were characterized: neutral glycoproteins, sialidase-sensitive sialomucin, sialidase-resistant sialomucin, and sulfomucin. In saline-instilled controls, most of the mucosubstance (75.7% of total) was neutral glycoprotein, and sulfomucin occupied only 13.2% of total. The newly produced mucosubstance after LPS instillation or OVA challenge contained higher amounts of sulfomucin and lower amounts of neutral glycoprotein ($p < 0.01$). LPS-induced mucosubstance contained more sulfomucin (70.1%) and less neutral glycoprotein (8.6%) than OVA-induced mucosubstance (sulfomucin 33.6%, neutral glycoprotein 41.8%, $p < 0.01$).

Increased mucus sulfation may be important for airway inflammation because of the increase in its negative charge. Mucin, the most plentiful high-molecular-weight polyanion on the respiratory surface, has been shown to react with cationic inflammatory proteins such as leukocyte elastase and lysozyme. The negatively charged sulfated carbohydrates are responsible for the inhibitory effects of mucin against these enzymes. Newly produced sulfomucin may play a role in protecting the mucosa against proteolysis by these cationic enzymes or by bacterial enzymes.

Lectin Histochemistry

We found that LPS-induced mucin contained more PNA-reactive and MAL-II-reactive mucin, compared with control and antigen-induced mucin. The amount of PNA-reactive mucosubstance increased significantly after LPS stimulation (64.8%), compared with saline instillation (3.5%) and OVA challenge (5.8%, $p < 0.01$). The amount of MAL-II-reactive mucosubstance also increased after LPS stimulation (75.8%), compared with saline instillation (19.1%) and OVA challenge (32.3%, $p < 0.05$). PNA reacts with galactose-N-acetyl galactosamine, and MAL-II reacts with α2,3-linked sialic acid-galactose. We found that these carbohydrate residues increased specifically in LPS-induced mucin.

These residues were reported to be potential sites for the attachment of many kinds of bacteria and viruses, promoting their trapping and removal by mucociliary clearance. The altered mucus may play an important role in host defense against bacterial infections, and it is interesting that these alterations did not occur in allergic inflammation in our study.

Conclusions

Respiratory mucus is heterogeneous in its carbohydrate structure. The alteration of carbohydrate chains of mucin in airway inflammation is an important event for host defense, causing entrapment of micro-organisms and neutralization of proteolytic enzymes.

References

1 Shimizu T, Hirano H, Shimizu S, et al: Differential properties of mucous glycoprotein in rat nasal epithelium. Am J Respir Crit Care Med 2001;164:366–371.

2 Shimizu T, Takahashi Y, Kawaguchi S, et al: Hypertrophic and metaplastic changes of goblet cells in rat nasal epithelium induced by endotoxin. Am J Respir Crit Care Med 1996;153:1412–1418.

3 Shimizu T, Hirano H, Majima Y, et al: A mechanism of antigen-induced mucus production in nasal epithelium of sensitized rats. Am J Respir Crit Care Med 2000;161:1648–1654.

Takeshi Shimizu, MD
Department of Otorhinolaryngology, Shiga University of Medical Science
Seta-tsukinowa
Otsu, Shiga 520-2192 (Japan)
Tel. +81 77 548 2261, E-Mail shimizu@belle.shiga-med.ac.jp

Harabuchi Y (ed): Recent Advances in Tonsils and Mucosal Barriers of the Upper Airways.
Adv Otorhinolaryngol. Basel, Karger, 2011, vol 72, pp 110–112

Nasal-Associated Lymphoid Tissue Immunity and Vaccine Development

Satoru Kodama · Masashi Suzuki

Department of Otolaryngology, Oita University Faculty of Medicine, Hazama-cho, Yufu, Oita, Japan

Abstract

Nasal vaccination is an effective therapeutic regimen for preventing upper respiratory infectious diseases. In the development of nasal vaccine, an appropriate adjuvant is required. In the present study, we examined the efficacy of fms-like tyrosine kinase receptor-3 ligand (Flt3L) as a mucosal adjuvant. Mice were immunized intranasally with Flt3L and P6 protein of nontypeable *Haemophilus influenzae* (NTHi), and P6-specific immune responses were examined. In addition, NTHi challenges were performed and the level of NTHi was quantified in nasal washes. Nasal vaccination with P6 and Flt3L induced an increase in the number of dendritic cells in nasal-associated lymphoid tissue. P6-specific nasal wash immunoglobulin (Ig)A and serum IgG titers were elevated significantly after nasal immunization. Enhanced NTHi clearance from the nasopharynx was also observed. These results indicate the potential of Flt3L as an effective mucosal adjuvant and suggest that nasal vaccination with P6 and Flt3L might be an effective regimen for the induction of NTHi-specific protective immunity.

Nontypeable *Haemophilus influenzae* (NTHi) is a major pathogen of upper respiratory infectious diseases (URI). Inhibition of NTHi colonization in the nasopharynx is considered effective in preventing diseases. P6 outer membrane protein of NTHi is a common antigen (Ag) among all NTHi strains and is a suitable candidate for a mucosal vaccine [1].

Nasal immunization is the most effective therapeutic regimen for inducing mucosal secretory immunoglobulin A (S-IgA) and systemic IgG responses. To elicit maximal levels of Ag-specific immune responses in both mucosal and systemic compartments, it is necessary to use an appropriate mucosal adjuvant. Cholera toxin (CT) is one of the most potent mucosal adjuvants in animal models but is toxic in humans [2]. Consequently, an alternative adjuvant would be necessary for the development of a mucosal vaccine.

Dendritic cells (DCs) are essential for the induction of Ag-specific immune responses; therefore, DC-targeted vaccination might be an effective strategy for the induction of specific immune responses. Fms-like tyrosine kinase receptor-3 (Flt3) ligand (Flt3L) mobilizes and stimulates myeloid and lymphoid progenitor cells, and DCs [1]. In the present study, we investigated the efficacy of nasal Flt3L application for the induction of protective immunity against NTHi in the nasopharynx, with the ultimate goal of developing a mucosal vaccine for preventing URI.

Materials and Methods

Immunization
Specific pathogen-free BALB/c mice were immunized intranasally with P6 10 μg and recombinant Flt3L 5 μg on days 0, 7 and 14 (P6+FL group). Control animals were immunized with P6 alone (P6 group). PBS administration without an antigen was used as negative control. The animals were sacrificed 1 week after the final immunization and samples were collected.

Flow Cytometry
To evaluate the effect of Flt3L application on nasal DCs, mononuclear cells (MNCs) were isolated from nasal-associated lymphoid tissue (NALT), and the number of CD11c+ DCs and DC subsets in NALT was analyzed by three-color flow cytometry, as previously described [1].

P6-Specific Antibody Assay
P6-specific antibody titers in nasal wash, and serum were determined by enzyme-linked immunosorbent assay (ELISA), as previously described [1].

For quantification of Ig-producing cells, MNCs were isolated from the nasal passage (NP), and NALT, and the numbers of P6-specific IgA-, IgG- and IgM-producing cells were determined by enzyme-linked immunospot (ELISPOT) assay, as previously described [1].

Nasal Challenge with Live NTHi
On day 21, live NTHi suspension (10^8 CFU) was injected into the nose. Twenty-four hours after the nasal challenge, mice were sacrificed and nasal wash samples were collected. The diluted samples were spread on chocolate agar plates for quantification of live bacteria. After overnight incubation at 37°C in 5% CO_2, NTHi colonies were counted.

Results

DCs in NALT
CD11c+ DCs markedly increased in NALT after immunization with P6 and Flt3L. In addition, the expression of MHC II, B7–1 and B7–2 on DCs was enhanced in P6+FL group.

P6-Specific Antibody Responses
P6-specific immune responses were induced by nasal immunization with P6 and Flt3L. The levels of IgA antibodies in the nasal wash were significantly elevated in the P6+FL group. Serum IgG antibodies were also elevated in this group. Low levels of the specific antibodies were detected in the P6 groups.

The number of P6-specific IgA antibody-producing cells increased markedly in NP of the P6+FL group. Fewer IgA antibody-producing cells were detected in the P6 groups.

NTHi Clearance from the Nasopharynx
Bacterial clearance was examined after nasal immunization. Enhanced NTHi clearance was observed in the P6+FL group as indicated by the reduced quantity of live NTHi in nasal washes. Although P6-specific antibodies were detected in nasal washes and serum from the P6 groups, these were insufficient to account for the protection against NTHi challenge.

Discussion

Nasal immunization is now considered an effective vaccination route for the induction of Ag-specific S-IgA responses in the upper respiratory tract [1, 2]. Nasal vaccination is thought to be an effective therapeutic regimen for preventing URI. Here, we have demonstrated that nasal vaccination with P6 and Flt3L induced a P6-specific immune response and enhanced the clearance of NTHi from the nasopharynx. The elevated levels of IgA in the nasal washes of the P6+FL group were associated with a specific, local B cell immune response, as indicated by a marked increase in the number of P6-specific IgA-producing cells in the NP. The sustained IgA-producing cellular response may be due to the activation of T cells by DCs.

Flt3L has been shown to play a central role in the proliferation and differentiation of early hematopoietic precursor stem cells. Flt3L also mobilizes and stimulates DCs. Mucosal administration of Flt3L with protein Ag induced Ag-specific systemic and mucosal immune responses [1]. In the present study, nasal application of Flt3L resulted in a significant increase in the number of DCs in NALT, which might have a stimulatory effect on local antibody production. DC-targeted vaccines have emerged as a promising strategy for inducing antitumoral cytotoxic T cells for the immunotherapy of cancer. The maturation state of DC is of critical importance for the success of vaccination; however, the most effective mode of maturation is still a matter of debate. Whereas immature DCs carry the risk of inducing tolerance, extensive stimulation of DCs may lead to DC unresponsiveness and exhaustion [1]. In the present study, we also showed an effect of Flt3L for DC development in NALT. Thus, nasal application of Flt3L might be an effective vaccination strategy for the induction of Ag-specific immune responses in the upper respiratory tract.

In conclusion, nasal vaccination with P6 and Flt3L induced a differential increase in the number of DCs and enhanced antibody production in the nasal mucosa but did not induce tolerance. These findings suggest that the nasal application of Flt3L might be a new strategy for nasal vaccination to prevent URI.

References

1 Kodama S, Hirano T, Noda K, Abe N, Suzuki M: A single nasal dose of fms-like tyrosine kinase receptor-3 ligand, but not peritoneal application, enhances nontypeable *Haemophilus influenzae*-specific long-term mucosal immune responses in the nasopharynx. Vaccine 2010;28:2510–2516.

2 Noda K, Kodama S, Umemoto S, Abe N, Hirano T, Suzuki M: Nasal vaccination with P6 outer membrane protein and a-galactosylceramide induces nontypeable *Haemophilus influenzae*-specific protective immunity associated with NKT cell activation and dendritic cell expansion in nasopharynx. Vaccine 2011;29:5068–5074.

Satoru Kodama, MD, PhD
Department of Otolaryngology, Oita University Faculty of Medicine
1–1 Idaigaoka, Hazama-cho
Yufu, Oita 879-5593 (Japan)
Tel. +81 97 586 5913, E-Mail satoruk@med.oita-u.ac.jp

Harabuchi Y (ed): Recent Advances in Tonsils and Mucosal Barriers of the Upper Airways.
Adv Otorhinolaryngol. Basel, Karger, 2011, vol 72, pp 113–115

Intranasal Therapy with CpG DNA Alone for the Control of Allergic Rhinitis

Motohiko Suzuki · Yoshihisa Nakamura · Tamami Matsumoto · Makoto Yokota · Nobuaki Ohno · Shingo Murakami

Departments of Otorhinolaryngology, Nagoya City University, Mizuho-ku, Nagoya, Japan

Abstract

Many people all over the world suffer from allergic rhinitis, induced by Th2 responses. CpG DNA, containing a central unmethylated C-G dinucleotide, promotes Th1 responses. Consequently, Th2 responses decrease. Systemic administration of CpG DNA could attenuate allergic rhinitis. However, studies investigating the effects of intranasal therapy with CpG DNA alone on allergic rhinitis are rare. Therefore, we estimated the effectiveness of intranasal administration of CpG DNA alone on allergic rhinitis compared with intradermal administration. Mice were sensitized intraperitoneally and challenged intranasally with *Cryptomeria japonica*. Therapy with CpG DNA alone was performed during the challenge, either intranasally or intradermally. Immunologic variables and nasal symptoms were examined. Intranasal administration of CpG DNA alone significantly reduced nasal symptoms, nasal eosinophilia, and the levels of IgE as well as IL-5 production from nasal lymphocytes and splenocytes, although intradermal administration of CpG DNA alone did not show a significant reduction. This study demonstrated that CpG DNA has effects not only on splenocytes but also on nasal lymphocytes, and that the intranasal administration of CpG DNA alone is useful in the management of allergic rhinitis.

CpG DNA, containing a central unmethylated C-G dinucleotide, induces Th1 responses characterized by the production of interferon-γ (IFN-γ) and IgG2a. Consequently, Th2 responses, characterized by the production of IgE, interleukin-4 (IL-4), and IL-5, decrease. It has been reported that co-administration of CpG DNA and allergens inhibited allergic rhinitis [1, 2].

Physicians often cannot identify the causative antigens. Many patients are suffering from sensitization with multiple antigens. Therefore, it should be important to investigate allergen-independent immunotherapy with CpG DNA alone. However, there have only been few reports on the investigation of the effects of CpG DNA alone on allergic rhinitis. Furthermore, there is another controversy whether intranasal administration of CpG DNA is as useful as corticosteroids for the control of allergic rhinitis.

In this study, we investigated the effect of local administration of CpG DNA alone on allergic rhinitis using mice sensitized with *Crypotmeria japonica* (Japanese cedar), a major allergen in Japan.

Materials and Methods

Reagents
C. japonica pollen was dissolved in phosphate-buffered saline. CpG DNA containing two CpG motifs (TCC ATG ACG TTC CTG ACG TT) was synthesized.

Animals
BALB/c mice (6 weeks of age) were used in this study. All mice were maintained under SPF conditions at the University animal facility.

Immunization Protocol
BALB/c mice were sensitized on days 0 and 7 by intraperitoneal injection with *C. japonica* pollen (0.5 mg) absorbed to alum (1 mg). Three weeks after the last sensitization, all mice were challenged intranasally on days 28–32 with *C. japonica* pollen (10 μg). On days 28, 29 and 30, mice received CpG DNA (10 μg) intranasally or intradermally 1 h after nasal challenge. The number of nasal rubbings was counted for 15 min immediately after the last nasal challenge. Mice were sacrificed 24 h after the last challenge.

Results

Nasal Symptom
To investigate the effect of CpG DNA on allergic rhinitis with Japanese cedar, we formed three groups (1) mice that had received intranasal therapy with CpG DNA alone (intranasal CpG therapy), (2) mice that had received intradermal therapy with CpG DNA alone (intradermal CpG therapy), and (3) mice that had received no therapy (controls). The number of nasal rubbing movements in mice received CpG therapy was significantly fewer compared with mice received no therapy or intradermal CpG therapy ($p < 0.01$). However, there is no significant difference between intradermal CpG therapy and the controls.

Local Eosinophilia
Intranasal CpG therapy reduced the numbers of eosinophils detected compared with no therapy or intradermal CpG therapy ($p < 0.01$), although we did not find a significant difference between no therapy and intradermal CpG therapy.

Levels of C. Japonica-Specific IgE
Mice that had received intranasal CpG therapy exhibited significantly lower levels of *C. japonica*-specific IgE compared to those mice that had received no therapy and mice that had received intradermal CpG therapy ($p < 0.01$). There was no significant difference in *C. japonica*-specific IgE between those that received intradermal CpG therapy and those that received no therapy.

Cytokine Production from Nasal Lymphocytes and Splenocytes
After intranasal CpG therapy, nasal lymphocytes produced significantly lower levels of IL-5 than controls ($p < 0.01$). Intranasal CpG therapy significantly decreased IL-5 production by splenocytes in mice, compared with intradermal CpG therapy or no therapy ($p < 0.01$). Levels of IL-4 released by splenocytes in mice receiving either intranasal or intradermal CpG therapy were below detectable levels, although splenocytes in the controls produced IL-4 ($p < 0.01$).

Discussion

Intranasal therapy with CpG DNA alone during allergen exposure reduced the severity of nasal symptoms, degree of nasal eosinophilia, level of IgE, and levels of IL-5 production from nasal lymphocytes and splenocytes. However, intradermal therapy with CpG DNA alone did not significantly inhibit nasal symptoms, nasal eosinophilia, level of IgE, and levels of IL-5 production from nasal lymphocytes and splenocytes. This suggested that intranasal (local) administration of CpG DNA alone is more effective than intradermal (systemic) administration of CpG DNA in the management of allergic rhinitis.

There has only been little documentation on the effects of CpG DNA on nasal lymphocytes. In this study, we showed that CpG DNA reduces

IL-5 production by nasal lymphocytes, suggesting that CpG DNA attenuates allergic rhinitis through a reduction of Th2 cytokines from nasal lymphocytes.

Although further studies are necessary, our finding may give hope that a new drug such as CpG DNA nasal spray will soon appear on the market.

References

1 Hussain I, Jain VV, Kitagaki K, Businga TR, O'Shaughnessy P, Kline JN: Modulation of murine allergic rhinosinusitis by CpG oligodeoxynucleotides. Laryngoscope 2002;112:1819–1826.

2 Tulic MK, Fiset PO, Christodoulopoulos P, Vaillancourt P, Desrosiers M, Lavingne F, Eiden J, Hamid Q: Amb a_1-immunostimulatory oligodeoxynucleotide conjugate immunotherapy decreases the nasal inflammatory response. J Allergy Clin Immunol 2004;113:235–241.

Motohiko Suzuki, MD, PhD
Department of Surgery, Otorhinolaryngology, Nagoya City University
1 Kawasumi, Mizuho-cho
Mizuho-ku, Nagoya, 467-8601 (Japan)
Tel. +81 52 853 8256, Fax +81 52 851 5300, E-Mail suzu-mo@med.nagoya-cu.ac.jp

Harabuchi Y (ed): Recent Advances in Tonsils and Mucosal Barriers of the Upper Airways.
Adv Otorhinolaryngol. Basel, Karger, 2011, vol 72, pp 116–120

Airway Bacterial Interactions and Impact on Host Immune Responses

Jennelle Kyd[a] · Ajay Krishnamurthy[a] · John McGrath[a] · Jessica Browne[a] · Fatemah Vahedi[a,b]

[a]Institute for Health and Social Science Research, School of Medical and Applied Science, CQ University Australia, Rockhampton, Qld., Australia; [b]Razi Vaccine & Serum Research Institute, Mashhad, Iran

Abstract

The dynamic interactions of the major respiratory microbial pathogens are complex. An understanding of the impact on naturally acquired immune responses to respiratory polymicrobial commensal bacteria is slowly evolving. Maintaining a micro-floral balance and the host's ability to respond to imbalances associated with disease is critical. Studies of acquired immune responses have found that both antibody and cellular immune responses are suppressed by the presence of multiple bacteria when compared with colonization by the single microbe. Microbes interact with the mucosal epithelium through a range of receptor-ligand interactions, including interactions with Toll-like receptors and adhesion molecules. Regulation of the inflammatory response associated with commensal colonization suggests a possible role for Treg cells in controlling the upper airway responses to bacterial microflora with both bacteria-bacteria and bacteria-host interactions affecting colonization and immune responses.

Human upper respiratory tract (URT) bacterial infections, like otitis media (OM) and exacerbations of chronic obstructive pulmonary disease (COPD), are of enormous and global socioeconomic importance. The major causative bacterial agents exist as opportunistic commensals in the nasopharynx. Clinical epidemiological studies consistently report a strong correlation between nasopharyngeal colonization and infection, yet experimentally there remains a poor understanding about how the microbial environment of commensals shift to that of pathogen. *Streptococcus pneumoniae*, nontypeable *Haemophilus influenzae* (NTHi) and *Moraxella catarrhalis* are obligate commensal flora of the human URT with Australian aboriginal children having one of the highest and earliest colonization rates in the world [1].

The colonization rates between the Australian aboriginal (highly susceptible to OM) and non-aboriginal infants differs significantly with carriage rates for *S. pneumoniae*, *M. catarrhalis* and NTHi in aboriginal children at 49, 50 and 41%, respectively, and 25, 25 and 11% for nonaboriginal children [1]. Some of this difference may be attributable to differences in socioeconomic conditions. Modeling of colonization patterns found there was a positive association between virus (rhinovirus and adenovirus) and bacteria, and significant positive associations between pairs of bacteria, in particular, *M. catarrhalis* with *S. pneumoniae* and *H. influenzae* at both the host and microbe levels [2].

Microbial Interactions with Epithelial Cells

Microbes and microbial products that contact the airway epithelia are sensed by pattern-recognition receptors (PRRs), such as the Toll-like receptors (TLRs) that are responsible for upregulating the host's immune response including eliciting inflammation. The relationships between PRRs and the microbial molecules enable the innate immune system to discriminate between 'self' and 'non-self'. Commensals have developed mechanisms that enable certain microbial molecules to trigger reactions that favour the bacterium through either molecular mimicry or induction of modulation of the cell's innate responses.

Bacterial phosphorylcholine (ChoP) on the lipooligosaccharides (LOS) of Gram-negative and lipoteichoic acid (LTA) of Gram-positive bacteria, is a ligand for PAFR, initiating anti-inflammatory pathways by way of negative regulation of TLR2, TLR4 and TLR9. This anti-inflammatory process of engagement is important to commensal bacteria. *M. catarrhalis* LOS has been shown to upregulate ICAM-1 expression [3]. Thus, microbes can differentially affect both expression and downstream signaling of PRRs.

TLRs are transmembrane receptors that recognize a range of lipopeptides, LOS/LPS and other moieties present on these bacteria as ligands. Recent studies have specifically focused on affects on downstream signaling. Molecular mimicry such as incorporation of host-derived sialic acid into NTHi LOS in part help to evade TLR4 stimulation, whereas NTHi surface lipoproteins, such as lipoprotein P6, activate NF-κB and p38 MAPK pathways via TLR2 [4]. The *M. catarrhalis* adhesin, UspA1, appears to counteract TLR2-induced immunity [5] through engagement with CEACAM1. The localization of CEACAM1 with TLR2 following binding by UspA1 caused recruitment of SHP-1, initiating negative feedback pathways that regulate TLR signaling and production of proinflammatory cytokines. Thus, the formation of the signaling complex that is composed of TLR2 and PI(3)K was abrogated, inhibiting the PI(3)K-Akt-NF-κB signaling pathway. SHP-1 initiates events that deactivate PI(3)K-Akt signaling through phosphorylation of the p85α subunit of PI(3)K. Bacterial binding to CEACAM1 may in part explain the hyporesponsiveness of epithelial cells during colonization [5].

S. pneumoniae can differentially regulate innate and adaptive humoral immunity through TLR2 interactions shaping an in vivo type 1 IgG response [6], whereas pneumococcal pneumolysin associates with TLR4 initiating an intracellular signaling cascade that activates NF-κB. Pneumolysin appears to be involved in the induction of the acquired immune response with pneumolysin-induced TLR4 signaling compensating for the TLR2 signaling deficiency during infection [7]. Bacteria express an array of molecular moieties that interact with many host cell structures that include β-glucan receptors, epidermal growth factor receptor, heparin-binding extracellular matrix proteins, mucins and others. Bacteria have evolved a high degree of potential redundancy within expressed molecules, highlighted by the capacity for numerous gene expression changes.

Microbial Interactions and Otitis Media

It is not known how microbe-microbe and microbe-host interactions amongst colonizing bacteria exert an influence on the host immune system that leads to recurrent disease in some individuals. A limitation to our experimental knowledge is that most animal models of OM focus on a single microbe or direct infection inoculation of the bulla. It is known that colonization and reduced immune responses relate to disease, but the specific mechanisms that induce

Table 1. *S. pneumoniae* OM in the middle ears of mice 14 days postnasal inoculation [9]

Nasal inoculation group (n = 25)	Incidence of bacterial otitis media, %	
	no antecedent viral infection	antecedent viral infection
S. pneumoniae	20	70
S. pneumoniae + NTHi	10	40
S. pneumoniae + *M. catarrhalis*	45	88

the immunological measures and susceptibility to OM are not defined.

The concept that bacterial-bacterial interactions may be important contributing factors in OM and respiratory infections has been the subject of only a few studies. When *H. influenzae* type b (Hib) and *S. pneumoniae* were co-inoculated nasally in BALB/c SCID or C3H/HeOuJ (TLR4-expressing) mice, the Hib rapidly outcompeted *S. pneumoniae* [8]. In contrast, our results using bacterial combinations of NTHi, *M. catarrhalis* and *S. pneumoniae* in BALB/c mice found that *S. pneumoniae* outcompeted the other two [9]. In these studies co-bacterial inoculation increased overall bacterial nasal colonization, and co-colonization with *M. catarrhalis* and *S. pneumoniae* significantly increased the incidence, duration and severity of OM associated with *S. pneumoniae* (table 1). These results are consistent with the data obtained from children and modeling studies that show the strong positive association between *M. catarrhalis* and *S. pneumoniae* [2].

Colonization and the Host Immune System

Otitis-prone children reportedly have: fewer total T and CD4+ T cells in adenoidal tissue [10], lower levels of total serum IgG_2 [11], lower serum specific antibody [12], lower lymphoproliferation of adenoidal lymphocytes (to the NTHi antigen, P6) [13], lower levels of IL-1β, IL-6 and TNFα in nasopharyngeal secretions [14], and variation in the genes *TNFA-863A, TNFA-376G, TNFA-238G, IL10–1082 A*, and *IL6–174G* [15]. In children, antibody to pneumococcal antigens appears to be regulated by adenoidal T-cell-derived IFN-γ and IL-10 [16], and poor CD4+ T cell responses to pneumolysin were associated with carriage of *S. pneumoniae* [17]. Protective immunity against *S. pneumoniae* colonization was CD4+ dependent, and more specifically Th17 cells/IL-17. Th17 cells from children's tonsils produced IL-17 in response to *S. pneumoniae*, but not IFN-γ or IL-4, was critical for protection and increased killing by neutrophils independent of antibody or complement [18]. Furthermore, protective immunity was not dependent on antibody, natural killer or CD8+ cells [19, 20].

Regulation of the Cellular Immune System

Bacteria induce distinct patterns of cytokine and leukocyte gene expression responses, demonstrating that differences in colonization patterns are likely to affect the host's responses to the polymicrobial environment. The immune system must be tightly regulated to balance antimicrobial inflammatory responses to prevent immune-mediated tissue destruction. Regulatory T cells (Treg) are critical to this process. Tregs can be CD4+ or CD8+ and are distinguished by expression of the transcription factor FoxP3. There are two functional types of Treg cells, naturally occurring and induced. CD4+CD25+FoxP3+ are naturally occurring in mice, differentiate in the thymus and account for about 5–10% of CD4+ T cells in the blood, lymph nodes and spleen [21]. Induced Tregs are generated from naïve T cells in the periphery after encounter with antigen presented by dendritic cells (DCs) that have been conditioned by epithelial cells in contact with microorganisms [22]. Cytokines such as IL-10 and TGF-β produced by Tregs are involved in suppression of T cell responses [21].

The recent discovery of Th17 cells as key inflammatory mediators of the mucosa is opening new insights into mucosal immunity and its regulation. It now appears that Th17 inflammatory cells can differentiate into regulatory T cells (Tregs) and back, depending on the cytokine milieu [23, 24]. Termed 'plasticity', this ability means that the balance between effective immunity (infection protection) and associated inflammatory tissue damage is managed. Further evidence that all T cells are transiently Treg during activation suggests that Treg plasticity may be an important regulatory mechanism for the immune system in general [25].

Conclusion

There is increasing realization that bacteria can control the immune system. Some bacterial species appear to promote survival by actively inducing Tregs via TLR signaling or mucosally conditioned DCs. Different micro-organisms induce different T cells responses. Thus, there is evidence from studies of different mucosal sites that commensalism and mucosal infections are a function of the nature of the colonizing species and Treg controlled immunity. It is not known whether the same applies in the upper airway with opportunistic commensals like *S. pneumoniae*, NTHi and *M. catarrhalis*. Such suppression may be critical in immune-failure in individuals that are susceptible to or suffer chronic respiratory infections such as OM and COPD.

References

1 Watson K, Carville K, Bowman J, et al: Upper respiratory tract bacterial carriage in aboriginal and non-aboriginal children in a semi-arid area of Western Australia. Pediatr Infect Dis J 2006;25:782–790.

2 Jacoby P, Watson K, Bowman J, et al: Modelling the co-occurrence of *Streptococcus pneumoniae* with other bacterial and viral pathogens in the upper respiratory tract. Vaccine 2007;25:2458–2464.

3 Xie H, Gu XX: *Moraxella catarrhalis* lipooligosaccharide selectively upregulates ICAM-1 expression on human monocytes and stimulates adjacent naive monocytes to produce TNF-alpha through cellular cross-talk. Cell Microbiol 2008;10:1453–1467.

4 Punturieri A, Copper P, Polak T, Christensen PJ, Curtis JL: Conserved nontypeable *Haemophilus influenzae*-derived TLR2-binding lipopeptides synergize with IFN-β to increase cytokine production by resident murine and human alveolar macrophages. J Immunol 2006;177:673–680.

5 Slevogt H, Zabel S, Opitz B, et al: CEACAM1 inhibits Toll-like receptor 2-triggered antibacterial responses of human pulmonary epithelial cells. Nat Immunol 2008;9:1270–1278.

6 Khan AQ, Chen Q, Wu ZQ, Paton JC, Snapper CM: Both innate immunity and type 1 humoral immunity to *S. pneumoniae* are mediated by MyD88 but differ in their relative levels of dependence on toll-like receptor 2. Infect Immun 2005;73:298–307.

7 Dessing MC, Florquin S, Paton JC, van der Poll T: Toll-like receptor 2 contributes to antibacterial defence against pneumolysin-deficient pneumococci. Cell Microbiol 2008;10:237–246.

8 Lysenko ES, Ratner AJ, Nelson AL, Weiser JN: The role of innate immune responses in the outcome of interspecies competition for colonization of mucosal surfaces. PLoS Pathogens 2005;1:1–9.

9 Krishnamurthy A, McGrath J, Cripps AW, Kyd JM: The incidence of *Streptococcus pneumoniae* otitis media is affected by the polymicrobial environment particularly *Moraxella catarrhalis* in a mouse nasal colonisation model. Microbes Infect 2009;11:545–553.

10 Wysocka J, Hassmann-Poznanska E, Kasprzycka E, Musiatowicz M: Lymphocyte subpopulations in the adenoids analyzed by flow cytometry. Wiad Lek 2001;54:418–423.

11 Freijd A, Oxelius V-A, Rynnel-Dagöö B: A prospective study demonstrating an association between plasma IgG2 concentrations and susceptibility to otitis media in children. Scand J Infect Dis 1985;17:115–120.

12 Yamanaka N, Faden H: Low serum IgG antibody levels specific for P6 of nontypeable *Haemophilus influenzae* in otitis prone children. J Pediatr 1993;122:212–218.

13 Kodama H, Fadden H, Harabuchi Y, Kataura A, Bernstein JM, Brodsky L: Cellular immune response of adenoidal and tonsillar lymphocytes to the P6 outer membrane protein of non-typeable *Haemophilus influenzae* and its relation to otitis media. Acta Otolaryngol 1999;119:377–383.
14 Lindberg K, Rynnel-Dagoo R, Sundqvist K: Cytokines in nasopharyngeal secretions; evidence for defective IL-1β production in children with recurrent episodes of acute otitis media. Clin Exp Immunol 1994;97:369–402.
15 Emonts M, Veenhoven RH, Wiertsema SP, et al: Genetic polymorphisms in immunoresponse genes TNFA, IL6, IL10, and TLR4 are associated with recurrent acute otitis media. Pediatrics 2007;120:814–823.
16 Zhang Q, Bernatoniene J, Bagrade L, et al: regulation of production of mucosal antibody to pneumococcal protein antigens by T-cell-derived gamma interferon and interleukin-10 in children. Infect Immun 2006;74:4735–4743.
17 Zhang Q, Bagrade L, Bernatoniene J, et al: Low CD4 T Cell immunity to pneumolysin is associated with nasopharyngeal carriage of pneumococci in children. J Infect Dis 2007;195:1194–1202.
18 Lu YJ, Gross J, Bogaert D, et al: Interleukin-17A mediates acquired immunity to pneumococcal colonization. PLoS Pathog 2008;4:e1000159.
19 Malley R, Srivastava A, Lipsitch M, et al: Antibody-independent, interleukin-17A-mediated, cross-serotype immunity to pneumococci in mice immunized intranasally with the cell wall polysaccharide. Infect Immun 2006;74:2187–2195.
20 Cao J, Gong Y, Li D, et al: CD4(+) T lymphocytes mediated protection against invasive pneumococcal infection induced by mucosal immunization with ClpP and CbpA. Vaccine 2009;27:2838–2844.
21 Mills KHG: Regulatory T cells: friend or foe in immunity to infection? Nat Rev Immunol 2004;4:841–855.
22 Iliev ID, Mileti E, Matteoli G, Chieppa M, Rescigno M: Intestinal epithelial cells promote colitis-protective regulatory T-cell differentiation through dendritic cell conditioning. Mucosal Immunol 2009;2:340–350.
23 Siegmund K, Ruckert B, Ouaked N, et al: Unique phenotype of human tonsillar and in vitro-induced FOXP3+CD8+ T cells. J Immunol 2009;182:2124–2130.
24 Lee YK, Mukasa R, Hatton RD, Weaver CT: Developmental plasticity of Th17 and Treg cells. Curr Opin Immunol 2009;21:274–280.
25 Pillai V, Ortega SB, Wang CK, Karandikar NJ: Transient regulatory T-cells: a state attained by all activated human T-cells. Clin Immunol 2007;123:18–29.

Prof. Jennelle Kyd
The Chancellery, CQ University Australia
Rockhampton, Qld. 4702 (Australia)
Tel. +61 7 4930 6731, E-Mail j.kyd@cqu.edu.au

Harabuchi Y (ed): Recent Advances in Tonsils and Mucosal Barriers of the Upper Airways.
Adv Otorhinolaryngol. Basel, Karger, 2011, vol 72, pp 121–125

Protection of Pneumococcal Infection by Maternal Intranasal Immunization with Pneumococcal Surface Protein A

Muneki Hotomi[a] · Masamitsu Kono[a] · Susan K. Hollingshead[b] · David E. Briles[b] · Noboru Yamanaka[a]

[a]Department of Otolaryngology, Head and Neck Surgery, Wakayama Medical University, Wakayama, Japan;
[b]Department of Microbiology, University of Alabama at Birmingham, Birmingham, Ala., USA

Abstract

Streptococcus pneumoniae is one of the important causative pathogens for both upper and lower respiratory tract infections during childhood. The current study was designed to evaluate the protection against fatal pneumococcal infections during the infant period by maternal immunization with pneumococcal surface protein A (PspA). Four-week-old females BALB/c mice were immunized with PspA and cholera toxin B (CTB) intranasally twice a week for 3 weeks. After mating, the 10-day-old offspring of these mice were intraperitoneally (i.p.) infected with *S. pneumoniae* to evaluate survival. Anti-PspA-specific IgG antibody was induced in the sera of mother and offspring. The survival times to death after systemic fatal pneumococcal infections were significantly extended among offspring delivered from PspA-immunized mothers than the controls. Current findings suggest that maternal intranasal immunization with PspA is an attractive procedure against pneumococcal infections in early childhood.

Streptococcus pneumoniae is responsible for a significant proportion of both upper and lower respiratory infectious diseases [1]. Pneumococci first colonize asymptomatically in the human nasopharynx and transmission to others is thought to be primarily from carriers. Children who colonized pneumococci in their nasopharynx in the first year of life were at an increased risk of developing acute otitis media (AOM) compared with children who remained free of pneumococci.

The efficacy of polysaccharide-based pneumococcal vaccines have some limitations due to the wide variety of capsular serotypes of pneumococci, while capsular polysaccharide vaccine against type B encapsulated *Haemophilus influenzae* has achieved tremendous success [2]. Efforts have been made to develop protein-conjugated polysaccharide vaccines containing up to 11 serotypes. However, children younger than 2 years of age usually have lower levels of pathogen-specific IgG antibody in their sera due to the age-related immaturity of immune responses [3]. Otitis-prone children also showed subnormal levels of serum IgG antibody against the causative pathogens [3–5]. Thus, it is important to induce effective protective immune responses against pneumococci during early childhood.

Pneumococcal surface protein A (PspA), a surface-exposed protein antigen of pneumococci, is a virulent factor and a highly immunogenic protein [6–10]. PspA is an attractive candidate for future protein-based pneumococcal vaccines. In this study, we evaluated the protection against pneumococcal infections during infant period by maternal intranasal immunization with PspA.

Materials and Methods

Experimental Design and Immunization Schedule

Four-week-old female BALB/c bjy mice were used in this experiment. Mice were immunized intranasally with rPspA (1 μg) mixed with cholera toxin B subunit (CTB) (List Biological Labs, Campbell, Calif., USA) (4 μg) on the Mondays and Fridays of 3 consecutive weeks. These immunizations included CTB for the first 2 weeks of immunization. During the last week, the last two immunizations, mice received antigen alone. Control mice received only CTB for the first 2 weeks and only saline for the last week.

After the final immunization, the female mice were mated with male mice for 2 weeks. Approximately 3 weeks after mating, offspring were obtained. Sera and milk were collected from the mothers and sera were collected from the offspring at birth (day 0) and 7 and 14 days after birth. At 10 days of age, the offspring were used as the systemic fatal pneumococcal infection model. All animal studies were conducted in accordance with and after approval of the Wakayama Medical University Animal Care and Use Committee.

Enzyme-Linked Immunosorbent Assay

Anti-PspA-specific IgG antibody in milk and sera of mothers and offspring were evaluated by ELISA. Briefly, 96-well microplates (MaxSorp, Nunc, Roskilde, Denmark) were coated with 50 μl of rPspA (2 μg/ml) in phosphate-buffered saline (PBS) overnight at 4°C. After washing three times with PBS containing 0.05% Tween 20 (PBS-T), the wells were blocked for 1 h with casein buffer (0.2% casein, 0.05% Tween 20 in PBS) at room temperature. Then, 50-μl samples diluted with casein buffer were incubated at 4°C overnight. After washing with PBS-T, the plate was incubated with 50 μl of biotynylated antimouse IgG antibody (1:3,000) (Southern Biotechnology Associates, Birmingham, Ala., USA) diluted in casein buffer for 2 h at room temperature. Then, after washing with PBS-T, the plate was incubated with alkaline phosphatase-conjugated streptavidin (1:4,000) (Southern Biotechnology Associates) for 2 h at room temperature. Color was developed with *p*-nitorophenyl phosphate (Sigma Chemical Co., St. Louis, Mo., USA) and the optical density of each well was measured by a spectrophotometer at 405 nm.

Systemic Infection Model

At 10 days of age, the offspring were inoculated intraperitoneally (i.p.) with pneumococcal cells at 1×10^4 CFUs in 100 μl of sterile PBS under anesthesia. *S. pneumoniae* TIGR4, serotype 4 strain, was grown at 37°C in Todd-Hewitt broth with 0.5% yeast extract (THY) until the mild log phase. After the intraperitoneal infection, the offspring were monitored for their death every 6–8 h. The survival periods were expressed as times from inoculations of pneumococci to death.

Statistics

Comparisons between the two groups were calculated by Student's t test. Statistical values were calculated with Prism 4 (GraphPad Software, La Jolla, Calif., USA).

Results

Anti-PspA-Specific IgG Antibody in Sera of Mother Mice and Offspring

Anti-PspA-specific IgG antibody levels were high at birth and maintained during the nursing periods in both sera and breast milk of PspA-immunized mothers, while the sera of the control mothers did not possess any of the specific IgG antibody (fig. 1). Offspring delivered from PspA-immunized mothers had similar levels of anti-PspA-specific IgG antibody in sera at birth (fig. 2).

Survival after Pneumococcal Infection

The median, 75% value, and 25% value of survival times of offspring delivered from PspA-immunized mothers were 32, 43 and 28 h, respectively. On the other hand, survival times of offspring delivered from control mothers were 16, 18 and 16 h, respectively (fig. 3). Times to death of PspA-immunized offspring were significantly prolonged compared with the controls ($p < 0.05$).

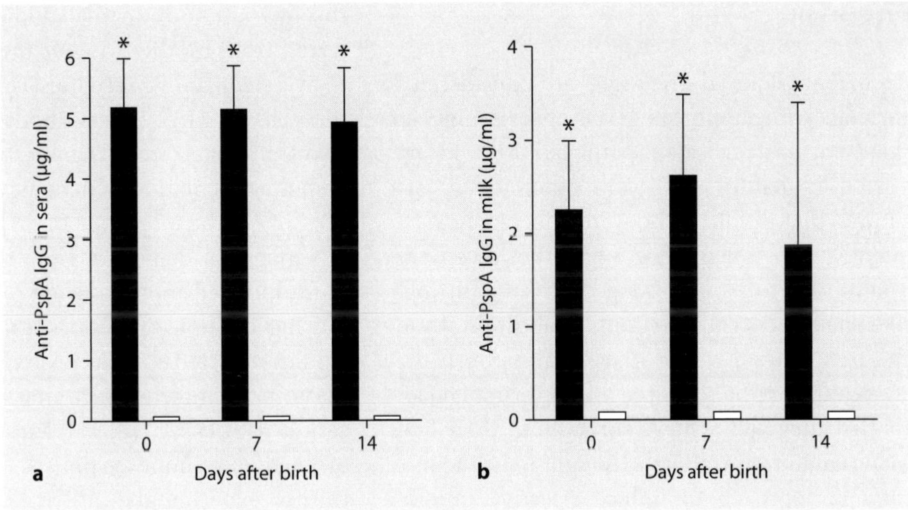

Fig. 1. Levels of anti-PspA-specific IgG antibody in mother's sera and breast milk. Results are expressed as mean ± SE of anti-PspA-specific IgG in mother's sera (**a**) and breast milk (**b**). Closed bar = Immunized mother; open bar = nonimmunized mother. * $p < 0.05$ compared with nonimmunized control by the Student's t test.

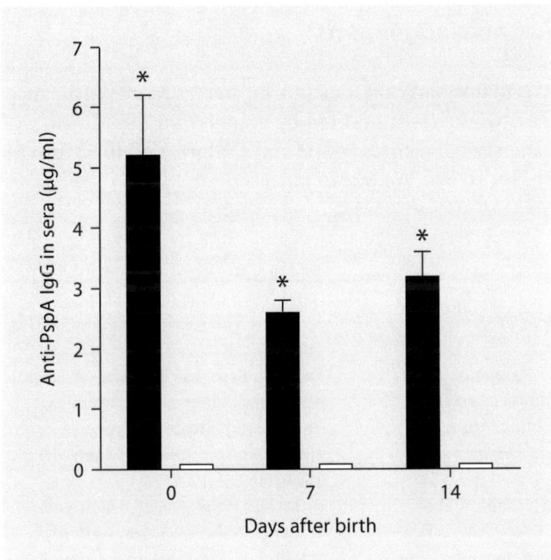

Fig. 2. Levels of anti-PspA-specific IgG antibody in offspring sera. Results are expressed as mean ± SE of anti-PspA-specific IgG in offspring sera. Closed bar = Immunized mother; open bar = nonimmunized mother. * $p < 0.05$ compared with nonimmunized control by the Student's t test.

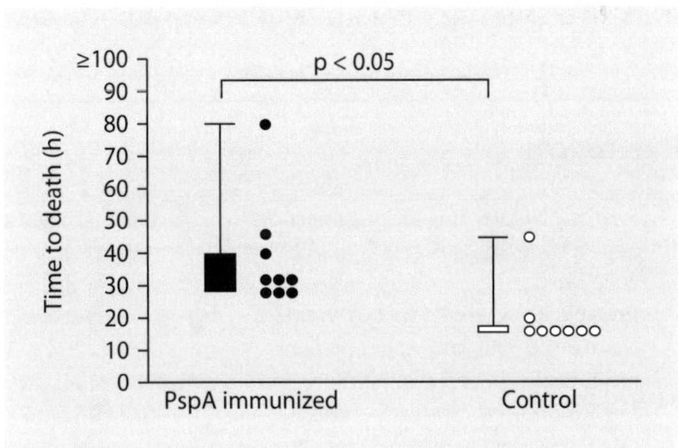

Fig. 3. Survival times of mice and offspring after systemic fatal pneumococcal infections. ● = Offspring delivered form PspA immunized mother mice; ○ = offspring delivered from nonimmunized mother mice. $p < 0.05$ compared with offspring delivered from nonimmunized control by the Student's t test.

Discussion

Recurrent bacterial infections are considered to correlate with subnormal levels of serum IgG antibody against causative pathogens due to age-related immaturity [3]. Virolainen et al. [10] showed that children who were infected most frequently with pneumococci had the lowest titer of antibody to PspA among children with invasive pneumococcal infections. In addition, young children below 2 years of age, no matter if they are healthy or not, show the lowest serum IgG levels that they will achieve throughout their lives. Maternal immunization is thought to be the most suitable approach to induce effective immune protection against pneumococcal infections.

Our previous study showed that maternal intranasal immunization with the outer membrane protein P6 of *H. influenzae* evoked anti-P6-specific IgG antibody in breast milk and sera of the mothers and this was then transferred to the offspring [11]. The present study further reports that induction of specific immune responses among offspring results in prolongation of survival times after lethal pneumococcal infections. The anti-PspA-specific IgG antibody in sera was transferred to the offspring via the placenta [12]. Differing from humans, mice colostrum/breast milk contains high amounts of IgG antibody and the IgG antibody in the mother's sera is transferred from mother to fetus through the placenta by a neonatal Fc receptor (FcRn) expressing in the yolk sac [13]. IgG antibody in breast milk is also transferred from the intestinal lumen to the systemic circulation in neonate mice by FcRn expressing in the intestine [14, 15].

Offspring delivered from PspA intranasally immunized mothers were protected from acquiring systemic pneumococcal infections. Some studies reported enhanced survival times of intraperitoneally infected mice after systemic immunization with PspA [16, 17]. PspA could also elicit protective immune responses from passive protection experiments with monoclonal antibodies to PspA [18, 19]. The current findings suggest that maternal immunization is an attractive procedure against pneumococcal infections in early childhood because transplacental immunoglobulin is transferred during pregnancy as well as after birth.

Acknowledgements

We thank Ms Yuki Tatsumi for her technical assistance. This work was supported by grants from the Ministry of Education, Science, Sports and Culture, and the Ministry of Health and Welfare in Japan.

References

1 Swartz MN: Attacking the pneumococcus – a hundred years' war. N Engl J Med 2002;346:722.

2 Prymula R, Peeters P, Chrobok V, Kriz P, Novakova E, Kaliskova E, Kohl I, Lommel P, Poolman J, Prieels JP, Schuerman L: Pneumococcal capsular polysaccharides conjugated to protein D for prevention of acute otitis media caused by both *Streptococcus pneumoniae* and nontypable *Haemophilus influenzae*: a randomized double-blind efficacy study. Lancet 2006;367:740–748.

3 Yamanaka N, Faden H: Antibody response to outer membrane protein of nontypeable *Haemophilus influenzae* in otitis-prone children. J Pediatr 1993;122:212–218.

4 Hotomi M, Yamanaka N, Saito T, Shimada J, Suzumoto M, Suetake M, Faden H: Antibody responses to the outer membrane protein P6 of non-typeable *Haemophilus influenzae* and pneumococcal capsular polysaccharides in otitis-prone children. Acta Otolaryngol. 1999;119:703–707.

5 Faden H, Bernstein JM, Brodsky L: Otitis media in children. I. The systemic immune response to nontypeable *Haemophilus influenzae*. J Infec Dis 1989;160:999–1004.

6 Briles DE, Hollingshead SK, Brooks-Walter A, Nabors GS, Ferguson L, Schilling M, Gravenstein S, Braun P, King J, Swift A: The potential to use PspA and other pneumococcal proteins to elicit protection against pneumococcal infection. Vaccine 2000;18: 1707–1711.

7 Briles DE, King JD, Gray MA, McDaniel LS, Swiatlo E, Benton KA: PspA, a protection-eliciting pneumococcal protein: immunogenicity of isolated native PspA in mice. Vaccine 1996;14:858–867.

8 Briles DE, Tart RC, Swiatlo E, Dillard JP, Smith P, Benton KA, Ralph BA, Brooks-Walter A, Crain MJ, Hollingshead SK, McDaniel LS: Pneumococcal diversity: considerations for new vaccine strategies with emphasis on PspA. Clin Micro Rev 1998;11:645–657.

9 Crain MJ, Waltman II WD, Turner JS, Yother J, Talkington DF, McDaniel LS, Gray BM, Briles DE: Pneumococcal surface protein A (PspA) is serologically highly variable and is expressed by all clinically important capsular serotypes of *Streptococcus pneumoniae*. Infect Immun 1990;58:3293–3299.

10 Virolainen A, Russell W, Crain MJ, Rapola S, Käyhty H, Briles DE: Human antibodies to pneumococcal surface protein A in health and disease. Pediatr Infect Dis J 2000;19:134–138.

11 Yamauchi K, Hotomi M, Billal DS, Suzumoto M, Yamanaka N: Maternal intranasal immunization with outer membrane protein P6 maintains specific antibody level of derived offspring. Vaccine 2006; 24:5294–5299.

12 Baril L, Briles DE, Crozier P, King JD, Hollingshead SK, Murphy TF, McCormick JB: Natural materno-fetal transfer of antibodies to PspA and to PsaA. Clin Exp Immunol 2004;135:474–477.

13 Ahouse JJ, Hagerman CL, Mittal P, Gilbert DJ, Copeland NG, Jekins NA, Simister NE: Mouse MHC class I-like Fc receptor encoded outside the MHC. J Immunol 1993;151:6067–6088.

14 Israel EJ, Patel VK, Taylor S, Marshak-Rothstein A, Semister NE: Requirement for a beta 2-microglobulin-associated Fc receptor for acquisition of maternal IgG by fetal and neonatal mice. J Immunol 1995;154:6246–6251.

15 Israel EJ, Taylor S, Wu Z, Mizoguchi E, Blumberg RS, Bhan A, Simister NE: Expression of the neonatal Fc receptor, FcRn, on human intestinal epithelial cells. Immunology 1997;92:69–74.

16 Ogunniyi AD, Folland RL, Briles DE, Hollingshead SK, Paton JC: Immunization of mice with combinations of pneumococcal virulence proteins elicits enhanced protection against challenge with *Streptococcus pneumoniae*. Infect Immun 2000;68:3028–3033.

17 Roche H, Ren B, McDaniel LS, Hakansson A, Briles DE: Relative roles of genetic background and variation in PspA in the ability of antibodies to PspA to protect against capsular type 3 and 4 strains of *Streptococcus pneumoniae*. Infect Immun 2003;71:4498–4505.

18 McDaniel LS, Sheffield JS, Delucchi P, Briles DE: PspA, a surface protein of *Streptococcus pneumoniae*, is capable of eliciting protection against pneumococci of more than one capsular serotype. Infect Immun 1991;59:222–228.

19 Tart R, McDaniel LS, Ralph BA, Briles DE: Truncated *Streptococcus pneumoniae* PspA molecules elicit cross-protective immunity against pneumococcal challenge in mice. J Infect Dis 1996;173:380–386.

Muneki Hotomi
Department of Otolaryngology, Head and Neck Surgery, Wakayama Medical University
811–1 Kimiidera, Wakayama-shi
Wakayama 641-8509 (Japan)
Tel. +81 73 441 0651, E-Mail mhotomi@wakayama-med.ac.jp

Harabuchi Y (ed): Recent Advances in Tonsils and Mucosal Barriers of the Upper Airways.
Adv Otorhinolaryngol. Basel, Karger, 2011, vol 72, pp 126–128

Heat-Shock Protein ClpL/HSP100 Increases Penicillin Tolerance in *Streptococcus pneumoniae*

Thao Dang-Hien Tran[a] · Hyog-Young Kwon[a] · Eun-Hye Kim[a] · Ki-Woo Kim[b] · David E. Briles[a,c] · Suhkneung Pyo[a] · Dong-Kwon Rhee[a]

[a]School of Pharmacy, Sungkyunkwan University, Suwon, and [b]School of Ecological and Environmental System, Kyungpook National University, Sangju, Korea; [c]Department of Microbiology, University of Alabama at Birmingham, Birmingham, Ala., USA

Abstract

Penicillin resistance and tolerance has been an increasing threat to the treatment of pneumococcal pneumoniae. However, no penicillin tolerance-related genes have been claimed. Here we show that a major heat shock protein ClpL/HSP100 could modulate the expression of a cell wall synthesis enzyme PBP2x, and subsequently increase cell wall thickness and penicillin tolerance in *Streptococus pneumoniae*.

Streptococcus pneumoniae is well known as a dominant cause of community-associated pneumonia, otitis media, septicemia and meningitis [1, 2]. Beta-lactam antibiotics are the most common treatment for pnemococcal pneumonia [3], but recently antibiotic resistance and tolerance has been an increasing threat to global health [4]. Therefore, uncovering the mechanism of resistance and tolerance is a good way to control this emerging threat. Although several genes related to penicillin tolerance in pneumococci have been identified [5], no genes have been claimed for this tolerance. We demonstrated that a major heat-shock protein ClpL/HSP100 (fig. 1) could modulate the expression of a cell wall synthesis enzyme PBP2x, and subsequently increase cell wall thickness and penicillin tolerance. Overexpression of ClpL in D39 increased the minimum penicillin concentration required to kill the bacteria, while a lack of ClpL in D39Δ*clpL* increased the penicillin susceptibility (fig. 2). Exposing pneumococci to penicillin causes a dose-dependent increase of the protein expression level of ClpL and PBP2x in the wild type, but a decrease of those in the D39Δ*clpL*. In addition, in the heat-shock condition, ClpL induced the expression of PBP2x both at the transcription and at the translation level, interacted with PBP2x in the cytosol, and colocalized with PBP2x at the cell wall fraction. Thus, ClpL appears to stimulate cell wall synthesis by inducing PBP2x, interacting with PBP2x, and facilitating translocation of PBP2x (fig. 3). This is the first demonstration that stress response could contribute to an increase of antibiotic tolerance.

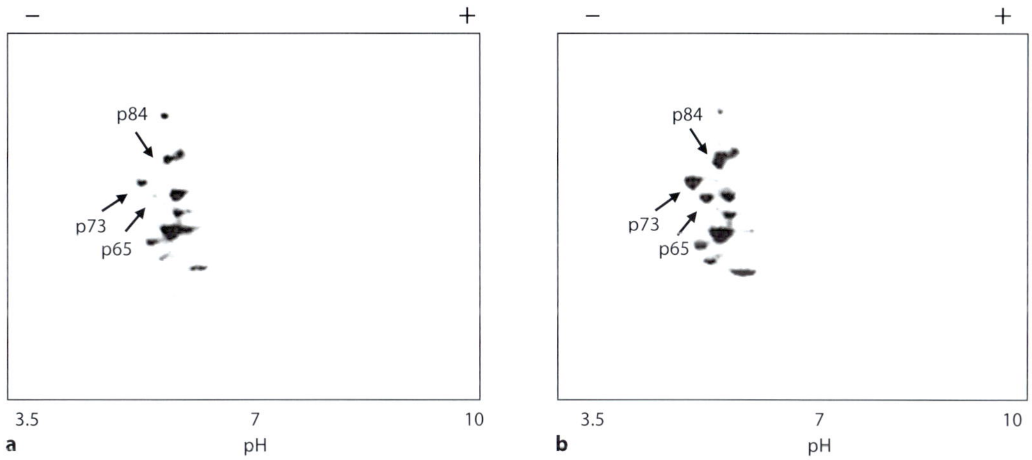

Fig. 1. Autoradiogram of the heat-shock proteins induced by heat shock in *S. pneumoniae* and analyzed by 2D-PAGE. Logarithmically growing cells were pulse-labeled with [^{35}S]-methionine while growing at either 30°C (**a**) or following a shift to 42°C for 30 min (**b**). Total cellular proteins were separated on an equilibrium isoelectric focusing gel followed by a 10% SDS-polyacrylamide gel and visualized by fluorography. The arrows indicate the major heat-induced proteins. p65; GroEL, p73; DnaK, p84; ClpL.

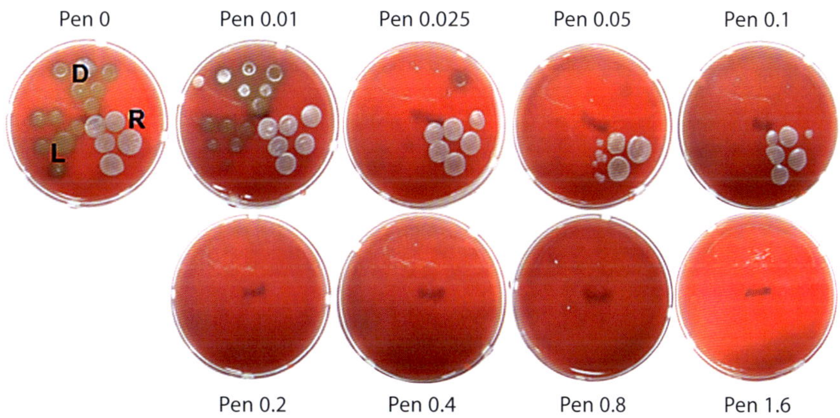

Fig. 2. D39ClpL overexpressing strain was resistant to penicillin. Bacteria were cultured in THY broth until OD 550 = 0.3, and were serially diluted to 10^{-3}, 10^{-4}, and 10^{-5}. 1 µl of each diluted culture (6 drops/plate) was dropped onto the plate containing appropriate concentration of penicillin (Pen) (µg/ml). The plates were then incubated overnight at 37°C in incubator. D = D39WT; L = D39Δ*clpL*; R = D39ClpL overexpressing strain.

Fig. 3. Model for how ClpL increases penicillin tolerance in stress. In nonstress conditions (upper half), exposure of D39 to penicillin leads to bacteria lysis. In stress, i.e. after exposure to heat and other stresses (lower half), ClpL is overexpressed, and subsequently PBP2x is induced. ClpL then functions as a molecular chaperone which first interacts with PBP2x in the cytosol, and then facilitates the translocation of PBP2x to the cell wall. Therefore, the cell wall becomes thicker which might contribute to the increase in penicillin tolerance.

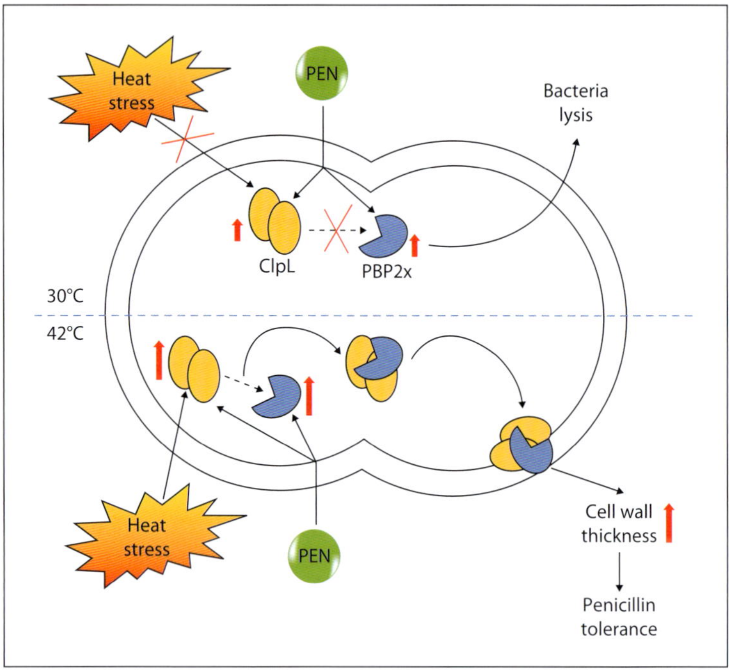

References

1 Fang GD, Fine M, Orloff J, et al: New and emerging etiologies for community-acquired pneumoniae with implications for therapy: a prospective multicenter study of 359 cases. Medicine (Baltimore) 1990;69:307–316.

2 Mandell LA, Wunderink RG, Anzueto A, Bartlett JG, Campbell GD, Dean NC, Dowell SF, File TM Jr, Musher DM, Niederman MS, Torres A, Whitney CG: Infectious Diseases Society of America/American Thoracic Society consensus guidelines on the management of community-acquired pneumonia in adults. Clin Infect Dis 2007;44(suppl 2):S27–S72.

3 Pernot L, Chesnel L, Le Gouellec A, Croize J, Vernet T, Dideberg O, Dessen A: A PBP2x from a clinical isolate of *Streptococcus pneumoniae* exhibits an alternative mechanism for reduction of susceptibility to beta-lactam antibiotics. J Biol Chem 2004;279:16463–16470.

4 Normark BH: Molecular epidemiology and mechanisms for antibiotic resistance in *Streptococcus pneumonie*; in Hakenbeck R, Chhatwal S (eds): Molecular Biology of Streptococci. Wymondham, Horizon Bioscience, 2007, pp 269–290.

5 Mitchell LS, Tuomanen EI: Molecular analysis of antibiotic tolerance in pneumococci. Int J Med Microbiol 2002;292:75–79.

Dong-Kwon Rhee, PhD
College of Pharmacy, Sungkyunkwan University
Suwon, 440–746 (South Korea)
Tel. +82 31 2907707, E-Mail dkrhee@skku.edu

Harabuchi Y (ed): Recent Advances in Tonsils and Mucosal Barriers of the Upper Airways.
Adv Otorhinolaryngol. Basel, Karger, 2011, vol 72, pp 129–131

Immunologic Impact of Tonsillopharyngitis Associated with Group A Streptococci

Edward L. Kaplan

Department of Pediatrics, University of Minnesota Medical School, Minneapolis, Minn., USA

Abstract

While very common clinically, group A streptococcal infections of the upper respiratory tract remain incompletely understood. Vital to clarifying these incompletely answered questions is the understanding of the immune responses associated with infection and the enigmatic 'carrier state'. An important aspect of this is understanding the differences between an immune response and a protective immune response. Several of these concerns are discussed.

Group A beta-hemolytic streptococci *(Streptococcus pyogenes)* are highly transmissible and have the capacity to spread rapidly and widely among susceptible individuals or in a susceptible population. Thus, it is not surprising that these infections are very common. The spectrum of these infections ranges from the relatively less dangerous group A upper respiratory tract 'carrier state' or streptococcal impetigo and skin colonization to the more serious and severe suppurative and nonsuppurative complications. The latter group includes systemic invasive infections with the resulting toxic shock syndrome, as well as rheumatic fever (resulting in rheumatic heart disease) and acute post-streptococcal glomerulonephritis. Streptococcal infections are very common throughout the world; they are largely endemic among school aged children. Epidemics are not infrequently reported. This organism remains problematic clinically, epidemiologically, and pathogenetically.

The purpose of this discussion is to examine some of the issues, many of which remain incompletely explained, relating to streptococcal upper respiratory tract infections and the resulting immune response. The relevance of this approach is justified by the fact that there remains no exact animal model for studying group A streptococcal infections and their sequelae. The human is the only known natural reservoir for group A beta-hemolytic streptococci. The group A streptococcus rarely, if ever, causes natural infection in animals. Parenthetically, this fact is often overlooked when attempting to study these infections in vivo; one wonders about the applicability of current animal models to infection in humans.

One of the most relevant in vivo ways that group A streptococcal infections can be studied is through observations on patients who represent the group A upper respiratory tract 'carrier state' [1]. For this discussion, true/bona fide group A upper respiratory tract infection is defined as the presence of this microbe in the human upper respiratory tract accompanied by immunologic recognition of its presence (i.e. a documented immune response). In contrast, the streptococcal 'carrier state' is defined as recovery of this organism from the upper respiratory tract, but the absence of a host immune response (as measured by antibodies to streptococcal somatic or extracellular antigens).

There are important epidemiologic and pathogenetic differences and therefore unique consequences of the streptococcal upper respiratory tract 'carrier state'. Individuals with bona fide infection demonstrate rapid multiplication of the organism in the upper respiratory tract, an immune response and the possibility of developing nonsuppurative sequelae. In contrast, assessment of individuals representing the carrier state reveals that there is slow streptococcal multiplication in the upper respiratory tract, and an immune response is absent [1]. Very rarely, if at all, do nonsuppurative sequelae occur in documented upper respiratory tract carriers. However, it is very difficult for the clinician to prospectively differentiate some patients with bona fide infection from many individuals who represent the 'carrier state'.

There are two important aspects to understanding of the immune response(s) to group A streptococcal upper respiratory tract infection (e.g. pharyngitis and tonsillitis). The first is that which only represents the immune response(s) to the streptococcal antigens by the host. This is most often determined clinically by measuring antibodies to commercially available group A streptococcal extracellular antigens such as streptolysin O and streptococcal nuclease B (DNAse B).

The other equally or perhaps more important immune responses are those which produce antibodies which convey protection to the host. The best example is the type-specific antibody to the M protein of the group A streptococcus; this opsonic antibody promotes phagocytosis and killing of the organism in vivo. This form of immunity has been demonstrated to persist for as long as four decades after infection by a specific type of group A streptococci [2]. At present, there is intense interest to identify other antigens which confer immunity to the infected host; this is required for an effective streptococcal vaccine.

Also important in understanding the group A streptococcal 'carrier state' and its role in clinical disease is the information demonstrating ingestion of group A streptococci by epithelial cells; this results in viable intracellular streptococci. It has been hypothesized that these intracellular streptococci may be responsible for the clinically problematic group A streptococcal upper respiratory tract carrier state [3]. Adequate understanding of this unique situation has not been achieved.

Recent studies have demonstrated the complexity of the immune response to streptococcal extracellular antigens [4]. One hundred and sixty children were followed prospectively for 104 consecutive weeks. Throat cultures were obtained every 4 weeks and also during any intercurrent illness. Serum was obtained from each subject every 13 weeks and also 4–6 weeks after any intercurrent illness. Throat cultures were processed by standard techniques and antibody titers by classical laboratory techniques [5].

While space does not allow in-depth discussion of the individual findings, analysis revealed examples of subjects with repeatedly positive throat cultures with the same streptococcal strains (homologous M/*emm* type) for almost 2 consecutive years who failed to demonstrate the expected antibody response to group A streptococcal extracellular antigens associated with true infection [4]. Indeed, antistreptolysin O (ASO) and antideoxyribonuclease B (anti-DNase B) titers actually fell during this prolonged period of observation. Additionally, these studies also demonstrated examples of individuals from whom group A streptococci were eradicated from the throat who maintained elevated antibody titers despite multiple negative throat cultures (no positive cultures) during periods of 6 months or more [4].

Such observations document the problems with interpretation and understanding of the immune response to streptococcal infections. Further studies are required to understand not only the phenomenon of asymptomatic streptococcal carriage, but whether the role of the nonimmune responding streptococcal carrier is capable of inducing suppurative and nonsuppurative sequelae such as rheumatic fever and acute glomerulonephritis. The clinical implications are obvious.

The incomplete understanding of the significance of the immune response to streptococcal extracellular (and presumably somatic) antigens is further revealed by recent observations regarding immune protection following documented infection. One recent study, for example, demonstrated that 20 individuals with documented streptococcal upper respiratory tract acquisition associated with symptomatic pharyngitis were not protected from acquiring a completely different pharyngitis-associated strain of streptococci within approximately 4 months [6]. These observations strongly suggest that natural upper respiratory tract infection does not convey broad (nonspecific) immunity. This observation is important to remember in the design of future streptococcal vaccine studies with unique antigens.

One might ask what these mentioned observations mean for the clinician and for the basic scientist. It is clear that our understanding of the qualitative and quantitative differences in production/stimulation of somatic and/or extracellular antibodies to group A streptococcal antigens is incomplete. Second, we know very little about persistence of known and also as yet unrecognized antibodies (either those that only represent past infection or those who both represent past infection and also confer immunity) following group A streptococcal infection. Third, we know relatively little about protective immunity with the exception of type specific antibody to M protein. Finally, our knowledge is also incomplete about the significance and the pathogenesis of the group A upper respiratory tract 'carrier state' and how/if this might influence the human immune status.

All of these are extremely important questions which require answers to more completely address the medical and public health aspects of group A streptococcal infection.

References

1 Kaplan EL: The group A streptococcal upper respiratory tract carrier state: an enigma. J Pediatr 1980;97:337–345.

2 Bencivenga JF, Johnson DR, Kaplan EL: Determination of group A streptococcal anti-M type-specific antibody in sera of rheumatic fever patients after 45 years. Clin Infect Dis 2009;49: 1237–1239.

3 Kaplan EL, Chhatwal GS, Rohde M: Reduced ability of penicillin to eradicate ingested group A streptococci from epithelial cells: clinical and pathogenetic implications. Clin Infect Dis 2006;43:1398–1406.

4 Johnson DR, Kurlan R, Leckman J, Kaplan EL: The human immune response to streptococcal extracellular antigens: clinical, diagnostic and potential pathogenetic implications. Clin Infect Dis 2010;50:481–490.

5 Johnson DR, Kaplan E: (World Health Organization Collaborating Center for Reference and Research on Streptococci; Minneapolis, Minn., USA) and Sramek J, Motlova J, Bicova R, Havlickova H, Havlicek J, Kriz P (World Health Organization Collaborating Center for reference and Research on Streptococci; Prague, Czech Republic): Laboratory Diagnosis of Group A Streptococcal Infections: A Laboratory Manual. World Health Organization, Geneva, 1996.

6 Kaplan EL, Wotton J, Johnson DR: Dynamic epidemiology of group A streptococcal serotypes associated with pharyngitis: implications for sequelae and vaccines. Lancet 2001;358:1334–1337.

Edward L. Kaplan, MD
Department of Pediatrics, University of Minnesota Medical School
Mail Code 296, 420 Delaware St. SE
Minneapolis, MN 55455 (USA)
Tel. +1 612 624 1112, Fax +1 612 626 6645, E-Mail kapla001@umn.edu

Harabuchi Y (ed): Recent Advances in Tonsils and Mucosal Barriers of the Upper Airways.
Adv Otorhinolaryngol. Basel, Karger, 2011, vol 72, pp 132–135

Influence of Waldeyer's Ring Hypertrophy on Snoring and Sleep Apnea

Desiderio Passàli[a] · Michele De Benedetto[b] · Maria Lauriello[c] · Francesco Maria Passàli[d]

[a]ENT Department Medical School University of Siena, Siena, [b]ENT Department, 'Vito Fazi' Hospital Lecce, Lecce, [c]Experimental Medicine Department Medical School, University of L'Aquila, L'Aquila, and [d]ENT Department Tor Vergata University Roma, Rome, Italy

Abstract

Severe adenotonsillar hypertrophy can be the main cause of nocturnal respiratory affections, as confirmed by the improvement of symptoms seen after adenotonsillectomy. Unsuccessful surgical treatment can be due to craniofacial morphological alterations. Hypotony of the pharyngeal muscles could also be responsible together with tonsil hypertrophy. In our study, we enrolled 125 patients (87 males and 38 females), aged from 3 to 8 years, suffering from chronic snoring. All the patients underwent adenotonsillectomy. The follow-up was carried out at 2, 4 and 6 months after the operation. Snoring and nocturnal apneas were no longer present in almost all the patients. Overnight polysomnography remains the gold standard diagnostic test for obstructive sleep apnea syndrome, but its feasibility in clinical practice is debated. Rhinomanometry, which gives an objective evaluation of ventilatory nasal function, acoustic rhinometry, which measures the cross-section in fixed nasal areas, and nasal mucociliary transport time can be considered useful tests to evaluate the cause of respiratory obstruction.

Obstructive sleep apnea syndrome (OSAS) cannot be left untreated. Evaluation of the individual pathophysiology gives the best opportunity to restore adequate upper respiratory ventilation by a rational choice between medical and surgical treatment [1].

Severe adenotonsillar hypertrophy is the most frequent cause of respiratory alterations in children: about 80% of children may benefit from the surgical procedure [2]. Nevertheless, the role of the pharyngeal obstruction in the pathogenesis of OSAS is still debated in literature.

According to Suen et al. [3], a severe adenotonsillar hypertrophy can be the only reason for nocturnal respiratory affections: this is confirmed by the improvement of symptoms and of the 'respiratory disturbance index' after adenotonsillectomy. However, adenotonsillar hypertrophy is not always accompanied by nocturnal obstructive disturbances and there is no clear relationship between the size of the adenoids/tonsils and apnea indexes. Therefore, according to some authors, other anatomopathological factors can influence the respiratory disturbances.

According to Shintani et al. [4, 5] maxillary and mandibular protrusion was significantly smaller in OSAS patients and the hyoid bone was significantly lower in an OSAS group than in a control group.

The effect of adenotonsillectomy on changes of position during sleep was evaluated by Choi et al. [6]. Forty-four polysomnograms from 22 children with OSAS were analyzed. By comparing the frequency of positional changes during sleep and the distribution of sleep positions before and after surgery, the authors concluded that adenotonsillectomy significantly improved all the respiratory parameters studied. The total number of positional changes during sleep ($p < 0.001$) and the positional change index ($p < 0.001$) decreased significantly. The proportion of sleep time spent in the supine position was significantly increased ($p = 0.001$), and the proportions spent in the lateral ($p = 0.003$) and upright ($p = 0.018$) positions were significantly decreased.

Adenotonsillar hypertrophy seems to be strictly linked to nocturnal respiratory disturbances; nevertheless, the obstruction in the condition of 'rest' does not always allow to evaluate or foresee the degree of obstruction during sleep when there is a physiological reduction of muscular tone, especially of the genioglossus muscle. Perhaps hypotony or alterations of the neural control of the pharyngeal muscles or a particular laxity of the ligaments can be responsible together with tonsil hypertrophy for the pharyngeal obstruction, as it sometimes occurs in very young children. The attempt to look for histological changes of the palatopharyngeal muscle that are typical for OSAS children was not successful. Vuono et al. [7] analyzed the palatophryngeal muscle in 34 oral-breathing children with hypertrophic tonsils and adenoids. The participants were divided into children without sleeping disorders (group I) and children with primary snoring (group II) or apnea (group III). The main histological findings (fiber size variability, perimysial connective tissue infiltration, intracytoplasmatic mitochondrial proliferation, internal architecture alteration) were similar in the three groups. The authors concluded that such changes could be a normal histological feature of this muscle rather than a sign of a neurogenic or myopathic pathology.

Since breast-fed babies' airways are very narrow, a reduction of a few millimeters can cause a 65% decrease in diameter, determining a remarkable obstruction. According to our experience, adenotonsillar hypertrophy remains one of the most frequent causes of respiratory disturbances in children, especially snoring, that sometimes can be followed by a real OSAS.

Personal Experience: Snoring and Adenotonsillectomy

In our study, we enrolled 125 patients (87 males and 38 females), aged from 3 to 8 years, suffering from chronic snoring. Clinical history elicited persistent and noisy day-night oral breathing. Particular attention was paid to other night disturbances such as apnea episodes, nocturnal awakening and enuresis and daytime disturbances such as sleepiness, hyperreactivity, aggressiveness, absentmindedness, and bad scholastic results.

Flexible optic fibers evaluation of the upper airways stenosis had been performed in all the children. In 65% of the patients snoring was not accompanied by nocturnal apneas. All the patients underwent adenotonsillectomy. The follow-up was carried out at 2, 4, and 6 months after the operation.

Snoring and nocturnal apneas were no more present in almost all the patient.

A second adenoidectomy was necessary in 2 children, because the increasing lymphoid activity was responsible for an incomplete surgical removal of the lymphoid tissue in the youngest patients (3 years old).

Etiopathogenesis and Diagnosis of Upper Respiratory Obstruction

According to our results, management of OSAS includes tonsillectomy and/or adenoidectomy to which most of the cases responded. Nevertheless, other risk factors and coexisting conditions should be investigated and treated prior to considering surgical treatment.

Ng et al. [8] reviewed the literature to evaluate the association between allergic rhinitis (AR) and OSAS in childhood. They concluded that allergic rhinitis affected approximately 40% of children and OSAS occurred in 2% of children. As AR is associated with nasal obstruction, enlargement of tonsils and adenoids, and an elongated face, it can be considered a risk factor for OSAS. The treatment of AR is helpful to decrease the severity of OSAS and prevent emergence of an elongated face, which is responsible for a smaller upper airway size.

Overnight polysomnography remains the gold standard diagnostic test for OSAS, but its feasibilty in clinical practice is debated because its use is complex and expensive. Furthermore, interpretation of its results is not unanimously agreed on. History and physical examination can still be considered useful diagnostic tools. A significant contribution to the clinical picture can be given by some tests, which are specific for evaluating nasal physiopathology.

Rhinomanometry gives an objective evaluation of the ventilatory function of the nose and the physiology of the rhino-pharyngo-tubal area. When anterior rhinomanometric examination reveals lower than normal values for nasal conductance, we carry out the nasal decongestion test (NDT). It allows to differentiate functional from structural stenosis and to address the patient to medical or surgical therapy. The NDT is performed as follows: (1) basal anterior active rhinomanometry (AAR), (2) nasal decongestant: 2 sprays in each nostril, (3) after 10 min control ARR. If this test proves negative (total nasal resistance unchanged), one might envisage the possibility of a surgical correction of the pathology, already revealed in the course of the objective examination and confirmed by X-ray examination.

Acoustic rhinometry is a relatively new method of using acoustic reflections from the airway to estimate their shape and the morphological changes induced by the congestion of the mucosa.

By comparing the acoustic wave reflected from the nasal cavity to the incident wave, this technique makes it possible to measure the cross-section in fixed areas at varying distances from the nostril. This method need more standardization such as the choice of the most suitable acoustic wave, the way of connecting the nosepiece to the nostril or the positioning of the head in respect to the incident wave. We perform acoustic rhinometry with the aid of an optometric craniostat [9].

The degree of involvement of the nasal mucosa in pathologic reactions is also well documented by the determination of the efficiency of nasal mucociliary transport (muco-ciliary transport time). All the above-mentioned methods are useful in the differential diagnosis between sleep apnea syndrome and other noises caused by the turbulence that inspired air causes when coming into contact with the walls of the nose and the pharynx.

Conclusions

Together with history and clinical examination, the above-mentioned tests are sensitive tools, even thought relatively aspecific. Surgery can restore the patency of the upper airways, contributing to contrast the neuromuscular hypotonia as a result of the effect of the surgical scar. Primary snoring and OSAS are a continuum, and surgery may be defined as a form of prevention against pathology with potential complications. As suggested by Ameli et al. [2], polysomnography cannot be carried out routinely due to the lack of specialized centers and because of its excessive cost. It could be prescribed only in unsuccessful adenotonsillectomies and for those children who have complicated presentations from the outset.

In any case, OSAS cannot be left untreated: evaluation of the individual pathophysiology gives the best opportunity to restore adequate upper respiratory ventilation by the rational choice between medical and surgical treatment.

References

1 Arens R, Marcus CL: Pathophysiology of upper airway obstruction: a developmental perspective. Sleep 2004;27:997–1019.

2 Ameli F, Brocchetti F, Semino L, Fibbi A: Adenotonsillectomy in obstructive sleep apnea syndrome: proposal of a surgical decision-taking algorithm. Int J Pediatr Otorhinolarylgol 2007;71:729–734.

3 Suen JS, Arnold JE, Brooks LG: Adenotonsillectomy for treatment of obstructive sleep apnea in children. Arch Otolaryngol Head Neck Surg 1995;125:525–530.

4 Shintani T, Asakura K, Kataura A: The effect of adenotonsillectomy in children with OSAS. Int J Pediatr Otorhinolaryngol 1998;44:51–58.

5 Shintani T, Asakura K, Kataura A: Adenotonsillar hypertrophy and skeletal morphology of children with obstructive sleep apnea syndrome. Acta Otolaryngol Suppl 1996;523:22–24.

6 Choi JH, Kim EJ, Choi J, Kim TH, Know SY, Lee SH, Shin C, Lee SH: The effect of tonsillectomy on changes of position during sleep in pediatric obstructive sleep apnea syndrome. Am J Rhinol Allergy 2009;23:e56–e58.

7 Vuono IM, Zanotelli E, de Oliveira AS, Fujita RR, Pignatari SS, Pizarro GU, de Cassia Pradelle-Hallinan ML, Moreira GA: Histological analysis of palatopharyngeal muscle from children with snoring and obstructive apnea syndrome. Int J Pediatr Otorhinolaryngol 2007;71:283–290.

8 Ng DK, Chan CH, Hwang GY, Chow PY, Kwok KL: A review of the role of allergic rhinitis in childhood obstructive sleep apnea syndrome. Allergy Asthma Proc 2006;27:240–242.

9 Passàli D, Bellussi L, Bianchini-Ciampoli M, De Seta E: Our experiences in nasal mucociliary transport time determination Acta Otolaryngol (Stockh.) 1984;97:319.

Prof. Desiderio Passàli
Via Anagnina, 718
IT–00118 Rome (Italy)
Tel. +39 3356102667, E-Mail desiderio.passali@passali.org

Harabuchi Y (ed): Recent Advances in Tonsils and Mucosal Barriers of the Upper Airways.
Adv Otorhinolaryngol. Basel, Karger, 2011, vol 72, pp 136–138

Tonsils Diseases, Past, Present and Future and the Impact in Clinical Practice in Brazil

Luiza Hayashi Endo

Campinas State University, Medical Sciences Faculty, São Paulo, Brazil

Abstract

A simplified review of the research carried out in Brazil on tonsils is presented: histopathological findings in children's tonsils with allergy, the detection of Epstein-Barr virus, herpes virus (SV1 e SV2, HHV8) and the correlation between tonsil hypertrophy and recurrence of infection is discussed. The role of allergy in children with tonsillitis and/or tonsil and adenoid hypertrophy are analyzed. After participating in the Tonsils Symposium in 1991, the knowledge of tonsils morphology, immunology and histopathology increased, triggering a change in clinical practice in Brazil.

As Professor of the Department of Otorhinolaryngology at the University of Campinas, since 1973, I focused on Pediatric Otolaryngology and, in 1986, had the opportunity to meet and work with Professor Keijiro Koga at the National Children's Hospital. This exceptional experience enabled me to establish this specialty in my country.

My goal was to learn more about diseases of the tonsils and adenoids (T&A) since at that time in Brazil nobody was doing any research into this area. My PhD brought up the discussion about tonsil histopathology [1].

Professor Koga introduced me to Professor Tabata who invited me to participate at the II International Symposium on Tonsils (IST) in Pavia, Italy. It was 1991 and I had my first contact with many researchers in T&A, mainly Japanese professors, and I could present my first paper: 'Allergic tonsillitis, a histopathological study' at this symposium [2].

Since then, the motivation to work in this new field increased and I prepared papers to present at the III IST to be held in Sapporo, Japan, but also to spread all the knowledge that I had received at this meeting to my fellow Brazilian ENT doctors.

The surgical treatment of T&A in children with hypertrophy and/or recurrent infections (without upper airway obstruction – UAO) and allergy was a controversial topic, but after our histopathological studies [3], comparing the response of T&A to anti-allergic medication, it could be well established to perform T&A surgery only when there was no good response after anti-histaminic therapy.

In Brazil, ENT doctors normally choose to follow and treat acute and chronic tonsillitis based on swab results without any previous knowledge of normal and chronic tonsillar flora, resulting in overuse of antibiotics. Things started to change in Brazil, especially after our studies in tonsils bacteriology, where we showed findings from patients with recurrent tonsillitis and those without infection that underwent surgery by UAO due to T&A

hyperplasia. These new findings about tonsils microflora helped prevent the misuse of antibiotics [4].

One question remains: Why do some children have more T&A infections than others? With a retrospective view, I found a study by Yamanaka and Kataura from 1984, suggesting a correlation between EBV and the recurrence of tonsillitis. This article inspired me to look for the detection of the T&A virus, beginning with Epstein-Barr virus (EBV) and the correlation with recurrent infections, using the in situ hybridization technique (ISH-EBER RNA). We searched for EBV in the tonsillar tissue of 42 patients with recurrent tonsillitis (RT) and 43 patients without infections but with tonsillar hyperplasia (TH), and we detected 29.4% positive cases. However, no statistical difference was found between the two groups. The conclusion was that tonsils of children can be colonized by EBV which may be implicated in both RT and TH [5].

By extending our study to include the adenoid tissue of 80 children (32 specimens from children 12–24 months of age and 48 from 25 months to 15 years of age) and using the same technique, our results showed that the presence of EBV in the adenoids (61%) was higher than in tonsils (29.4%) [6].

We also searched for the frequency of EBV expression in the adenoids of children in a lower age group (1–2 years). It was also intended to establish which lymphoid subsets were involved in this infection. Among 21 adenoid tissue samples, 7 (33%) were positive for EBV and in almost all cases they were also CD20-positive, confirming the preferential infection of B lymphocytes by EBV, which in some instances can downregulate the expression of CD20 [7].

Another point of interest was the possible relation between herpes simplex virus (HSV) and acute pharyngotonsillitis. Continuing our studies detecting for viruses in T&A, we searched for HSV-1 and HSV-2 by ISH in 21 adenoids and 15 tonsil tissue from children with hyperplasia, with age 2–12 years. None of 36 cases was positive for the HSV-1 and HSV-2 in T&A, either in lymphoid, stroma or epithelial cells as those seen in positive control. HSV does not seem to be implied in T&A hyperplasia. These organs apparently do not harbor the latent virus, or the viral load is too low to be detected without amplification methods [8].

We also looked for herpesvirus type 8 (HHV8) in children's tonsils (181) and adenoids (162) by immunochemistry (IHC) and in situ hybridization (ISH).

In 20 cases (6.8%) HHV8 was detected by ISH, whereas only 2 of them were concomitantly positive by IHC [9].

We also compared a possible correlation between the presence of EBV and HHV8. We compared 38 tonsil and 2 adenoid tissue samples of children up to 14 years of age and cases previously positive for HHV8 by ISH as they belong to the same *y-herpesvirus* subfamily and share some biological characteristics. HHV8 was detected in 19 tonsils and 1 adenoid. The other 19 tonsils and 1 adenoid taken from the HHV8-negative group were selected by pairing age and gender of patients with the HHV8-positive group. EBV was similarly detected in the groups negative and positive for HHV8, suggesting a different spread mechanism [10].

The study in T&A during these years allowed me to show these findings to my ENT and pediatric Brazilian colleagues through many lectures at medical meetings. I also published many chapters in books of basic study printed by the International Federation of ENT Societies (IFOS), Pediatric Brazilian Society, Brazilian Otorhinolaryngology Society, Inter-American Association of Pediatric Otorhinolaryngology and the São Paulo Pediatric Society.

I am very grateful to Japanese professors, mainly Professors Keijiro Koga, Toshihide Tabata and Akikatsu Kataura, and others who succeeded them in tonsils research for the opportunity to grow up in the knowledge of Waldeyer's ring.

Today and for the future, I am challenging and preparing new Brazilian researchers to be part of this wonderful team.

References

1 Endo LH, Prigenzi LS, Lorand-Metze IL: Tonsillectomy: critical clinical approach based on histological analysis. Folha Med (Brazil) 1989;99:141–145.
2 Endo LH, Vassallo J, Moreira SRL: Allergic tonsillitis: histopathological study. Adv Otolaryngol 1992;47:41–45.
3 Endo LH, Altemani A, Chone CT, Idagawa, E: Histopathological comparison between tonsil and adenoid response to allergy. Acta Otolaryngol (Stock) 1996;(suppl 523):17–19.
4 Endo, LH, Carvalho, DS, Sakano E, Baracat EC, Reis M, Moraes de Oliveira U: Panorama global da bacteriologia das amígdalas palatinas de crianças. Rev Bras ORL 1998;64:553–558.
5 Endo LH, Ferreira D, Montenegro MCS, Pinto AG, Vassallo J: Detection of Epstein-Barr vírus in tonsillar tissue of children and the relationship with recurrent tonsillitis. Int J Otorhinolaryngol 2001;58:9–15.
6 Endo LH, Sakano E, Camargo LA, Ferreira DR, Pinto GA, Vassallo J: Detection of Epstein-Barr vírus in children's adenoids by in situ hybridization. Int Congr Ser 2003;1257:157–160.
7 Endo LH, Vassallo J, Sakano E, Brousset P: Detection of Epstein-Barr vírus and subsets of lymphoid cells in adenoid tissue of children under two years of age. Int J Otorhinolaryngol 2002;66:223–226.
8 Vassallo J, Camargo LA, Chagas CA, Pinto GA, Endo LH: Search for herpesvirus 1 and 2 by in situ hybridization in tonsils and adenoids. Int J Otorhinolaryngol 2005;69:345–349.
9 Chagas CA, Endo LH, Sakano E, Pinto GA, Brousset P, Vassallo J: Detection of herpersvirus type 8 (HHV8) in children's tonsils and adenoids by immunochemistry and in situ hybridization. Int J Otorhinolaryngol 2006;70:65–72.
10 Chagas CA, Endo HE, Santos WLC, Pinto GA, Sakano E, Brousset P, Vassallo J: Is there a correlation between the detection of human herpesvirus 8 and Epstein-Barr virus in Waldeyer's ring? Int J Otorhinolaryngol 2006;70:1923–1927.

Luiza Hayashi Endo, PhD, MD
Departamento Otorrinolaringologia, Faculdade de Medicina, Universidade Estadual de Campinas – UNICAMP
Av. José Bonifácio 2240
13093–241 Campinas, SP (Brazil)
Tel. +55 19 3252 4241, E-Mail luiza.endo@kingslamb.com.br

Harabuchi Y (ed): Recent Advances in Tonsils and Mucosal Barriers of the Upper Airways.
Adv Otorhinolaryngol. Basel, Karger, 2011, vol 72, pp 139–141

Clinical Scoring System of Acute Pharyngotonsillitis

Akihisa Togawa · Muneki Hotomi · Shinji Tamura · Noboru Yamanaka

Department of Otolaryngology, Head and Neck Surgery, Wakayama Medical University, Wakayama, Japan

Abstract

Objectives: The aim of this study was to evaluate clinical outcomes of acute pharyngo-tonsillitis by a scoring system and the impact of causative pathogens. **Methods:** The patients with acute pharyngotonsillitis were evaluated for causative pathogens and her clinical symptoms and pharyngotonsillar finding by a clinical scoring system were assessed. **Results:** *Streptocococcus pyogenes* were identified at 13.6%. Thirty-one viruses were also identified by PCR. The numbers of total white blood cells and the levels of C-reactive protein showed a significant positive correlation with clinical scores ($p < 0.001$) and were significantly higher in cases with *S. pyogenes*. The clinical scores rapidly improved after the antimicrobial treatments in moderate cases and severe cases. **Conclusion:** A clinical scoring system represents the severity of acute pharyngotonsillitis and is useful for evaluating clinical course of the illness.

Acute pharyngotonisillits is one of the most frequent respiratory infectious diseases. To investigate clinical and microbial features of acute pharyngotonsillitis, we organized a nationwide prospective surveillance study group named the Pharyngotonsillitis Study Group (PhaTONS) in Japan. The aims of this prospective study were to evaluate the causative pathogens of adult acute pharyngotonsillitis in comparison with clinical features of the infectious disease [1]. Some cases of pharyngotonsillitis are caused by viral infections and are self-limiting by only symptomatic treatments, whereas sometimes bacterial infection takes part in this disease resulting in severe symptoms and complications such as peritonsillar abscess which need treatment with antimicrobial agents. To save medical costs and avoid complications, the appropriate usage of antimicrobial agents against acute pharyngotonsillitis would be essential.

We conducted a prospective study between May 2004 and June 2005.

214 patients with acute pharyngo-tonsillitis were assessed for clinical symptoms and pharyngotonsillar findings by a clinical scoring system (table 1) and were also evaluated for causative pathogens.

They were 114 males and 100 females, ranging in age between 16 and 79 years, median 34 years.

Patients were classified into three groups according to their total score as mild (less than 3), moderate (4–8) and severe (higher than 9).

In this study, 33 (15.4%) cases were classified into the mild group, 121 (56.5%) into the moderate group, and 60 (28.0%) into the severe group.

Table 2. A Clinical scoring system for acute pharyngo-tonsillitis

	Clinical scores		
	0	1	2
Symptoms			
Difficulties in daily life	not so annoying	annoying, but can work	absence from work
Sore throat/swallowing pain	discomfort	sore, but can swallow	difficult to swallow
Fever	<37.5°C	37.0–38.5°C	<38.6°C
Pharyngo-tonsillar findings			
Pharyngeal erythema or swelling	mild	moderate	marked
Tonsillar erythema or swelling	mild	moderate	marked
Presence of exudates or plugs in tonsils	none	scattered	whole tonsil

A total of 234 pathogenic bacteria were identified in 157 (73.4%) of 214 patients. The microorganisms detected in patients with acute pharyngotonsillitis were *Streptococcus pyogenes* (29 isolates, 13.6%), hemolytic streptococci (35 isolates, 16.4%), *Haemophilus influenzae* (52 isolates, 24.3%), and others (71 isolates, 33.2%). There was no significant difference in distribution of bacteria between acute tonsillitis and pharyngitis.

31 viruses were identified by PCR. Major viruses were adenovirus (10 of 205 cases, 4.9%), and hMPV (human metapneumovirus) (13 of 206 cases, 6.3%). Among the 206 cases in which both bacterial culture and virus PCR were performed, bacteria alone were identified in 128 cases (62.1%), virus alone were identified in 7 cases (3.4%), and both bacteria and virus were identified in 23 cases (11.2%). In 48 cases (23.3%), neither bacteria nor virus was identified.

Both severities of disease and inflammatory parameters were compared with pathogens. Although *S. pyogenes* together with hemolytic streptococci, *H. influenza, Haemophilus haemolyticus, Staphylococcus aureus, Streptococcus pneumonia* and *Moraxilla catarrhalis* were frequently identified among patients with acute pharyngotonsillitis, we could not find any differences in the clinical scores among those pathogens.

The numbers of total WBC at the first visit were significantly higher in cases with *S. pyogenes* than in cases with other pathogens. The levels of CRP were also significantly higher in cases with *S. pyogenes* than in cases with *S. aureus* and *M. catharrhalis* ($p < 0.05$). There was no difference among other pathogens.

The total number of WBC at the first visit showed a positive correlation with clinical scores ($r = 0.482$, $p < 0.001$). The levels of CRP at the first visit also showed a positive correlation with clinical scores ($r = 0.571$, $p < 0.001$).

Of 33 mild cases, 21 (63.6%) patients were followed up without antibiotics and showed gradual improvement of their scores, whereas 12 (36.4%) patients were treated with oral antimicrobial agents (AMPC: 12.1%, LVFX: 15.2%, CFPN: 9.1%) due to exacerbation of the disease.

Of 121 moderate cases, 120 (99.2%) patients were treated with antimicrobial agents and 87 patients (71.9%) were treated with AMPC (66 patients, 54.5%) or LVFX (21 patients, 17.4%).

All severe cases were treated with antimicrobial agents. Seven patients (11.7%) were treated with AMPC and 14 patients (23.3%) were treated with LVFX. In the severe cases, 22 patients (36.7%) were treated with parenteral antimicrobial agents. Among those 22 patients, 12 (20.0%) were treated with CTRX.

The clinical scores of moderate and severe cases decreased significantly after antimicrobial treatment ($p < 0.01$). In contrast to the moderate and severe cases, the mild cases showed a decrease in their scores regardless of the antimicrobial treatment.

The current findings strongly suggest that the clinical scoring system will be valuable to determine the severity of the disease and for the appropriate usage of antimicrobial agents.

Acknowledgements

We greatly thank Prof. Edward L. Kaplan, MD (Department of Pediatrics, the University of Minneapolis, Minn., USA) for his superb suggestions on this paper. This work was organized by a nationwide surveillance group for adult acute pharyngotonsillitis (Pharyngotonsillitis Study Group: PhaTONS). We greatly thank all members of the PhaTONS.

Reference

1 Suzumoto M, Hotomi M, Billal DS, Fujihara K, Harabuchi Y, Yamanaka N: A scoring system for management of acute pharyngo-tonsillitis in adults. Auris Nasus Larynx 2009;36:314–320.

Akihisa Togawa
Department of Otolaryngology, Head and Neck Surgery, Wakayama Medical University
811–1 Kimiidera
Wakayama, 641-8509 (Japan)
Tel. +81 73 441 0651, E-Mail togawa@wakayama-med.ac.jp

Harabuchi Y (ed): Recent Advances in Tonsils and Mucosal Barriers of the Upper Airways.
Adv Otorhinolaryngol. Basel, Karger, 2011, vol 72, pp 142–145

Clinical Guideline on Adenotonsillectomy: The Italian Experience

Luisa M. Bellussi[a] · Paola Marchisio[b] · Enrico Materia[c] · Francesco M. Passàli[d]

[a]ENT Clinic University of Siena, Siena, [b]Department of Maternal and Pediatric Sciences, University of Milan Fondazione IRCCS Ca' Granda Ospedale Maggiore Policlinico Milan, Milan, [c]Public Health Agency Lazio-Sanità Roma, Roma, and [d]ENT Department Tor Vergata University Roma, Roma, Italy

Abstract

Five years after publishing the document on 'The clinical and organizational appropriateness of tonsillectomy and adenoidectomy' in 2003, a multidisciplinary group of experts came together again to update this document and to publish a guideline with grading of evidences and recommendations. Major revisions of the previous document were addressed to: (1) the diagnosis and indications for adenotonsillectomy in presence of OSAS in children, (2) the analysis of advantages of new surgical techniques in terms of effectiveness, costs or the risk of postsurgery bleeding and recurrences, and (3) the efficacy of perioperative management in reducing the incidence and duration of post-operative events. In fact, in the last years, a relevant number of evidence became available on the above-mentioned items making the need for a continuing updating of guidelines tangible. As a premise to the guideline, it is stressed how the previous document impact was prominent: the decrease of total number of tonsillectomy in Italy was evident and accompanied by a decrease of variations in the regional rates. Besides the document contributed to strengthen the multidisciplinary collaboration, especially between pediatricians and otorhinolaryngologists, and to divulge the Evidence-Based Medicine culture.

Five years after publishing the Italian document on 'The clinical and organizational appropriateness of tonsillectomy and adenoidectomy' in 2003, a multidisciplinary group of experts, including general practitioners, otorhinolaryngologists, pediatricians, anesthesiologists, infectiologists, neurologists as well as representatives of parents and caregivers, came together again to update this document.

In Italy, tonsillectomy and adenoidectomy are the most common surgical operations performed in children. However, the rate of these surgical procedures, ranging from 3.5 to 19.0 per 10,000 in the year 2000 in different regions of our country, seems to vary independently from geographic and climatic factors being rather related to socioeconomic factors or uncertainties regarding clinical indications. The aim of the document published in 2003 [1] was to find the most shared indications based on appropriateness and effectiveness criteria. The literature search included systematic reviews and protocols either developed by the Cochrane collaboration or not, existing guidelines and documents covering the period from 1990 to 2002. It should be stressed that the document was not aimed at providing graded recommendations per se, but instead at offering only suggestions and advice for clinical practice. Grading of evidence level was established from I to VI according to the criteria suggested by the Italian National Programme for Clinical Guidelines. Dissemination of the document included: mailing to health care givers, publications on national and international journals, symposia and educational courses organization to inform and involve colleagues, opinion leaders, and scientific societies. The document was also on-line on the web site of different societies.

The first important result of the document was the impact on clinical practice; the rate of tonsillectomy has decreased: from 2000 to 2004 about 4,000 cases less were registered as a whole and the lowest level was reached in 2003, year of the document publication [2, 3]. Also, the trend in geographical variations of standardized rates has changed showing a more uniform distribution among Northern, Central and Southern regions in accordance with climatic variability (fig. 1). This trend was coupled with changes in indications for performing adenotonsillectomy: more surgical procedures for obstructive cases, less for recurrent infection. The trend was confirmed by an epidemiological multicentric investigation performed in otorhinolaryngology units in different Italian regions [4].

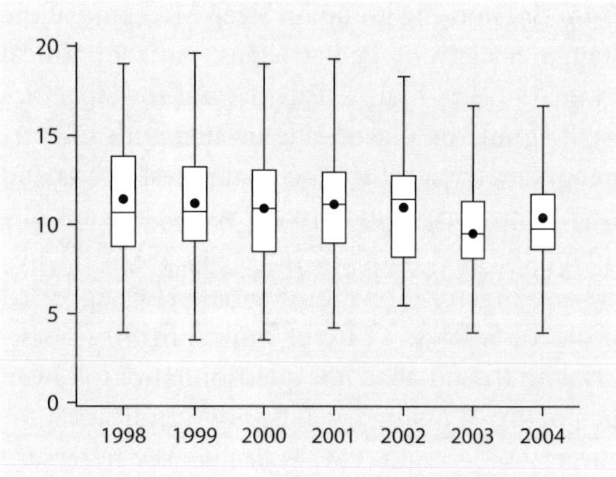

Fig. 1. Distribution of tonsillectomy standardized rates per region in Italy during the years 1998–2004.

Following a previous agreement, the working group met again to update the document publishing a guideline which was aimed at ensuring that tonsillectomy and adenoidectomy are not only clinically appropriate, but also safe and are carried out in a suitable health care setting. Appropriateness and safety in the guideline published in April 2008 are, thus, treated side by side from the title, not forgetting organizational issues and local health system.

Major revisions of the previous document were addressed to: (1) the diagnosis and indications for adenotonsillectomy in presence of obstructive sleep apnea syndrome (OSAS) in children according to an integrated clinical and instrumental approach; (2) the analysis of the advantages of new surgical techniques in terms of effectiveness, costs or the risk of post surgery bleeding or recurrences, and (3) the efficacy of perioperative management in reducing the incidence and duration of postoperative events.

Generally speaking, in fact, in the last years a relevant number of clinical studies and new evidence became available on the above-mentioned items making the need for a continuing updating of guidelines tangible.

Focusing on OSAS, the first document stated that: 'Adenotonsillectomy should be performed in children with significant OSAS. Since at that time there wasn't a single set of universally accepted criteria for evaluating and managing OSAS in children it was suggested that the decision should be based on clinical evaluation (day time sleepiness, load snoring, dispnea/apnea and open mouth breathing). Clinical evaluation was also considered sufficient for: (1) diagnosing full-blown OSAS, (2) excluding cases not requiring additional instrumental diagnosis or surgery, (3) diagnosing obstructive forms associated to other causes such as obesity, craniofacial malformations or hypothyroidism. A comment to this suggestion arrived immediately after the document publication from the working group on Sleep Medicine of the Italian Society of Pediatricians. As the clinical evaluation has high sensitivity, but low specificity it should be placed side by side with nocturnal ossimetry, a reliable screening test cheap and easy to perform. Nocturnal PSG is, without any doubt, the gold standard, but is limited by technical and organizational difficulties. The suggested protocol follows: a careful clinical history possibly with the aid of ad hoc questionnaires followed by nocturnal ossimetry; if positive, indication for surgery. Overnight, PSG is in this way necessary only in doubtful cases or in negative cases and in presence of symptoms.

Considering recurrent tonsillitis, more than to the indications for surgery, in case of recurrent/chronic tonsillitis the attention should be addressed to overcome the emerging problems of biofilm formation and bacterial internalization.

Concerning the surgical techniques and given the lack of evidence for justifying partial tonsillar ablation, total bilateral tonsillar removal seems to be indicated even for treating obstructive forms in children; in fact if tonsillotomy with intracapsular techniques results in lower postsurgical morbidity (pain, nausea and vomiting, return to normal activities) the risk of tonsillar residual or recurrent tissue is higher.

Comparing several surgical techniques available in the last years with traditional 'cold' dissection, we should analyze as outcomes the time required for surgery, intra-operative bleeding, post operative morbidity as well as the risks and costs for the health care system. The most updated data on this topic are the results of the English register of the National Prospective Tonsillectomy Audit [5] and the systematic review by Mowatt et al. [6]. According to these reviews, the risk of postsurgery bleeding is 3 times higher with bipolar diathermy compared to cold dissection, whereas the return to theater is 3 times more frequent with plasma dissection compared to cold dissection; contrasting results are reported regarding time required for surgery, postoperative pain and return to oral intake. As far as the attitude on this topic and the clinical reality in our country, in 2008 a paper was published on the official journal of our national society demonstrating that the radiofrequency based plasma dissection is superior to cold dissection with sutures as regard postoperative pain, analgesic use and the return to normal diet. However, the authors clearly state that this procedure should be considered a completely new surgical method which needs adequate training before obtaining benefits for the surgeon and the patient [7].

Managing tonsillectomy patient foresees a long list of preoperative, perioperative and in the immediate period after surgery procedures which should be carefully evaluated and weighted in collaboration with other specialists first of all anesthesiologists especially in children at risk for severe OSAS. Different ENTs in our country are adopting common protocols for the perioperative management of tonsillectomy children on line with the guideline and with the data from the literature.

In Italy, 1-day surgery (i.e. day surgery followed by 1 night hospital stay) seems to be the most suitable option for performing tonsillectomy with/without adenoidectomy, in both children and adults with no clinical and social contraindications. After the first document publication, this modality was adopted in several ENT Departments in our country, but still differences between northern and southern regions are observed related to organizational local realities and problems. On the other hand, a careful revision of the literature has demonstrated that this modality is still appropriate, provided that contraindications are kept steady and security rules implemented [8, 9].

The experience of drawing up a guideline could be summarized as follow: as its effect could tone down over the time, there is always the need for a steady revision: guidelines are really effective if adequately implemented and multidisciplinary combined interventions are the most effective.

References

1 Italian National Programme for Clinical Guidelines (PNLG) Address Document: The clinical and organisational appropriateness of tonsillectomy and/or adenoidectomy. Available at http://www.pnlg.it

2 Materia E, Di Domenicantonio R, Baglio G, et al: Epidemiology of tonsillectomy and/or adenoidectomy in Italy. Pediatr Med Chir 2004;26:179–186.

3 Materia E, Rossi L, Di Domenicantonio R, et al: Impatto del documento PNLG sugli interventi di adenotonsillectomia. Rapporto Osservazionale, 2007.

4 Motta G, Casolino D, Cassiano B, et al: Adenotonsillar surgery in Italy. Acta Otorhinolaryngol Ital 2008;28:1–6.

5 National Prospective Tonsillectomy Audit: Final report London: The Royal College of Surgeons of England, 2005. Available at www.rcseng.ac.uk

6 Mowatt G, Cook JA, Fraser C, et al: Systematic review of the safety of electrosurgery for tonsillectomy. Clin Otolaryngol 2006;31:95–102.

7 Di Rienzo Businco L, Coen Tirelli G: Paediatric tonsillectomy: radiofrequency based plasma dissection compared to cold dissection with sutures. Acta Otorhinolaryngol Ital 2008;28:67–72.

8 Brigger MT, Brietzke SE: Outpatient tonsillectomy in children: a systematic review. Otolaryngol Head Neck Surg 2006;135:1–7.

9 Singarelli S, Berni A, Coppo G, et al: Day surgery, one-day surgery: the experience of an ENT unit in a 250 bed hospital. Acta Otorhinolaryngol Ital 2005;25:365–369.

Luisa Maria Bellussi
Via Anagnina, 718
IT–00118 Roma (Italy)
Tel. +39 3477944777, Fax +39 0679844154, E-Mail l.bellussi@virgilio.it

Harabuchi Y (ed): Recent Advances in Tonsils and Mucosal Barriers of the Upper Airways.
Adv Otorhinolaryngol. Basel, Karger, 2011, vol 72, pp 146–148

Diversity of Mucosal Immune Responses in Upper Respiratory Organs and Its Application for Mucosal Vaccine

Yuichi Kurono · Keiichi Miyashita · Takaho Makise · Hiromi Nagano

Department of Otolaryngology, Faculty of Medicine, Kagoshima University, Kagoshima, Japan

Abstract

Mucosal vaccine has been considered a promising strategy to prevent upper respiratory infections. As the immunization routes to induce mucosal immune responses, oral, intranasal, and sublingual immunizations are proposed for clinical application. Recently, it has been reported that transcutaneous immunization is also capable of inducing mucosal immune responses. However, it still remains unclear which route is the most effective to induce mucosal immune responses in upper respiratory organs. In order to investigate the differences in the immune responses among several mucosal immunizations, mice were immunized with phosphorylcholine (PC) together with cholera toxin (CT) as mucosal adjuvant intranasally, sublingually, and transcutaneously, and the mucosal as well as systemic immune responses were compared. PC-specific IgA antibody titers in saliva and nasal wash were increased by intaranasal as well as sublingual immunization to the same levels. However, IgE levels induced by mucosal immunization were remarkably reduced by sublingual immunization. Transcutaneous immunization increased mucosal IgA responses, although the levels were lower than those induced by intaranasal and sublingual immunization. Those results suggest that sublingual immunization might be superior to the other immunizations in inducing PC-specific mucosal immune responses in upper respiratory tract.

Since intranasal influenza vaccine developed in United States showed remarkable effects in preventing not only influenza but also following occurrence of acute otitis media [1], mucosal vaccine has been considered a promising strategy to prevent upper respiratory infections. As the immunization routes to induce mucosal immune responses, oral, intranasal, and sublingual immunizations are proposed for clinical application [2, 3]. Recently, it has been reported that transcutaneous immunization is also capable of inducing mucosal as well as systemic immune responses [4]. However, it still remains unclear which route is the most effective to induce mucosal immune responses in upper respiratory organs.

In the present study, mucosal immune responses against phosphorylcholine (PC), a structural component of a wide variety of Gram-positive and Gram-negative bacterium, was investigated by intranasal, sublingual, and transcutaneous immunization. The availability of

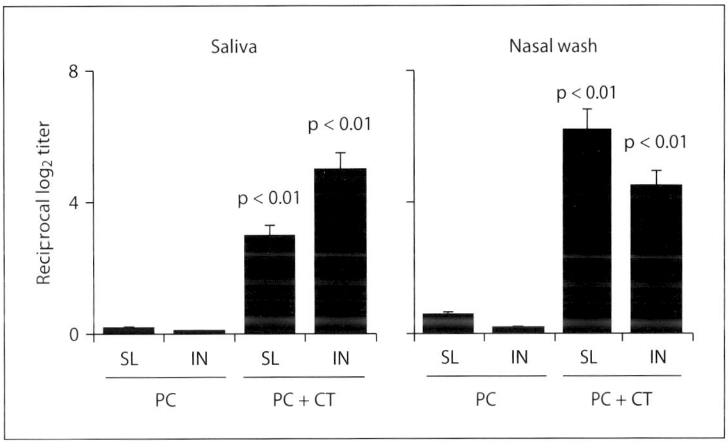

Fig. 1. Anti-PC IgA responses by intranasal (IN) and sublingual (SL) immunization. PC = Phosphorylcholine; CT = cholera toxin.

PC as mucosal vaccine and the usefulness of the mucosal and transcutaneous immunization with PC were discussed.

Materials and Methods

BALB/c 6-week-old female mice were immunized intranasally, sublingually, and transcutaneously with PC and cholera toxin (CT) as a mucosal adjuvant. In transcutaneous immunization, a dorsal portion or the skin was shaved and a cotton patch soaked with the antigen was attached for 24 h. Nasal wash, saliva, serum and mucosal specimens were collected on day 7 after the final immunization. PC-specific antibody activities in those samples were examined by ELISA and ELISPOT assay.

Results

Intranasal Immunization with PC

Intranasal immunization with PC together with CT induced increased levels of PC-specific IgA in saliva and nasal wash, and PC-specific salivary IgA and serum IgG were cross-reactive with all strains of *Streptococcus pneumoniae* and *Haemophilus influenzae*. Moreover, clearance of both bacteria from the nasal cavity was significantly enhanced by intranasal immunization with PC [5].

Sublingual Immunization with PC

Sublingual immunization with PC together with CT increased PC-specific IgA in saliva and nasal wash in the same levels induced by intranasal immunization with PC and CT. (fig. 1) PC-specific IgG in serum was also increased. The pattern of IgG subclasses was almost same in both intranasal and sublingual immunization, and Th2-type responses, such as IgG1 and IgG2b, were dominant in both groups. However, IgG2a level was significantly higher in sublingual immunization than intranasal immunization, suggesting that the Th1-type immune response is stronger in sublingual immunization. Further, sublingual immunization with PC did not increase IgE levels as observed in intranasal immunization.

IgE Production by Intranasal Immunization with PC

Intranasal administration of bacterial antigen might affect olfactory and the other central nervous systems. Recently, it has been reported that intranasal vaccination with inactivated influenza intranasal vaccine frequently induced Bell's palsy [6]. Those findings indicate the importance of the study regarding side reactions of mucosal vaccine. Since mucosal immunization induces Th2-type immune responses, the production of

IgE and the occurrence of type I allergy are concerned. In fact, intranasal immunization with CT induced an increased level of IgE in serum. However, intranasal immunization with PC did not induce IgE production and even reduced the lgE level increased by CT. In order to investigate the mechanism of PC in reducing IgE production, mice were sensitized with OVA after intranasal immunization with PC and serum IgE levels were compared. In results, IgE levels were remarkably increased after intranasal sensitization with OVA. However, the levels were significantly lower in mice intranasally immunized with PC when compared to mice having no previous immunization with PC.

Transcutaneous Immunization with PC
According to the method reported by Koizumi et al. [4], the immune responses induced by transcutaneous immunization with PC was investigated. PC was administered with CT transcutaneously three times every week. Although the responses were not remarkable, serum and salivary IgG and nasal wash IgA levels were increased after the immunization.

Conclusions

The present study demonstrates that mucosal immune responses in the upper respiratory tract vary according to the route and antigen used for immunization. Among several vaccinations, sublingual immunization might be superior to the other immunizations in inducing PC-specific mucosal immune responses in the upper respiratory tract. Further investigation is needed for the development of transcutaneous vaccination.

References

1 Belshe RB, Mendelman PM: Safety and efficacy of live attenuated, cold-adapted, influenza vaccine-trivalent. Immunol Allergy Clin North Am 2003; 23:745–767.
2 Kurono Y, Yamamoto M, Fujihashi K, Kodama S, Suzuki M, Mogi G, McGhee JR, Kiyono H: Nasal immunization induces *Haemophilus influenzae*-specific Th1 and Th2 responses with mucosal IgA and systemic IgG antibodies for protective immunity. J Infect Dis 1999;180:122–132.
3 Song JH, Nguyen HH, Cuburu N, Horimoto T, Ko SY, Park SH, Czerkinsky C, Kweon MN: Sublingual vaccination with influenza virus protects mice against lethal viral infection. Proc Natl Acad Sci USA 2008;105:1644–1649.
4 Koizumi Y, Kurita-Ochiai T, Yamamoto M: Transcutaneous immunization with an outer membrane protein of *Porphyromonas gingivalis* without adjuvant elicits marked antibody responses. Oral Microbiol Immunol 2008;23:131–138.
5 Tanaka N, Fukuyama S, Fukuiwa T, et al: Intranasal immunization with phosphorylcholine induces antigen specific mucosal and systemic immune responses in mice. Vaccine 2007;25:2680–2687.
6 Mutsch M, Zhou W, Rhodes P, et al: Use of the inactivated intranasal influenza vaccine and the risk of Bell's palsy in Switzerland. N Engl J Med 2004;350:896–903.

Yuichi Kurono
Department of Otolaryngology, Faculty of Medicine, Kagoshima University
8–35–5 Sakuragaoka
Kagoshima 890-8520 (Japan)
E-Mail u196kuro@m2.kufm.kagoshima-u.ac.jp

Harabuchi Y (ed): Recent Advances in Tonsils and Mucosal Barriers of the Upper Airways.
Adv Otorhinolaryngol. Basel, Karger, 2011, vol 72, pp 149–152

Nasal Submucosal Administration of Antigen-Presenting Cells Induces Effective Immunological Responses in Cancer Immunotherapy

Yoshitaka Okamoto[a] · Akira Fujikawa[a] · Motoyoshi Kurosaki[a] · Kazuki Yamasaki[a] · Daijyu Sakurai[a] · Shigetoshi Horiguchi[a] · Toshinori Nakayama[b]

[a]Department of Otorhinolaryngology, Head and Neck Surgery, Graduate School of Medicine, Chiba University Hospital, and [b]Department of Immunology, Graduate School of Medicine, Chiba University, Chiba, Japan

Abstract

Human NKT cells are known to have strong antitumor activities and to be activated by specific ligand, α-galactosylceramide (αGelCer). We examined the migration pattern of αGalCer-pulsed DCs and the immune responses after administration by different routes. DCs injected into nasal submucosa quickly migrated to the lateral neck lymph rather than the lateral lymph nodes. The absolute number of NKT cells and the IFN-γ-producing cells increased in peripheral blood after injection of the DCs into nasal submucosa. We conducted a phase I study with αGalCer-pulsed DCs administered in nasal submucosa of patients with head and neck cancer, and evaluated safety and feasibility. The results showed that nasal submucosal administration of α GalCer pulsed DCs was safe and a smaller number of these DCs could exhibit significant immune responses and some positive clinical effects. In additional study, the use of the intra-arterial infusion of activated NKT cells and the submucosal injection of α-GalCer-pulsed DCs has been shown to induce significant antitumor immunity and had beneficial clinical effects in the management of advanced head and neck squamous cell carcinoma. The NKT cell-based cancer immunotherapy may be helpful in management of head and neck cancer and needs to be explored in further detail.

Cancer immunotherapy could be expected to be one of the combined modalities as an adjuvant for cancer therapy; however, its efficacy still needs to be improved.

Natural killer T (NKT) cells represent a unique lymphocyte subpopulation. After activation, humanVα24NKT cells show a strong anti-tumor activity against various malignant tumors both in vivo and in vitro. α-Galactosylceramide (α-GalCer) is known to be an exogenous ligand and activate NKT cells [1, 2].

Recently dendritic cells (DCs) have been shown to play a crucial role in the induction of the primary T cell-dependent immune response and DC-based cancer immunotherapy has shown to induce significant immunological responses and some clinical effects in the patients with a variety of cancer, such as gastric cancer, prostate cancer and colon cancer [3]. However, the desirable administration route of the tumor antigen pulsed DCs to induce effective antitumor response were still unknown. Most head and neck cancer arise from upper respiratory or digestive mucosa and the neck lymph nodes are well known as the draining regional lymph nodes. The intramucosally administered DCs may be expected to migrate to the regional lymph nodes and effectively induce mucosal antitumor responses.

Materials and Methods

The number of NKT cells in the peripheral blood, IFN-γ production and proliferation capacity were analyzed before and after 50 Gy radiation therapy in 12 patients with stage IV head and neck squamous cell carcinoma. The cytotoxic activity of NKT cells was also examined in vitro.

The migration pattern of DCs and the immune responses after administration by different routes were examined in the patients with head and neck cancer using indium-labeled DCs and single photon emission computed tomography (SPECT) images. Anti-tumor immune responses in the peripheral blood were also examined.

A phase I study with α-GalCer-pulsed DCs administered in the nasal submucosa of patients with head and neck cancer was conducted to evaluate the safety and feasibility of the treatment. Nine patients with unresectable or recurrent head and neck cancer received two treatments one week apart, of 1×10^8 of α-GalCer-pulsed autologous DCs into the nasal submucosa.

A Phase I study was designed with the intra-arterial administration of in vitro expanded Vα24 NKT cells to patients with recurrent refractory head and neck squamous cell carcinoma, in combination with nasal submucosal injection of α-GalCer-pulsed DCs mentioned just before. Eight patients received superselective transcatheter intra-arterial infusion of activated Vα24 NKT cells into tumor-feeding arteries and nasal submucosal injections of α-GalCer-pulsed DCs twice with a 1-week interval.

Results

The number of NKT cells was the same after radiation therapy as before. The IFN-γ production from exogenous ligand, α-GalCer, stimulate NKT cells collected just after radiotherapy was impaired after stimulation with exogenous ligand, but the proliferative responses of these NKT cells was enhanced in comparison to those collected before radiation therapy. These proliferated NKT cells had significant antitumor activities in the cytotoxic assay [4].

DCs injected into nasal submucosa and oral floor migrated to lateral neck lymph nodes and submandibular lymph nodes [5]. Nasal mucosal administration induced elevation of NKT cell number and IFN-γ-producing cell number but oral mucosa did not [6].

The nasal submucosal administration of α-GalCer-pulsed DCs for patients with head and neck cancer was safe and a small number of these DCs without inconvenience of apheresis with no adverse effects could exhibit significant immune responses and some positive clinical effects [7].

The use of the intra-arterial infusion of activated Vα24 NKT cells and the submucosal injection of αGalCer-pulsed DCs has been shown to induce significant antitumor immunity and had beneficial clinical effects in the management of advanced head and neck squamous cell carcinoma [8].

Discussion

To improve the survival and QoL of the patients with head and neck cancer, the development of new treatment strategies is of critical importance.

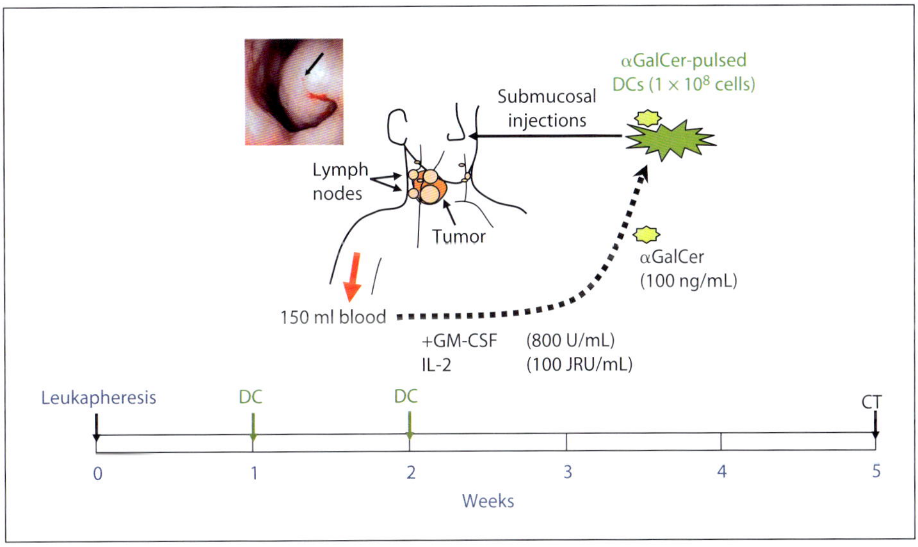

Fig. 1. Study protocol. Primary endpoint: to confirm the safety profile. Secondary endpoint: to detect the NKT cell-specific immune responses: to validate the antitumor effect.

NKT cells are relatively resistant to radiation and immunotherapy with NKT cells might be suitable for effective immunotherapy of head and neck cancer as a new treatment modality. As most head and neck cancer arises from mucosa in the upper respiratory or digestive tract, the submucosal administration of α-GarCer-pulsed DCs might be an effective treatment modality for head and neck cancer. In addition, a superselective administration of activated effector cells to the cancer-feeding artery is possible and can provide an efficient targeting to the cancer tissue inducing effective antitumor responses.

Further studies to certify and to improve the clinical benefits are required.

References

1 Schuler G, Schuler-Thurner B, Steinman RM: The use of dendritic cells in cancer immunotherapy. Curr Opin Immunol 2003;15:138–147.

2 Taniguchi M, Harada M, Kojo S, Nakayama T, Wakao H: The regulatory role of Valpha14 NKT cells in innate and acquired immune response. Annu Rev Immunol 2003;21:483–513.

3 Kawano T, Cui J, Koezuka Y, Toura I, Kaneko Y, Motoki K, Ueno H, Nakagawa R, Sato H, Kondo E, Koseki H, Taniguchi M: CD1d-restricted and TCR-mediated activation of valpha14 NKT cells by glycosylceramides. Science 1997;278:1626–1629.

4 Horiguchi S, Matsuoka T, Okamoto Y, Sakurai D, Kobayashi K, Chazono H, Hanazawa T, Tanaka Y: Migration of tumor antigen-pulsed dendritic cells after mucosal administration in the human upper respiratory tract. J Clin Immunol 2007;27:598–604.

5 Kobayashi K, Tanaka Y, Horiguchi S, Yamamoto S, Nakayma T, Sugimoto A, Okamoto Y: The effect of radiotherapy on NKT cells in patients with advanced head and neck cancer. Cancer Immunol Immunother 2010;59: 1503–1509.

6 Kurosaki M, Horiguchi S, Yamasaki K, Kunii N, Nakayama T, Okamoto Y: Migration and immunological reaction after administration of αGalCer-pulsed antigen presenting cells into different sites of patients with head and neck cancer. Cancer Immunol Immunother 2011;60:207–215.

7 Uchida T, Horiguchi S, Tanaka Y, Yamamoto H, Kunii N, Motohashi S, Taniguchi M, Nakayama T, Okamoto Y: Phase I study of alpha-galactosylceramide-pulsed antigen presenting cells administration to the nasal submucosa in unresectable or recurrent head and neck cancer. Cancer Immunol Immunother 2008;57:337–345.

8 Kunii N, Horiguchi S, Motohashi S, Yamamoto H, Ueno N, Yamamoto S, Sakurai D, Taniguchi M, Nakayama T, Okamoto Y: Combination therapy of in vitro-expanded natural killer T cells and alpha-galactosylceramide-pulsed antigen-presenting cells in patients with recurrent head and neck carcinoma. Cancer Sci 2009;100:1092–1098.

Yoshitaka Okamoto
Department of Otolaryngology, Head and Neck Surgery
Graduate School of Medicine, Chiba University Hospital
1–8–1 Inohana, Chuo-ku
Chiba 260-8670 (Japan)
Tel. +81 43 226 2578, Fax +81 43 227 3442, E-Mail yokamoto@faculty.chiba-u.jp

Harabuchi Y (ed): Recent Advances in Tonsils and Mucosal Barriers of the Upper Airways.
Adv Otorhinolaryngol. Basel, Karger, 2011, vol 72, pp 153–156

Respiratory Syncytial Virus Infection and the Tight Junctions of Nasal Epithelial Cells

Hiroyuki Tsutsumi[a] · Takashi Kojima[d] · Satoshi Hirakawa[a] · Tomoyuki Masaki[b] · Tamaki Okabayashi[c] · Shinichi Yokota[c] · Nobuhiro Fujii[c] · Tetsuo Himi[b] · Norimasa Sawada[d]

Departments of [a]Pediatrics, [b]Otolaryngology and [c]Microbiology and [d]2nd Department of Pathology, Sapporo Medical University School of Medicine, Sapporo, Japan

Abstract

Respiratory syncytial virus (RSV) primarily infects upper respiratory tract cells, mainly nasal epithelial cells. The tight junctions of nasal epithelial cells are thought to perform important innate immune function against foreign materials including respiratory viruses. We investigated in vitro the relationship of RSV infection and the tight junctions of primary nasal epithelial cells which had been transfected with human telomerase reverse transcriptase (hTERT) to prolong cell life. Nasal epithelial cells developed tight junctions when cultured in medium containing fetal bovine serum, and these cells showed apparent resistance to RSV infection compared to control cells. RSV could infect these cells from apical but not basolateral side, suggesting that only apical side possess RSV receptor or a mechanism for absorbing RSV particles. Importantly, RSV infection of the cells enhanced the expression of tight junction proteins occludin, claudin-4 and ZO-1. These findings suggest that RSV infection induces polarity in the infected cells. This polarity could facilitate cellular secretion of propagated RSV, thereby spreading the infection.

Respiratory syncytial virus (RSV) is now recognized as the most important viral agent of serious pediatric respiratory tract disease worldwide, i.e. acute bronchitis, bronchiolitis and pneumonia. RSV first establishes infection in nasopharyngeal epithelial cells and initiates replication. Against it, the epithelial barrier of the nasal mucosa plays a crucial role in host defense against respiratory viral infection. This barrier is regulated in large part by tight junctions. This time, we investigated the correlation of RSV infection and tight junctions of nasal epithelial cells in vitro.

An in vitro RSV Infection System in hTERT-Transfected Human Nasal Epithelial Cells Established by Us

The mechanisms regulating tight junction barrier in nasal epithelial cells remain unclear because the proliferation of epithelial cells in primary culture are limited. We established an in vitro RSV infection system in hTERT-transfected human cells [1].

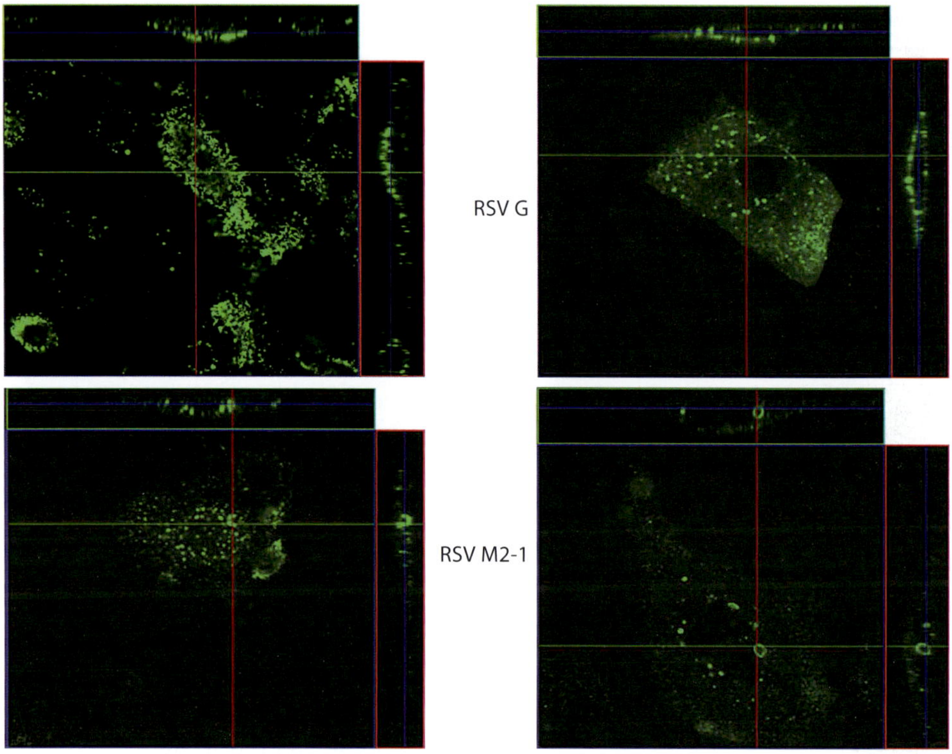

Fig. 1. Staining of RSV-infected nasal epithelial cells with anti-RSV F, G, NP and M2–1 antibodies (findings with the confocal microscope).

Surgically removed nasal epithelial cells were digested by enzyme and transfected with the hTERT gene to prolong life span. RSV (Long strain) can infect and propagate successfully in these nasal epithelial cells, and this was confirmed by FA staining with RSV-specific MAbs (fig. 1) [2, 3]. F and G envelope proteins exist in cytoplasm just under a cytoplasmic membrane of apical side. On the other hand, NP, M2–1 nucleocapsid proteins exist in cytoplasm around the nucleus.

Tight Junctions Perform a Barrier Function against RSV Infection

Nasal epithelial cells develop tight junctions shown by ZO-1 immunostaining, when cultured in medium containing fetal bovine serum (FBS) (fig. 2a). RSV (Long strain) was inoculated at MOI of 1 and incubated 24 h. The cells with developed tight junctions showed apparent resistance to RSV infection compared to control cells (fig. 2b), which implies a protective effect of the tight junction against RSV infection.

RSV Can Only Infect hTERT-Transfected Human Nasal Epithelial Cells from the Apical Side

Do tight junctions work as the only barrier against RSV? Is RSV unable to infect the nasal cell from the basolateral side? To settle these questions, an experiment of RSV infection to the cells with developed tight junctions was performed in a double chamber. RSV could infect the nasal epithelial cells only apical side (data not shown), suggesting that only

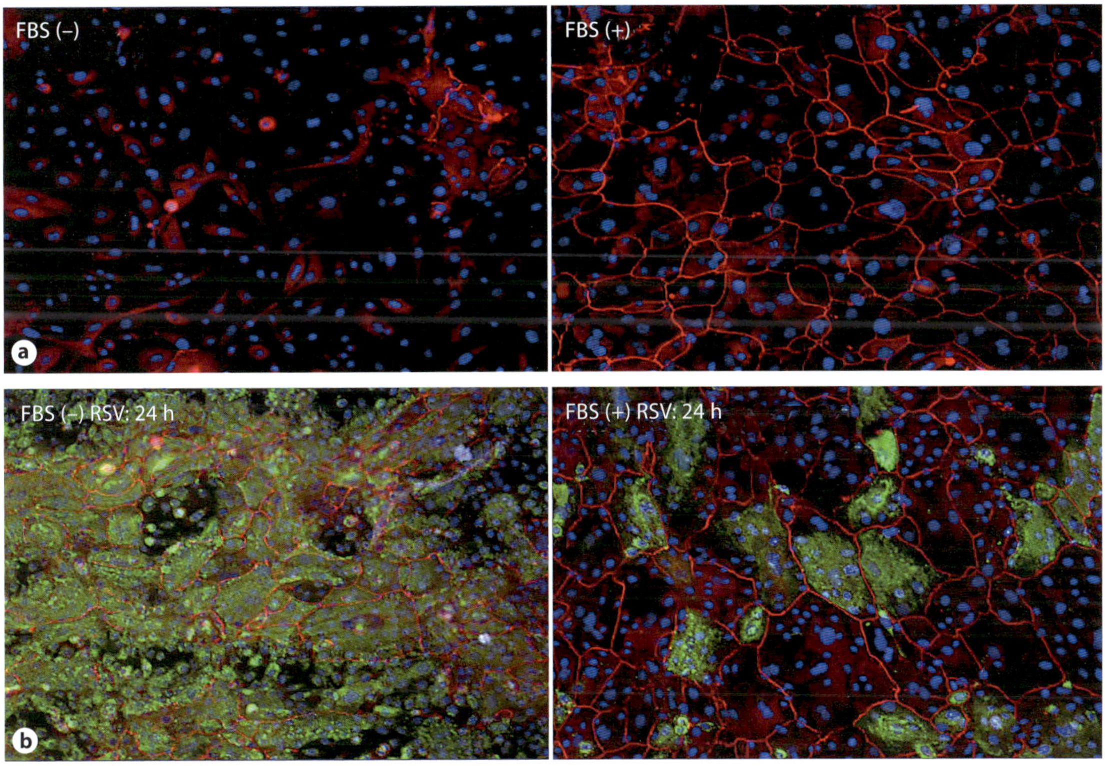

Fig. 2. Staining of nasal epithelial cells cultured with or without FBS with anti-ZO-1 antibody (**a**), and staining of RSV-infected nasal epithelial cells with anti-ZO-1 and anti-RSV F antibodies (**b**).

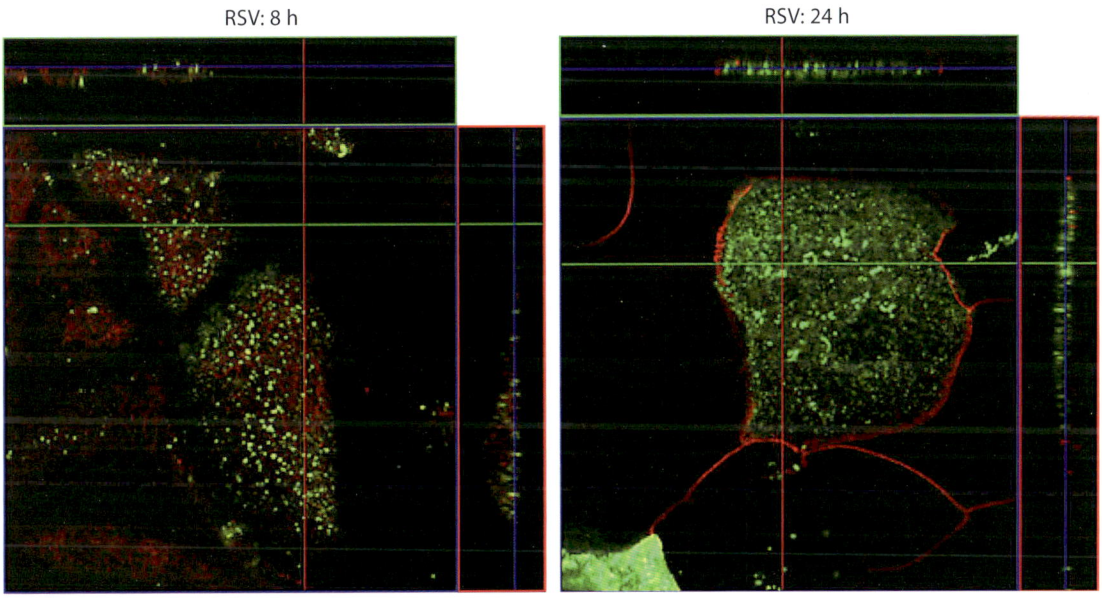

Fig. 3. Staining of RSV-infected nasal epithelial cells with anti-ZO-1 and anti-RSV G antibodies (findings with the confocal microscope).

apical side possess RSV receptor or a mechanism for absorbing RSV particles. The development of tight junctions polarizes nasal cells, which in turn may restrict the virus entry system to the apical side.

RSV Infection Develops Tight Junctions of Human Nasal Epithelial Cells

On the other hand, we confirmed that RSV infection itself gradually develops several tight junctions of nasal cells. Figure 3 shows that tight junctions developed with time after RSV inoculation, in proportion to progress of RSV infection. After all, RSV infection of nasal epithelial cells induces polarity of the cells and may induce the system by which propagated RSV can be secreted from the apical side of the infected cells to spread infection efficiently to adjacent cells. The mechanisms of these phenomena are now being investigated at protein and gene level.

References

1 Kurose M, et al: Induction of claudins in passaged hTERT-transfected human nasal epithelial cells with an extended life span. Cell Tissue Res 2007;330:63.

2 Nagai K, et al: Three antigenic variant groups in human respiratory syncytial virus subgroup B isolated in Japan. Arch Virol 1993;128:55.

3 Masaki T, et al: An NF-κB signaling pathway via PKCδ regulates replication of respiratory syncytial virus in polarized normal human nasal epithelial cells. Mol Biol Cell 2011 May 11 [Epub ahead of print].

Hiroyuki Tsutsumi
Department of Pediatrics, Sapporo Medical University School of Medicine
S-1, W-16, Chuo-ku
Sapporo, 060-8543 (Japan)
Tel. +81 11 611 2111, E-Mail tsutsumi@sapmed.ac.jp

Harabuchi Y (ed): Recent Advances in Tonsils and Mucosal Barriers of the Upper Airways.
Adv Otorhinolaryngol. Basel, Karger, 2011, vol 72, pp 157–159

A Novel Immune Evasion Mechanism of LMP-1, an EBV-Primary Oncogene, in Nasopharyngeal Carcinoma

Tomokazu Yoshizaki

Division of Otolaryngology, Head and Neck Surgery, Graduate School of Medical Science, Kanazawa University, Takaramachi, Kanazawa, Japan

Abstract

Nasopharyngeal carcinoma is an Epstein-Barr virus (EBV)-associated tumor. Viruses that are associated with malignant transformation have evolved unique mechanisms to interfere with this interaction to evade antiviral T cell responses. EBV exploits many immune evasive strategies to successfully establish a latent infection in B cells. CD8+ T cell responses to LMP-1 are generally very low and rarely detected in healthy virus carriers. Activation of the NF-kB pathway by EBV-LMP-1 leads to an upregulation of the MHC class I antigen-processing pathway. Paradoxically, LMP-1 itself induces a subdominant CD8+ T cell response and appears to have evolved to avoid immune recognition. An expression of LMP-1 in human cells enhanced the *trans*-presentation of CD8+ T cell epitopes; however, *cis*-presentation of LMP-1-derived epitopes was severely impaired. Deletion of the first transmembrane domain of LMP-1, which prevented self-aggregation, significantly enhanced the *cis*-presentation of T cell epitopes from this protein, whereas it lost its ability to upregulate *trans*-presentation. These results delineate a novel mechanism of immune evasion, which renders a virally encoded oncogene inaccessible to the conventional MHC class I pathway limiting its *cis*-presentation.

Epstein-Barr virus (EBV) exploits many immune evasive strategies to successfully establish a latent infection in B cells and epithelial malignant tumors such as nasopharyngeal carcinoma (NPC). Analysis of the role of individual EBV latent antigens in the regulation of antigen-processing genes indicated that latent membrane protein-1 (LMP-1) was sufficient to upregulate the expression of transporters associated with antigen processing and *trans*-presentation of MHC class I-restricted epitopes in B cells [1]. Subsequent studies demonstrated that the immunomodulatory effects of LMP-1 are mediated through C-terminal activator regions (CTAR1 and CTAR2), which are involved in the induction of nuclear factor-κB (NF-κB). At the same time, LMP-1 promotes invasion and metastasis through these intracellular activation domains [2–4]. Paradoxically, the population of CD8+ T cells that responded to LMP-1 is generally very low and rarely detected in healthy virus carriers, suggesting that LMP-1 may limit its *cis*-presentation through the MHC class I pathway. We have delineated a mechanism by which LMP-1 limits its self-presentation without compromising its ability to modulate *trans*-presentation of the CD8+ T cell epitope [5, 6].

To assess *trans*-presentation of LMP-1, we transfected multiple LMP-1 sequences to epithelial cell lines. Although all LMP-1 variants upregulated the expression of MHC class I on a human epithelial cell line, C33A, considerable activation of LMP-1-specific T cells was only evident after incubation with peptide-sensitized cells. In contrast, LMP-1 expression in C33A cells enhanced *trans*-presentation of CD8+ T cell epitopes from another EBV-encoded membrane protein, LMP-2A. Collectively, these results suggested that, despite its capacity to upregulate *trans*-presentation via the MHC class I pathway, LMP-1 limits its self-presentation to CD8+ T cells.

Much of the data presented are based on either stable or transient expression of LMP-1. To confirm these observations, we assessed the endogenous presentation of LMP-1 epitopes in EBV-transformed LCLs. Although activation of LMP-2A-specific T cells was evident after incubation with HLA-matched LCLs, very low levels of activation of T cells specific for multiple LMP-1-encoded peptide epitopes was observed. Activation of LMP-1-specific T cells could be detected after incubation with peptide-sensitized LCLs.

To investigate the mechanism for this immune evasion, we tested a series of LMP-1 expression vectors with mutations in the CTAR1 and/or CTAR2 domain as well as a deletion mutant commencing at the second methionine of LMP-1 (Δ1–43LMP-1-GFP), which removes the first trans-membrane domain. This domain has been shown to have an immunomodulatory effect, and Δ1–43LMP-1 has been used for expanding LMP-1-specific T cells. Although mutations within the CTAR domains had no impact on the presentation of LMP-1 epitopes, deletion of the first trans-membrane domain enhanced endogenous presentation of HLA class I-restricted epitopes. Consistent with previous studies, intracellular localization analysis using fluorescent microscopy revealed that, although full-length LMP-1 and its CTAR mutants formed large aggregates in the perinuclear region, Δ1–43LMP-1-GFP lost its ability to aggregate. This enhanced presentation was not the result of increased expression of Δ1–43LMP-1-GFP compared with full-length LMP-1. These observations indicate that, although the NF-κB signaling domains had no impact on the *cis*-presentation of LMP-1 epitopes, aggregation of this protein (a critical requirement for *trans*-presentation) limits its accessibility to the MHC class I processing machinery.

The data presented in this meeting indicate that, in addition to constraining its *cis*-presentation through aggregation, epitopes encoded within LMP-1 protein are most probably destroyed by cellular proteasomes, providing a dual strategy by which LMP-1 limits self-presentation to CD8+ T cells [7].

Acknowledgement

In addition to the author, this work was contributed by Corey Smith, Naohiro Wakisaka and Rajiv Khanna.

References

1 Rowe M, Khanna R, Jacob CA, et al: Restoration of endogenous antigen processing in Burkitt's lymphoma cells by Epstein-Barr virus latent membrane protein-1: coordinated up-regulation of peptide transporters and HLA-class I antigen expression. Eur J Immunol 1995;25:1374–1384.

2 Yoshizaki T, Sato H, Furukawa M, Pagano J: The expression of matrix metalloproteinase 9 is enhanced by Epstein-Barr virus latent membrane protein 1. Proc Natl Acad Sci USA 1998;95:3621–3626.

3 Wakisaka N, Kondo S, Yoshizaki T, Murono S, Furukawa M, Pagano JS: Epstein-Barr virus latent membrane protein 1 induces synthesis of hypoxia-inducible factor 1{alpha}. Mol Cell Biol 2004;24:5223–5234.

4 Kondo S, Seo SY, Yoshizaki T, Wakisaka N, Furukawa M, Joab I, Jang KL, Pagano JS: EBV latent membrane protein 1 up-regulates hypoxia-inducible factor 1alpha through Siah1-mediated down-regulation of prolyl hydroxylases 1 and 3 in nasopharyngeal epithelial cells. Cancer Res 2006;66:9870–9877.

5 Khanna R, Burrows SR: Role of cytotoxic T lymphocytes in Epstein-Barr virus-associated diseases. Annu Rev Microbiol 2000;54:19–48.

6 Smith C, Cooper L, Burgess M, et al: Functional reversion of antigen-specific CD8+ T cells from patients with Hodgkin lymphoma following in vitro stimulation with recombinant polyepitope. J Immunol 2006;177: 4897–4906.

7 Smith C, Wakisaka N, Crough T, Peet J, Yoshizaki T, Beagley L, Khanna R: Discerning regulation of *cis*- and *trans*-presentation of CD8+ T-cell epitopes by EBV-encoded oncogene LMP-1 through self-aggregation. Blood 2009;113:6148–6152.

Tomokazu Yoshizaki
Division of Otolaryngology, Head and Neck Surgery
Graduate School of Medical Science, Kanazawa University
13–1 Takaramachi
Kanazawa 920-8641 (Japan)
E-Mail tomoy@med.kanazawa-u.ac.jp

Harabuchi Y (ed): Recent Advances in Tonsils and Mucosal Barriers of the Upper Airways.
Adv Otorhinolaryngol. Basel, Karger, 2011, vol 72, pp 160–163

Otitis Media and Tonsils – Role of Adenoidectomy in the Treatment of Chronic Otitis Media with Effusion

Keehyun Park

Department of Otolaryngology, Ajou University School of Medicine, Suwon, South Korea

Abstract

Innate immunity involves the first line of the mucosal defense system. Homeostatic defense of the middle ear and Eustachian tube is maintained in part by molecules related to the innate immunity. The middle ear and tonsils are the organs related to the innate immunity. Recent attention has focused on the possibility that chronic otitis media and adenotonsillitis may represent a chronic infective state such as evidenced in conditions secondary to biofilms or small colony variants. The role of biofilms in the persistence of chronic mucosal-based ENT-related infections was first recognized in otitis media and adenotonsillitis. The efficacy of adenotonsillectomy on otitis media with effusion (OME) has been demonstrated by several randomized and controlled studies. It was speculated that tonsil and adenoid may play a role as an infectious focus to OME. In summary, patients suffering from recurrent or chronic OME may benefit from adenoidectomy due to the removal of an infectious source in the nasopharynx rather than the removal of a large adenoidal mass.

Otitis media is one of the most common diseases in childhood. The three major pathogens responsible for acute otitis media and otitis media with effusion (OME) are *Streptococcus pneumoniae, Haemophilus influenzae* and *Moraxella catarrhalis*. Nasopharyngeal colonization of these pathogens is associated with the development of otitis media. Three requirements are needed for otitis media to take place: bacterial adherence on the nasopharynx, bacterial entry to the middle ear via the Eustachian tube, and bacterial replication in the middle ear.

This chapter about the relationship between otitis media and tonsil was reviewed according to the following points:

1. The tonsil and middle ear are the organs related to the innate immunity.
2. Chronic adenotonsillitis and otitis media are a biofilm infection.
3. The adenoid leads to mechanical or inflammatory obstruction of the Eustachian tube: the role of adenoidectomy in the management of chronic OME.

Tonsil and Middle Ear as the Organs Related to the Innate Immunity

Homeostatic defenses of the middle ear and Eustachian tube are maintained in part by molecules related to the innate immunity, mucins, surface active substances, and aquaporins. The molecules related to the innate immunity are lysozyme, lactoferrin, defensin, collectin, Toll-like receptor, superoxide dismutase, etc.

Expression of β-defensin in human middle ear mucosa was noted by immunohistochemistry and RT-PCR [1]. β-Defensin 1 was expressed in both normal and inflamed middle ear mucosa, but β-defensins 2 and 3 were found only in the inflamed mucosa. Expression of β-defensin 1 in human palatine tonsil was also noted by in situ hybridization and RT-PCR [2]. We could show that β-defensin 1 is expressed in normal human tonsil and middle ear mucosa.

Expression of superoxide dismutase (SOD) was investigated as a protective system of the palatine tonsil and adenoid against O_2^- [3]. The immune reaction for cupper zinc superoxide dismutase (CuZnSOD) was diffusely expressed in the epithelial cells and subepithelial inflammatory cells of the adenoid. However, an immune reaction was rarely expressed in the germinal center of the palatine tonsil. Expression of CuZnSOD m-RNA was also noted by RT-PCR. Its activity significantly increased in the adenoids of OME patients. This result indicated that the pediatric adenoids and tonsils showed a site-specific CuZnSOD distribution. Another investigation of SOD was the comparison of its activity between the OME group and the non-OME group. Adenoids of the patients of the OME group showed higher ratio of SOD than those of the patients without OME. The ratio in tonsils between two groups was not significantly different. This result indicated that when considering the close anatomical location between the adenoid and Eustachian tube, there may be a close relationship between the increased level of O_2^- that leads to a CuZnSOD increase in the adenoid, and the development of otitis media. These studies about SOD demonstrated the potential clinical role of free radical scavengers in the pediatric adenoids and tonsils.

Chronic Adenotonsillitis and Otitis Media as a Biofilm Infection

Bacteria have historically been thought of as isolated organisms; however, it is now clear that the vast majority of bacteria exist in complex communities, attached to surfaces, known as biofilms. Biofilms are increasingly recognized as playing a role in diseases of otolaryngologic interest [4]. Bacterial biofilm is a common cause of persistent infections. Both chronic adenotonsillitis and otitis media were already confirmed as a biofilm infection. Al-Mazrou et al. [5] showed infected adenoid covered with biofilms, and an adenoid in child with obstructive sleep apnea syndrome did not show biofilms. Post [6] made biofilms through experimental otitis media induced by *H. influenza* in chinchilla. He also confirmed biofilms on the tympanostomy tube removed from a child with otorrhea. Effects of tympanostomy tube insertion in the management of chronic OME are that reventilation increases oxygen tension potentially altering the biofilm phenotypes, and suctioning of the effusion mechanically disrupts and debulks the biofim, and finally host middle ear mucosal defenses are restored.

Role of Adenoidectomy in the Management of Chronic OME

Clinical practice guideline on OME from the American Academy of Pediatrics, Family Medicine and Otorhinolaryngology, Head and Neck Surgery in 2004 [7] indicated that adenoidectomy should not be performed unless a distinct indication exists. The National Institute for Health and Clinical Excellence in United Kingdom in 2008 [8] also indicated that adjuvant adenoidectomy is not recommended in the absence of persistent and frequent upper respiratory symptoms. Anyway, adenoidectomy in the surgical management of chronic OME is seen

Table 1. Repeat tympanostomy tube insertion according to previous procedures

Group (previous procedures)	Repeat/total cases	%
1 T-tube Insertion only	289/1,425	20.3
2 T-tube insertion + adenoidectomy	16/525	3.0
3 T-tube insertion + adenotonsillectomy	113/6,700	1.7
Total	418/8,650	4.8

T = Tympanostomy.
p = 0.000 Pearson χ^2 test, group 1 vs. group 2; p = 0.000 Pearson χ^2 test, group 1 vs. group 3; p = 0.024 Pearson χ^2 test, group 2 vs. group 3.

Table 2. Comparison of adenoid size through TBCT scan (total 98 cases with congenital cholesteatoma under age of 10 were analyzed)

Group	Number of cases	Adenoid size, mm
With OME	37	25.2±3.86
Without OME	61	23.2±2.85

$p > 0.05$.
TBCT = Temporal bone computed tomography; OME = otitis media with effusion.

as a second-line treatment. However, some randomized and controlled trial [9] indicated that having adenoidectomy or adenotonsillectomy at the time of first tympanostomy tube insertion was associated with reduced risk of repeat tympanostomy tube insertion. The low complication rates for adenoidectomy and short hospital stays make adjunctive adenoidectomy a potentially cost-effective first-line management option for chronic OME.

We studied retrospectively the role of adenotonsillectomy in chronic OME treatment (table 1) [unpubl. data]. There were 8,650 children less than 10 years of age who underwent at least one tympanostomy tube insertion procedure from 1994 to 2008. Among 8,650 children, repeat tympanostomy tube insertion was done in 418 (4.8%), We analyzed 418 repeat surgery cases. This result showed that having adenoidectomy or adenotonsillectomy surgery together with tympanostomy tube insertion at the same time reduced repeat tympanostomy tube insertion.

Our other retrospective study (table 2) was the comparison of the adenoid size between OME group and non-OME group through the temporal bone computed tomography (TBCT) [unpubl. data]. We analyzed 98 children with congenital cholesteatoma under age of 10 who were taken TBCT scan from 1994 to 2008. Among 98 cases, 37 cases were associated with OME. Between OME and non-OME groups, the adenoid size was compared. The adenoid size was investigated via the axial section of the TBCT scan. In the axial view, the largest length of the soft tissue between the clivus and mucosal surface was recorded. In this study, adenoid size between OME group and non-OME group was not statistically significant.

In summary, having adenoidectomy or adenotonsillectomy procedure together with tympanostomy tube insertion at the same time can reduce repeat tympanostomy tube insertion. Also, it is indicated that adenoidectomy at first tympanostomy tube insertion is cost-effective and low-risk procedure to reduce the community cost of repeat tympanostomy tube insertion.

We can summarize that children suffering from recurrent or chronic OME may benefit from adenoidectomy due to the removal of an infectious source in the nasopharynx rather than the removal of a large adenoidal mass.

References

1 Moon SK, Lim DJ: Expression of β-defensins in the human middle ear mucosa. Korean J Otolaryngol 2004;47:103–107.

2 Chae SW, Lee SH, Cho JH, Lee HM, Choi G, Hwang SJ: Expression of human β-defensin 1 mRNA in human palatine tonsil. Acta Otolaryngol 2001;121:414–418.

3 Park SN, Yeo SW, Park KH, Chung MK, Lee HY, Chae S: Superoxide dismutase in pediatric palatine tonsils and adenoids and its related clinical parameters. Am J Otolaryngol 2003;24:323–327.

4 Macassey E, Dawes P: Biofilms and their role in otolaryngological disease. J Laryngol Otol 2008;122:1273–1278.

5 Al-Mazrou KA, Al-Khattaf AS: Adherent biofilms in adenotonsillar diseases in children. Arch Otolaryngol Head Neck Surg 2008;134:20–23.

6 Post JC: Direct evidence of bacterial biofilms in otitis media. Laryngoscope 2001;111:2083–2094.

7 Rosenfeld RM, Culpepper L, Doyle KJ, Grundfast KM, Hoberman A, Kenna MA, Lieberthal AS, Mahoney M, Wahl RA, Woods, JR CR, Yawn B: Clinical practice guideline: otitis media with effusion. Otolaryngol Head Neck Surg 2004;130(suppl):95–118.

8 National Institute for Health and Clinical Excellence: Surgical Management of Otitis Media with Effusion in Children. London, NiCE, 2008. See http://nice.org.uk/Guidance/CG60 (accessed 10 March 2010).

9 Kadhim AL, Spilsbury K, Semmens JB, Coats HL, Lannigan FJ: Adenoidectomy for middle ear effusion: a study of 50,000 children over 24 years. Laryngoscope 2007;117:427–433.

Keehyun Park, MD, PhD
Department of Otolaryngology, Ajou University School of Medicine
5 Woncheon-dong, Yeongtong-gu
Suwon 443–721 (South Korea)
Tel. +82 31 219 5000, Fax +82 31 216 6380, E-Mail parkkh@ajou.ac.kr

Harabuchi Y (ed): Recent Advances in Tonsils and Mucosal Barriers of the Upper Airways.
Adv Otorhinolaryngol. Basel, Karger, 2011, vol 72, pp 164–169

Otitis Media and Immunological Alterations of Waldeyer's Ring

Pasquale Cassano · Michele Cassano

Department of Otorhinolaryngology, University of Foggia, Foggia, Italy

Abstract

In the literature, correlations between adenoids and middle ear disorders have been widely discussed over the years. Adenoids fundamentally influence inflammation/infections of the middle ear through 3 factors: obstructive, inflammatory/infective, and immunologic. The authors carefully analyze each of these factors reviewing the opinion of the most important researches in the field. The important role of immunological (T cells and Ig), infective (micro-organisms and bacterial biofilms) and allergic factors as predisposing factors for otitis media leads one to consider the importance of a medical treatment oriented to correction of the infective and immunological disorders in children with OM, without adenoids hypertrophy.

The correlations between Waldeyer's ring disorders and middle ear (ME) disorders are very complex and therefore have been discussed widely in the literature over the years. In particular, the role carried out by the adenoids in the pathogenesis of otitis media is very interesting.

Adenoids fundamentally influence inflammation/infections of the ME through 3 factors: obstructive, inflammatory/infective and immunological problems. If we consider these aspects very carefully, it becomes evident that the different points are closely linked: in fact, obstruction supports the inflammation and consequently the infection, inflammation promotes hypertrophy of the structures of Waldeyer's ring, in particular adenoids, and consequently the obstruction of the nasopharynx cavum, immunological disorders are at the same time cause and consequence of the inflammation/infection. Therefore, there is a vicious circle, which progressively causes a dangerous dysfunction of the ME, injuring the function and the anatomic integrity.

However, it is advisable to consider the 3 factors individually.

A mechanical obstruction of the Eustachian tube (ET) has to be taken into consideration in recurrent secretory otitis media. The causes are different: adenoids, palatotubal insufficiency, persistent cartilaginous collapse of the tube, rhinopharyngeal tumors, etc. In children, the adenoid is undoubtedly the most important.

Many authors, particularly in the past, consider the mechanical obstruction to be due to hypertrophic adenoids, especially when developed laterally, an important pathogenic factor for otitis. In 1998, Wright et al. [1] underlined this situation, having found a strong correlation between otitis media with effusion (OME) and lateral adenoids abutting the torus tubarius. The clinical relevance of this finding is that it may allow the prediction of children with OME, who will benefit most from undergoing adenoidectomy. More recently, our experience also confirmed this opinion. In a recent study, we correlated the degree of adenoidal obstruction with locoregional pathologies. With regard to otitis, we found a high correlation between gravity of obstruction and incidence of otitis [2].

However, over the years the most common opinion is that mechanical obstruction of the adenoids is just one of the etiological factors for otitis. In particular, an ongoing inflammatory/infective process, namely adenoiditis, can spark off and keep up middle ear disorders. First of all, there is an inflammatory stenosis of the ET with insufficient ventilation of ME.

Nevertheless, the role of micro-organisms, present on the surface or in the deep crypts of the adenoid tissue, is undoubtedly much more important. Most researches evidenced that the adenoids represent a reservoir for bacteria, which played a significant role in the pathogenesis of otitis media. The nasopharynx is normally colonized by nonvirulent bacteria, such as viridians streptococci, nonhemolytic streptococci, *Neisseria, Prevotella*, anaerobic species, which establish equilibrium in the ecosystem of this area, inhibiting growth of potential pathogens with bacterial interference. Some studies established that in deep culture of adenoids examined post-operatively (much more important and significant deep culture than surface culture), the presence of saprophyte micro-organisms (normal flora) is lower in patients with bilateral chronic OME than in patients without ME disorders, especially with regard to some aerobic (*Neisseria*) and anaerobic (*Prevotella, Peptostreptococcus*) micro-organisms [3]. Other studies demonstrated a lower incidence also of AHS in the nasopharynx of children with OM, rOMA and OME [4]. The lower presence of natural flora obviously involves a potential aggression of pathogens. Otopathogens have essentially been identified in *Streptococcus pneumoniae*, non-typeable *Haemophilus influenzae* and *Moraxella catarrhalis*; they cause 75% of the infections. The development of OM begins in the nasopharynx, in which the above-named bacteria are often present also in healthy people. During periods of upper respiratory illness, and during episodes of OM in particular, colonization by middle ear pathogens increases significantly. This increase is especially evident among children who are prone to recurrent episodes of OM. In the study by Faden et al. [4], the correlation between frequencies of pathogen colonization and episodes of OM has been carefully considered. The authors demonstrate that *M. catarrhalis* was the first respiratory pathogen to colonize infants and the most prevalent pathogen throughout infancy. *S. pneumoniae* was next in frequency, followed by nontypeable *H. influenzae*. Furthermore, early colonization may be a risk factor for first infection and as well as recurrent disease.

In the last few years, some researches revealed the presence of bacterial biofilms on the adenoid surface, and so an inflammatory purulent process can be present also during asymptomatic periods. Experimental studies demonstrated that biofilms are present also in middle ear during OME, providing further evidence linking bacteria to this disease. Because the bacteria likely exist in their nonplanktonic form, this helps to explain the difficulty on initial investigators in demonstrating a bacterial presence in this disease. Zuliani et al. [5] evidenced in a group of bacterial patients with CRS or OM that nearly 95% of surface of adenoidectomy specimens were covered by natural bacterial biofilms, while specimens from controls patients revealed very little coverage. The presence of biofilms suggests long-term colonization and could support the notion that the chronic illness, in nasopharynx and next organs, paranasal sinus and middle ear may be secondary to bacterial infection in a nonplanktonic form, which has been shown to be difficult to erad icate with current antimicrobial therapies [5].

In conclusion, inflammation/infections of the adenoids are an important predisposing factor for OM (OME or AOM).

Fortunately, the Waldeyer's ring is characterized by a strong defensive system, which in adenoids in particular includes immunologic and nonimmunologic defenses against viral and bacterial micro-organisms. Only the impairment of these defenses and/or increase in bacterial resistances may lead to colonization/persistence of pathogenic bacteria on the mucosa and even an adenoid/tonsil surfaces.

The lymphoid tissue is not apparent in early infancy, as it gradually becomes hypertrophic and hyperplasic, acquiring its greatest relative mass between 2 and 5 years of age; during puberty, it undergoes an involution until, eventually, it is greatly reduced in older adults. Thus, Waldeyer's ring develops mostly during childhood when the oronasopharyngeal space is not yet completely developed. These considerations may explain why inflammation of tonsils and adenoids, with subsequent obstructive hypertrophy, is one of the oldest and most common pediatric problems.

One of the most important defense elements is a nonimmunological factor, i.e. the bacterial-mucin interaction in the nasopharynx. Mucins in the nasopharyngeal mucus may function as receptor molecules for bacteria and thus play an important role in the colonization of the nasopharynx. This bacterial-mucin interaction is not only specific but is important in preventing adherence of the organism to the surface of the epithelium and in this way prevents colonization of the epithelial surface which usually precedes penetration and potential infection. Comprehension of this interaction between bacterial and purified mucin may be a strategy to the prevent colonization of potential pathogens that cause otitis media and sinusitis in children.

The immunological factors of the adenoidal tissue are very important in promoting acute or chronic otitis.

Adenoids are organized in deep crypts outlined with a specialized lympho-epithelium designed for entrapping foreign material: indeed, the lymphoepithelium consists not only of epithelial cells but also of lymphocytes, macrophages, and dendritic cells. At a deeper level, the lymphoid tissue is characterized by the presence of follicular germinal centers and interfollicular areas. Each adenoid consists of 50–60% B lymphocytes, 40% T lymphocytes and approximately 3% plasma cells. Through B lymphocytes, the adenoids contain a secretory immune system: they represent a secretive immunological organ that contributes directly to regional surface protection by providing local secretory Ig, in particular Ig-A.

IgA comprises approximately 15–20% of serum antibody, and it is the major antibody in the intestinal mucosae, as well as in saliva, colostrums, trachea and the urogenital organs. In particular, secretory IgA (sIgA) on the mucosal surface plays an important role in immunity. The adenoid is the primary organ involved in the sIgA-dependent immunity in the upper respiratory tract. IgA precursor cells are formed in the adenoids and sent from there to reactive tissues and organs. Reductions in IgA in serum may occur in patients easily susceptible to recurrent infection, including those with recurrent otitis media. Eun et al. [6] found that staining with antibody to IgA was significantly lower in children with OME or CRS than in children who only had adenoid hyperplasia. The reduction in IgA was probably not due to increased IgA clearance due to inflammatory reactions; rather, the reduced susceptibility to infection was probably caused by the reduction of IgA.

About 70–75% of immunoglobulin in the serum of normal individuals is IgG. As children get older, IgG synthesis increases in adenoid lymphocytes, but is lower in the adenoids of children with OME compared to those without OME. IgM is the first antibody synthesized during a primary immune reaction, and in present primarily in blood vessels. Eun et al. [6] found that staining for IgM was similar in children with adenoids hypertrophy, OME and CRS. At the time of surgical treatment for OME or CRS, these diseases have become chronic; thus, IgM, which is associated with acute inflammatory reactions, is unlikely to be involved.

IgD is a minor constituent of serum, and IgD, like IgM, acts as an antigen-specific receptor on mature B cells. Eun et al. [6] observed no differences among the three groups (OME, CRS and adenoid hypertrophy) in staining for antibody to IgD, suggesting that IgD does not mediate specific effects on adenoid immunity.

BCL-6 and BLIMP-1 are factors involved in antibody synthesis by B lymphocytes.

Eun et al. [6] found that BLIMP-1 expression in adenoid tissues was lower in both the OME and CRS groups than in the adenoid hyperplasia group, but only the difference between the CRS and adenoid hyperplasia groups was statistically significant, perhaps because the number of OME patients was small or inflammation in the adenoids was involved in the development of OME. The reduced expression of BLIMP-1 in the OME and CRS group was associated with the reduction in IgA-secreting cells, thus decreasing immunity to viruses, bacteria, and other antigens, and increasing the likelihood of OME or CRS. In contrast to BLIMP-1 expression, the expression of BCL-6 was not elevated in the OME or CRS groups, and there were no between-group differences. These findings suggest that reduction in IgA synthesis following the reduced expression of BLIMP-1 in the adenoid of children with OME and CRS might be associated with the development of OME and CRS [6].

Regarding the effector T cells, the localization and function of effector T lymphocytes is crucial for the generation of an effective immune response. In particular, CD8+ T lymphocytes can mobilize two main mechanisms: cytolysis and production of cytokines, chemokines, and microbicidal molecules. Several authors did not find statistically significant differences in the helper-suppressor T cells (CD4/CD8) ratio between children with AH only and children with associated AH and infection of the adenoids and/or OME. Only Brodsky and Koch found slightly greater number and percentage of CD8-positive T lymphocytes in children with chronic adenoid infection compared to children with AH, as evidenced in the study of Mattila and Tarkkanen [7].

However, Avanzini et al. [8] demonstrated that children with recurrent otitis media showed significant lower percentage of CD8+ producing IFN- γ cells in adenoids than children with <3 otitis per year. It is well known that IFN-γ is a Th1 cytokine and that it is truly important in host defense against viral infections and in killing intracellular pathogens by inducting of cellular antiviral proteins and macrophage activation. The most important findings of this study are the children with recurrent otitis show detective IFN-γ production in adenoid-derived CD8+ T cells. These results agree with those published by Bernstein and co-workers, who have demonstrated that in children presenting with recurrent otitis that there is a relative decreased in the synthesis of Th1 cytokines, IL-2 and IFN-γ, in comparison with peripheral blood lymphocytes. In addition, they propose that it is likely that IFN-γ reduction is proportional to the number of otitis events affecting the child per year. As a consequence of reduced IFN-γ production, patients show an increased susceptibility to infectious viral diseases, which often precede upper respiratory tract infections, with a possible consequential increase in replication of pathogenetic bacteria in the adenoidal tissue.

Previous studies also suggested that adenoid mast cells have a role in the pathogenesis of OME based on increased mast cell population as well as increased blood and adenoid histamine in patients with OME. A study of Ulualp et al. [9] showed that patients with combined OME and chronic adenoiditis have a greater number of adenoid mast cells with less granules in the cytoplasm compared to patients with isolated chronic adenoiditis. Cytoplasm granules of mast cells contain potent mediators of inflammation. These mediators mainly act as chemotactic agents, inflammatory agents, inflammatory activators, and spasmogens. Spasmogens such as prostaglandin

D_4, leukotrienes C_4, and D_4 cause mucosal edema and secretion. Although histamine induces edema of Eustachian tube function and OME, it should be emphasized that possible contribution of mast cells in the pathogenesis of OME is not limited exclusively to the release of histamine. Arachidonic acid metabolites such as prostaglandins and leukotrienes have important roles in the pathogenesis of OME. The most obvious stimulus for mediator release from adenoid mast cells would be an antibody-mediated allergic disease. Although the relationship of OME with allergic disease has been implicated, the laboratory evidence remains controversial. In the otitis media-prone child the need for allergy evaluation was suggested if the child has any of the following: a positive family history for allergy and/or asthma, symptom triggers such as pets and indoor allergens or symptoms coincident with allergen, pale and bobbly appearance of nasal mucosa, and response to antiallergy medical therapy.

As regards correlations between allergy, adenoiditis and OME, the studies of Marseglia et al. [10] demonstrated that the risk to develop OME become higher when these two conditions (allergy and adenoiditis) are concomitant and the patients are younger.

Finally, an important role in the immunological response behind the development of otitis media seems to be expressed by Toll-like receptors (TLR1), present in the adenoids of young children. Toll-like receptors are a component of innate pattern recognition receptors, which produce proinflammatory cytokines and chemokines and natural antimicrobial molecules, the alpha and beta defenses upon ligation. Several studies have demonstrated the ability of nasopharyngeal palatine tonsils to produce proinflammatory molecules, which may be a consequence of TLR signaling in these tissues. A recent study by Granath et al. [11] demonstrated that the mRNA levels for TLR7 were increased among the children with a history of OME, confirming the role in the immunologial response behind the development of OME in children.

In conclusion, in the vicious circle of the correlations between adenoids and ME disorders inflammation/infective and immunological factors play an important role as much as hypertrophy and consequent nasopharynx obstruction. So, correction of these factors is fundamental, also in the cases with important hypertrophy requiring surgical treatment (adenoidectomy). Otherwise, we can have a postoperative failure in the results concerning otitis media, as in our experience.

On the other hand, these considerations suggest that adenoidectomy is sometimes useless, without concomitant adenoids hypertrophy. This opinion has been expressed by several authors, even if refused by others. We agree with the former opinion and prefer medical treatment oriented to correction of the infective and immunological disorders in children with OM, without adenoid hypertrophy.

References

1 Wright ED, Pearl AJ, Manoukian JJ: Laterally hypertrophic adenoids as a contributing factor in otitis media. Int J Pediatr Otorhinolaryngol 1998;45:207–214.

2 Cassano P, Gelardi M, Cassano M, Fiorella ML, Fiorella R: Adenoid tissue rhinopharyngeal obstruction grading based on fiberendoscopic findings: a novel approach to therapeutic management. Int J Pediatr Otorhinolaryngol 2003;67:1303–1309.

3 Almac A, Elicora SS, Yumuk Z, Dundar V, Willke A: The relationship between chronic otitis media with effusion and surface and deep flora of hypertrophic adenoids. Int J Pediatr Otorhinolaryngol 2009:17.

4 Faden H, Waz MJ, Bernstein JM, Brodsky L, Stanievich J, Ogra PL: Nasopharyngeal flora in the first three years of life in normal and otitis-prone children. Ann Otol Rhinol Laryngol 1991;100:612–615.

5 Zuliani G, Carron M, Gurrola J, Coleman C, Haupert M, Berk R, Coticchia J: Identification of adenoid biofilms in chronic rhinosinusitis. Int J Pediatr Otorhinolaryngol 2006;70:1613–1617.

6 Eun YG, Park DC, Kim SG, Kim MG, Yeo SG: Immunoglobulins and transcription factors in adenoids of children with otitis media with effusion and chronic rhinosinusitis. Int J Pediatr Otorhinolaryngol 2009:10.

7 Mattila PS, Tarkkanen J: B- and T-lymphocyte subpopulations in the adenoids of children with otitis media. APMIS 1996;104:698–704.

8 Avanzino AM, Castellazzi AM, Marconi M, et al: Children with recurrent otitis show detective IFN-γ-producing cells in adenoids. Pediatr Allergy Immunol 2008;19:523–526.

9 Ulualp SO, Sahin D, Yilmaz N, Anadol V, Peker O, Gursan O: Increased adenoid mast cells in patients with otitis media with effusion. Int J Pediatr Otorhinolaryngol 1999;49:107–114.

10 Marseglia GL, Pagella F, Caimmi D, Caimmi S, Castellazzi AM, Poddighe D, Klersy C, Ciprandi G: Increased risk of otitis media with effusion in allergic children presenting with adenoiditis. Otolaryngol Head Neck Surg 2008;138:572–575.

11 Granath A, Uddman R, Cardell LO: Increased TLR7 expression in the adenoids among children with otitis media with effusion. Acta Otolaryngol 2010;130:57–61.

Dott. Cassano Michele
via Crispi 34/C
IT–70123 Bari (Italy)
Tel. +39 0881 736282, E-Mail m.cassano@unifg.it

Harabuchi Y (ed): Recent Advances in Tonsils and Mucosal Barriers of the Upper Airways.
Adv Otorhinolaryngol. Basel, Karger, 2011, vol 72, pp 170–175

Role of Nontypeable *Haemophilus influenzae* in Otitis Media and Chronic Obstructive Pulmonary Disease

Yasmin Thanavala · Amit A. Lugade

Department of Immunology, Roswell Park Cancer Institute, Buffalo, N.Y., USA

Abstract

In both infants and adults, infections with non-typeable *Haemophilus influenzae* (NTHI) results in morbidity and mortality. NTHI strains are the leading cause of bacterial otitis media infections (both acute and recurrent) in young children and are also responsible for chronic obstructive pulmonary disease (COPD) exacerbations in current and former smokers. The realization that NTHI causes serious infections in humans has generated interest in the study of the pathogenesis associated with this bacterium and also stimulated considerable efforts towards the evaluation of candidate vaccines that will elicit protective immunity. As NTHI is exclusively a human pathogen and has not been associated with any diseases in other mammals, special efforts have been necessary to establish animal models of NTHI infection to generate useful data on the pathogenesis of infection and efficacy of potential vaccines. This article provides a brief summary of the role of NTHI in disease and the work that has been accomplished by us and several other investigators.

Nontypeable *Haemophilus influenzae* (NTHI) is a Gram-negative bacterium that is part of the normal flora present in the nasopharynx of humans. The nasopharynx is situated at the interface between the nose, ear, larynx, and lower respiratory tract, thereby providing easy access for pathogens in the nasopharynx to colonize and initiate infections in both the upper and lower respiratory tracts [1]. In children, the linkage of the nasopharynx with the middle ear via the Eustachian tube is responsible for the spread of NTHI in otitis media.

Despite the presence of six capsular serotypes, the nonencapsulated or nontypeable strains of *H. influenzae*, along with the capsular serotype b strains, are responsible for the majority of *H. influenzae* infections. Infections associated with the type b strains are spread via the bloodstream and cause invasive disease such as meningitis and pneumonia. In contrast, NTHI strains are spread via the mucosal route and are responsible for mucosal infections such as otitis media, sinusitis, and conjunctivitis [2]. NTHI (along with *Streptococcus pneumoniae* and *Moraxella catarrhalis*) is also commonly found in the sputum of chronic obstructive pulmonary disease (COPD) patients with acute and recurrent exacerbations [3].

Encapsulated *H. influenzae* strains are generally more virulent than the nonencapsulated strains owing to the presence of the carbohydrate capsule, which is essential for virulence. The serotype b strains are fundamentally a clonal population and since the licensure of the type b polysaccharide-protein conjugate vaccine in 1990, invasive *H. influenzae* disease has been nearly eliminated in developing countries [4]. No such protective vaccine exists for NTHI strains, partly owing to the fact that the nontypeable strains exhibit enormous genetic diversity. Progress has been made been in developing effective vaccines for NTHI, including the recent clinical trial outcomes of PHiD-CV (Synflorix^{TM}, GlaxoSmithKline) which will be briefly discussed below. This short review will focus on the role of NTHI in two important diseases, otitis media and COPD, and the status of vaccine development for this pathogen.

Otitis Media

In the developing world, visits to the physician's office are commonplace for children with otitis media. Approximately 3 in 4 children develop an episode of acute otitis media by 3 years of age, with one-third of these children experiencing recurrent infections. Children having four or more episodes of otitis media in a year and eight months of middle ear effusion are defined as otitis prone [5]. Beyond a simple earache, the regimen of antibiotics prescribed to treat otitis media accounts for nearly 42 days of treatment time in the first year of life and 49 days in the second year of life [6]. While efforts have been made in several countries to curtail the use of antibiotics in order to diminish the selective pressure driving antibiotic resistance, the impact on the incidence of otitis media has been limited [6].

Infection of the middle ear with NTHI and *M. catarrhalis* are well-documented causes of otitis media in children. Widespread use of the pneumococcal polysaccharide vaccine results in serotype-specific immunity to *S. pneumoniae*, another causative agent of otitis media, and has diminished this pathogen's involvement in this disease, leading to increasing proportion of otitis media caused by NTHI and *M. catarrhalis* [7]. The pathogenesis begins with the spread of NTHI from the nasopharynx to the middle ear. Middle ears of otitis-prone children are colonized with NTHI at higher rates than nonprone children, further underscoring the need for an effective vaccine to curtail infections. PCR of middle ear fluids for bacterial DNA suggests that NTHI is responsible for a large proportion of acute otitis media that is culture negative and may be present in a nonculturable state such as a biofilm [8].

NTHI is exclusively a human pathogen and has not been associated with any diseases in other mammals. Thus, animal models of NTHI infection are very limited and need to be critically evaluated in order to generate useful data on the pathogenesis of infection or efficacy of potential vaccines. Select experimental models, such as the chinchilla model of otitis media, have provided invaluable data on the pathogenesis and immune response to NTHI. The chinchilla Eustachian tube is anatomically similar to human and its structure permits serial sampling of middle ear fluids without damaging the tympanic membrane [9]. Although otitis media does not naturally occur in chinchillas, NTHI can be introduced into the ear and results in an infection pattern with several features similar to that observed in the human disease. This model has allowed several investigators to define the pathogenic events initiating otitis media precisely and testing of potential vaccine antigens. In fact, passive transfer of human anti-protein D antibodies generated by polysaccharide-protein D conjugate vaccines into chinchillas protected the animals from NTHI-induced otitis media [10]. Demonstration of protective responses in the chinchilla model therefore provides strong rationale to proceed with testing of vaccine antigens in clinical trials.

Chronic Obstructive Pulmonary Disease

It is estimated that over 16 million people suffer from COPD in the United States alone and that the prevalence of this disease is increasing each year [11]. Complications from COPD are listed as the fourth most common cause of death. This disease is responsible for the expenditure of approximately USD 15 billion in direct costs of medical care and impacts the health care system to the tune of 10 million physician office visits and 2 million hospitalizations. COPD is characterized by irreversible airway obstruction in patients concomitantly suffering from chronic bronchitis and/or emphysema. Tobacco smoke is recognized as a crucial factor in the development and pathogenesis of COPD and exposure to smoke results in increased vulnerability to many infections and airway diseases [12]. Tobacco smoking suppresses the immune system and is an established risk factor for several diseases including lung cancer, highlighted by the fact that a person with COPD has a 4–6 times greater risk of developing lung cancer.

COPD is characterized by intermittent disease exacerbation. Exacerbations in COPD patients can vary from mild to severe, sometimes requiring hospitalization and involving respiratory failure associated with significant mortality. Bacteria are always present in the upper airways; however, in the absence of lung disease the tracheobronchial tree is maintained sterile. Tobacco smoke causes airway inflammation and impairment of mucociliary clearance. Impaired mucociliary clearance can be the result of disruption of normal ciliary activity, enhanced mucus secretion and airway epithelial injury. Once there is impaired mucocilliary clearance, potential respiratory pathogens gain a foothold in the lower respiratory tract and then persist in the respiratory tract by further impairing mucociliary clearance because of their products (including proteins, peptidoglycans, lipo-oligosaccharide and nucleic acids). Even though the potential contribution of bacterial infection to the etiology, pathogenesis and clinical course of COPD could be identified, the precise role of bacterial infection was a source of some controversy for several decades. With improved technologies, the causal contribution of bacterial infections to exacerbations of COPD is now widely accepted, accounting for at least 50% of all exacerbations [11]. NTHI, *M. catarrhalis*, and *S. pneumoniae* are the three most common bacterial pathogens that cause respiratory tract infections in COPD patients. Bacteria, by invading and persisting in respiratory tissue, induce inflammation of the lower airway, promote hypersensitivity, cause immigration of neutrophils and activate eosinophils and macrophages. Bacteria and bacterial products serve as the most effective activators of inflammatory conditions characterized by the abundance of local and systemic mediators (chemokines and cytokines). The key initiators of these reactions are lung macrophages, resident dendritic cells and bronchial epithelial cells. Additionally, acquisition of new strains of NTHI is associated with COPD exacerbations; therefore, this susceptible population would also benefit from a vaccine to prevent lower respiratory tract infections of NTHI [3].

It is now generally accepted that COPD is an inflammation-mediated disease but a clear understanding of the inflammatory changes during an exacerbation of COPD is yet to emerge. As bacterial colonization of the lung in COPD patients results in a chronic inflammatory condition, we established a murine model of chronic pathogen-mediated inflammation by repeatedly delivering intact, live NTHI intratracheally into the lungs and following chronic exposure to the bacteria we evaluated the effects on lung pathology [13]. The lungs of mice exposed to NTHI for 4 weeks exhibited peribronchial inflammation highlighted by cuffs of immune cells around airway and vascular spaces. We noted that the lymphocytes appeared to be organized into aggregates, which resemble the morphology commonly observed with bronchial-associated lymphoid tissue (BALT) and were distributed throughout the lung, including some regions in which lymphocytes infiltrated the bronchio-epithelia. The lymphoid aggregates also strongly resembled those observed in the lungs of advanced stage COPD patients (GOLD Stage 3–4) [14].

Pathogenesis of NTHI Infection

A variety of adhesion molecules on the surface of NTHI allows the pathogen to adhere to a broad spectrum of receptors expressed by cells in the human mucosa and respiratory tract [15]. The bacterium has been shown to adhere to epithelial cells and macrophages via mucin, CEACAM1, and PAF-R. Additionally, extracellular matrix molecules, including vitronectin and laminin, are critical for colonization in the respiratory tract. Many strains of NTHI encode high molecular weight adhesions for adherence to sialylated proteins of the respiratory tract thereby initiating colonization. Upon colonization in the respiratory tract, NTHI evades innate clearance mechanisms by various methods including secretion of IgA protease [16]. Interaction of NTHI with respiratory epithelial cells up-regulates a vast number of genes from different functional families, in both the pathogen and the host cell. Upregulation of mucin transcription by epithelial cells is a topic of study for novel treatments, since mucin production is seen in otitis media and COPD bacterial exacerbations [17].

Based on its ability to bind to mucin and adherence to epithelial cells, NTHI was generally considered an extracellular mucosal pathogen. However, immunofluorescence microscopy of bronchial biopsies from COPD patients with stable disease or with recent exacerbations has revealed an intracellular niche of NTHI within epithelial cells and macrophages [18]. These findings suggest that intracellular NTHI may play an important role in exacerbations of COPD, especially in cases in which the bacterium is undetected in expectorated sputum. Biofilms of NTHI are present in the middle ear of infected chinchillas and presumably in the ears of children with otitis media. Bacteria growing in a biofilm are more resistant to host clearance mechanisms and antibiotics than planktonic bacteria. Various studies have reported that approximately 30% of NTHI strains produce β-lactamase thereby providing amoxicillin and ampicillin resistance [19]. Additionally, innate immune mechanisms, such as expression of TLRs, play an important role in recognition and clearance of NTHI. Importantly, presence of T cells specific for a lipoprotein expressed in the outer membrane of NTHI is associated with reduced episodes of COPD exacerbations [20].

Vaccine Development

Capsular polysaccharide antigens have been utilized successfully for vaccines against *H. influenzae* type b strains, but unfortunately NTHI is noncapsular and therefore other molecules expressed in various structures of the bacteria must be tested for vaccine potential. Major efforts have been directed against identifying outer-membrane proteins and lipo-oligosaccharides from NTHI that are surface-exposed and conserved among the various strains. The other consideration for the vaccine must be the immunogenicity of the antigen and its ability to induce protective responses against the intact bacteria. Several molecules from the outer membrane of NTHI, such as lipoprotein D, OMP5, Pil A peptides, and lipoprotein P6, fit the criteria for candidate vaccine antigens and have also been validated for protection in chinchilla models [21].

The most exciting progress for the development of a vaccine to prevent NTHI infections has been with the advent of the 10-valent lipoprotein D conjugate vaccine (PHiD-CV) under the brandname Synflorix^{TM}. It comprises ten pneumococcal serotypes (1, 4, 5, 6B, 7F, 9V, 14, 18C, 19F, and 23F) conjugated to NTHI lipoprotein

D as a protein carrier. In a randomized, double-blinded, prospective, placebo controlled trial, the vaccine demonstrated 57% efficacy for pneuomococcal otitis media and 35% efficacy for *H. influenzae* otitis media [22]. Further work lies ahead to improve efficacy of this promising vaccine.

Our own work suggests that the nature of the vaccine antigen is critical for immunogenicity. Lipoprotein P6 is highly conserved among NTHI strains and its immunogenicity is dependent on the expression of an amino-terminal tri-palmitoyl residue. The presence of this lipid motif affects its solubility for vaccine administration but removal of this motif severely limits its immunogenicity during in vivo vaccine testing in mouse models [23]. The lipid motif is critical for activation of innate and adaptive immune cells, thus efforts are focused on maintaining immunogenicity while improving solubility for aqueous administration. Combined with other vaccine antigens, there is great promise for a protective vaccine for NTHI.

Acknowledgements

This work was supported by AI069379 from NIAID to YT.

References

1 García-Rodríguez JA, Fresnadillo Martínez MJ: Dynamics of nasopharyngeal colonization by potential respiratory pathogens. J Antimicrob Chemother. 2002;50(suppl S2):59–73.
2 Hardy GG, Tudor SM, St Geme JW 3rd: The pathogenesis of disease due to non-typeable *Haemophilus influenzae*. Methods Mol Med. 2003;71:1–28.
3 Sethi S, Murphy TF. Bacterial infection in chronic obstructive pulmonary disease in 2000: a state-of-the-art review. Clin Microbiol Rev 2001;14: 336–63.
4 Musser JM, Kroll JS, Moxon ER, Selander RK: Evolutionary genetics of the encapsulated strains of Haemophilus influenzae. Proc Natl Acad Sci USA 1988;85:7758–62.
5 Faden H: The microbiologic and immunologic basis for recurrent otitis media in children. Eur J Pediatr. 2001;160:407–413.
6 Vergison A, Dagan R, Arguedas A, Bonhoeffer J, Cohen R, Dhooge I, Hoberman A, Liese J, Marchisio P, Palmu AA, Ray GT, Sanders EA, Simões EA, Uhari M, van Eldere J, Pelton SI: Otitis media and its consequences: beyond the earache. Lancet Infect Dis. 2010;10: 195–203.
7 Casey JR, Pichichero ME: Changes in frequency and pathogens causing acute otitis media in 1995–2003. Pediatr Infect Dis J 2004;23:824–828.
8 Ehrlich GD, Veeh R, Wang X, Costerton JW, Hayes JD, Hu FZ, Daigle BJ, Ehrlich MD, Post JC: Mucosal biofilm formation on middle-ear mucosa in the chinchilla model of otitis media. JAMA. 2002;287:1710–1715.
9 Bakaletz LO: Chinchilla as a robust, reproducible and polymicrobial model of otitis media and its prevention. Expert Rev Vaccines 2009;8:1063–1082.
10 Novotny LA, Jurcisek JA, Godfroid F, Poolman JT, Denoël PA, Bakaletz LO: Passive immunization with human anti-protein D antibodies induced by polysaccharide protein D conjugates protects chinchillas against otitis media after intranasal challenge with *Haemophilus influenzae*. Vaccine 2006;24:4804–4811.
11 Sethi S, Murphy TF. Infection in the pathogenesis and course of chronic obstructive pulmonary disease. N Engl J Med. 2008;359:2355–2365.
12 Janson C, Chinn S, Jarvis D, Zock JP, Torén K, Burney P, European Community Respiratory Health Survey: Effect of passive smoking on respiratory symptoms, bronchial responsiveness, lung function, and total serum IgE in the European Community Respiratory Health Survey: a cross-sectional study. Lancet 2001;358:2103–2109.
13 Lugade AA, Vethanayagam RR, Nasirikenari M, Bogner PN, Segal BH, Thanavala Y: Nrf2 regulates chronic lung inflammation and B cell responses to non-typeable *Haemophilus influenzae*. Am J Respir Cell Mol Biol 2011;epub Jan 7.
14 Hogg JC, Chu F, Utokaparch S, Woods R, Elliott WM, Buzatu L, Cherniack RM, Rogers RM, Sciurba FC, Coxson HO, Paré PD: The nature of small-airway obstruction in chronic obstructive pulmonary disease. N Engl J Med 2004;350:2645–2653.
15 St Geme JW 3rd: Molecular and cellular determinants of non-typeable *Haemophilus influenzae* adherence and invasion. Cell Microbiol 2002;4:191–200.
16 Vitovski S, Dunkin KT, Howard AJ, Sayers JR. Nontypeable *Haemophilus influenzae* in carriage and disease: a difference in IgA1 protease activity levels. JAMA 2002;287:1699–1705.
17 Wang B, Lim DJ, Han J, Kim YS, Basbaum CB, Li JD: Novel cytoplasmic proteins of nontypeable *Haemophilus influenzae* up-regulate human MUC5AC mucin transcription via a positive p38 mitogen-activated protein kinase pathway and a negative phosphoinositide 3-kinase-Akt pathway. J Biol Chem 2002;277:949–957.

18 Bandi V, Apicella MA, Mason E, Murphy TF, Siddiqi A, Atmar RL, Greenberg SB: Nontypeable *Haemophilus influenzae* in the lower respiratory tract of patients with chronic bronchitis. Am J Respir Crit Care Med 2001;164: 2114–2119.
19 Tristram S, Jacobs MR, Appelbaum PC: Antimicrobial resistance in *Haemophilus influenzae*. Clin Microbiol Rev 2007;20:368–89.
20 Abe Y, Murphy TF, Sethi S, Faden HS, Dmochowski J, Harabuchi Y, Thanavala YM: Lymphocyte proliferative response to P6 of *Haemophilus influenzae* is associated with relative protection from exacerbations of chronic obstructive pulmonary disease. Am J Respir Crit Care Med 2002;165:967–971.
21 Murphy TF, Bakaletz LO, Smeesters PR: Microbial interactions in the respiratory tract. Pediatr Infect Dis J 2009;28(10 suppl):S121–6.
22 Prymula R, Peeters P, Chrobok V, Kriz P, Novakova E, Kaliskova E, Kohl I, Lommel P, Poolman J, Prieels JP, Schuerman L: Pneumococcal capsular polysaccharides conjugated to protein D for prevention of acute otitis media caused by both *Streptococcus pneumoniae* and non-typeable *Haemophilus influenzae*: a randomised double-blind efficacy study. Lancet 2006;367:740–748.
23 Lugade AA, Bianchi A, Pradhan V, Elkin G, Murphy TF, Thanavala Y: Lipid motif of a bacterial antigen mediates immune responses via TLR2 signaling. Plos one 6:e19781.

Yasmin Thanavala, PhD
Dept of Immunology, Roswell Park Cancer Institute
Buffalo, NY 14263 (USA)
Tel. +1 716 845 8536, E-Mail yasmin.thanavala@roswellpark.org

Harabuchi Y (ed): Recent Advances in Tonsils and Mucosal Barriers of the Upper Airways.
Adv Otorhinolaryngol. Basel, Karger, 2011, vol 72, pp 176–178

Recent Changes in Nasopharyngeal Flora of Children in Japan

Tatsuya Hayashi · Tomoki Yoshizaki · Kenzo Ohara · Saeko Yoshida · Takumi Kumai · Yasuaki Harabuchi

Department of Otolaryngology- Head and Neck Surgery, Asahikawa Medical University, Asahikawa, Hokkaido, Japan

Abstract

We investigated the relationship between nasopharyngeal flora of pediatric patients and antibiotic consumption in a local community in Japan between 2000 and 2009 retrospectively. There was a clear relationship between the lower annual consumption rate of cephalosporins and the lower annual prevalence of non-susceptible strains of *Streptococcus pneumoniae* (SP). High prevalence of BLNAR (β-lactamase nonproducing ampicillin-resistant *Haemophilus influenzae*) has been one of the bacteriological features of Japan.

Surveillance of nasopharyngeal bacterial pathogens of acute otitis media (AOM) in Japan showed an increase in prevalence of nonsusceptible strains of SP and *Haemophilus influenzae* (HI) reached over 70 and 50%, respectively, around 2000 in Japan. Another feature of bacteriological profile in Japan is that about 90% of nonsusceptible strains of HI are those of BLNAR (β-lactamase nonproducing ampicillin-resistant HI). Excessive usage of cephalosporins has been considered a main cause of the increase. In order to spread appropriate uses of antibacterial agents, the guideline for pediatric patients with AOM issued in 2006 and revised in 2009 in Japan. This guideline recommends a wait-and-see policy for the first 3 days in mild cases and amoxicillin as the first-line antibiotic [1].

At Nemuro Municipal Hospital, we have been treating children with AOM by almost the same treatment mode as the guideline since 2001, i.e. before the guideline was published.

The purpose of this study is to clarify the recent changes in the prevalence of nonsusceptible strains of AOM pathogens obtained from the nasopharynx along with changes in antibiotic choice before the introduction of heptavalent conjugate pneumococcal vaccine (PCV7) to Japan.

Material and Methods

Consumption of β-Lactams

The gross weight of each prescribed antibiotic for children that was provided as a form of granule and/or syrup was obtained from the pharmacy database. A defined daily dose system was used to compare the annual consumption of each β-lactam [2].

Nasopharyngeal Bacteriology

A retrospective study of nasopharyngeal flora from pediatric patients with upper and/or lower respiratory tract infections treated at Nemuro Municipal Hospital between 2000 and 2009 was performed. Strains of SP with MIC to penicillin G being 0.06 μg/ml or under was defined as PSSP, between 0.12 and 1.0 μg/ml as PISP, and 2 μg/ml or over as PRSP, respectively. Strains of HI without producing β-lactamase with MIC to ampicilin (ABPC) being 4 μg/ml or over were defined as BLNAR, 2 μg/ml as low BLNAR, and 1 μg/ml or under as BLNAS (β-lactamase nonproducing ABPC susceptible). β-Lactamase-producing strains of HI were classified as BLPAR (β-lactamase-producing, ABPC-resistant strains).

Results

Annual Consumption of β-Lactams for Children

After the pediatricians and otolaryngologists at Nemuro Municipal Hospital decided to use AMPC as the first-line therapy in 2001, the proportion of annual consumption of cephalosporins in all β-lactams for children decreased from 79% in 1999 to 28% in 2009.

Annual Changes in Prevalence of Nonsusceptible Strains (table 1)

In 2001, only 25% (90 strains) of 362 SP strains were PSSP, and 59 and 17% were PISP and PRSP, respectively. After we changed our method of choosing antibiotics, the prevalence of PSSP increased up to 53% of all isolated SP, and that of PRSP decreased by 16.5%.

The prevalence of BLNAS had been decreasing in all strains of HI, and that of low BLNAR+BLNAR had been increasing until 2007 from 62 to 30 and 38 to 70%, respectively. However, the prevalence of BLNAR decreased a little in 2008 and 2009.

Table 1. Changes in prevalence of susceptible and non-susceptible strains of *S. pneumoniae* and *H. influenzae*

	2001	2007	2009
S. pneumoniae			
PSSP	90 (25%)		411(53%)
PISP	212 (59%)		358 (46%)
PRSP	60 (17%)		4 (0.5%)
H. influenzae			
BLNAS	330 (62%)	223(30%)	320 (41%)
low BLNAR	85 (16%)	167 (22%)	135 (17%)
BLNAR	114 (22%)	359 (48%)	303 (39%)
BLPAR	0 (0%)	0 (0%)	17 (2%)

Discussion

Before the Japanese version of the AOM guideline was issued, we started using a similar treatment algorithm to the guideline and succeeded in reducing the prevalence of nonsusceptible strains of SP by about 30%. Though the key to success was AMPC as the first-line antibiotic, another factor might have been that Nemuro is a geographically isolated community with a population of 32,000 and a limited number of clinicians who prescribe antibiotics for children.

On the other hand, we still have the continued issues concerning the high prevalence of BLNAR. The reason why the proportion of BLNAR has not shown an obvious decrease might be that the antibiotics we use, such as cefditoren pivoxil (CDTR-PI), do not have sufficient efficacy to kill them and may select BLNAR in the nasopharynx in spite of showing the lowest MIC value to BLNAR of all the oral antibiotics available in Japan [3]. In addition, we do not think the decrease in the prevalence of nonsusceptible strains of SP has reached its goal.

In 2010, PCV7 has become available in Japan, i.e. over 10 years after the USA or other developed countries. We are expecting a good efficacy of this vaccine in Japan. However, we have already known that the use of the vaccine has led to an increase in the rate of AOM due to nonvaccine serotypes [4]. Therefore, there must be no change in the importance of an appropriate use of antibiotics even in the multivalent vaccine era.

References

1 Japan Otological Society, Japan Society for Pediatric ORL, Japan Society of Infectious Diseases in Otolaryngology: Clinical practice guideline for pediatric acute otitis media (in Japanese). Otol Jpn 2006;16:1–34.

2 WHO: ATC/DDD index 2010. http://www.whocc.no/atc_ddd_index/.

3 Takahata S, Kato Y, Sanbongi Y, Maebashi K, Ida T: Comparison of the efficacies of oral beta-lactams in selection of *Haemophilus influenzae* transformants with mutated ftsI genes. Antimicrob Agents Chemother 2008;52:1880–1883.

4 Eskola J, Kilpi T, Palmu A, Jokinen J, Haapakoski J, Herva E, Takala A, Kayhty H, Karma P, Kohberger R, Siber G, Makela PH: Efficacy of a pneumococcal conjugate vaccine against acute otitis media. N Engl J Med 344:403–409.

Tatsuya Hayashi
Department of Otolaryngology- Head and Neck Surgery, Asahikawa Medical University
Midorigaoka Higashi 2–1–1–1
Asahikawa, Hokkaido 078-8510 (Japan)
Tel. +81 166 68 2554, Fax +81 166 68 2559, E-Mail thayashi@asahikawa-med.ac.jp

Harabuchi Y (ed): Recent Advances in Tonsils and Mucosal Barriers of the Upper Airways.
Adv Otorhinolaryngol. Basel, Karger, 2011, vol 72, pp 179–224

Mucosal Defense Mechanism and Vaccine

From Tonsils to NALT: Historical Perspective of Evolution of Inductive Lymphoid Tissue in the Nasopharynx

Pearay L. Ogra

University at Buffalo, School of Medicine and Biomedical Sciences; and Women and Children's Hospital, Buffalo, New York, N.Y., USA

The salivary glands, the palatine tonsils and other glandular tissues in the Waldeyer's ring in man have had a long-standing and often controversial association with the functional integrity of the upper respiratory tract and or development of disease. About one hundred years ago, plasma cells were first observed in tonsillar tissues. Since then, tonsillectomy and adenoidectomy (T&A) has been routinely recommended for the treatment and control of chronic recurrent pharyngeal and tonsillar infections. However, during the early part of 20th century, numerous clinical and epidemiologic studies clearly established a causal relationship between T&A and the significantly higher (4- to 6-fold) risk of development of Bulbar poliomyelitis. Although a number of possible mechanisms may underlie such association, studies carried out in early 1970s demonstrated a striking decline in poliovirus specific nasopharyngeal antibody responses after T&A and in subjects with prior history of T&A, following intranasal immunization with polio vaccines. Subsequently, a number of elegant investigations by other investigators defined the basic immunologic framework and function aspects of palatine tonsils in man. These include the demonstration of follicular germinal centers, mantle zones of lymphoid follicles, the extra follicular areas and the reticular crypt epithelium on the surface in constant contact with external environment. The tonsillar epithelium was shown to contain a significant number of dendritic cells (DC), M cells, memory B cells and scattered B and T cells. The formation of the germinal centers begins shortly after birth, secondary to the activation by environmental antigens, and plasma cells appeared in tonsils by 2–3 weeks of age. Unlike Peyer's patches, tonsils exhibited considerable in situ differentiation to plasma cells. The germinal centers (which typically arise during T cell-dependent B cell responses) were observed to generate plasma blasts and plasma cells of both IgG and IgA isotypes. There was, however, a predominance of IgG isotype (60–70% for IgG vs. 15–20% for IgA). Recent studies have shown that tonsils function as an effective inductive site for mucosal immune responses and exhibit features similar to gut associated lymphoid tissue (GALT), bronchus-associated lymphoid tissue (BALT) and other inductive sites. These include clonal B cell activation, affinity maturation of B cell receptors and selection of binding, B cell differentiation for memory and plasma cells, induction of j-chain genes, and expression and activation of specific homing receptors and selective delivery and homing of antigen sensitized B and T cells to effector mucosal sites. Recent studies in the rat, mouse and hamster have shown the presence of organized lymphoid tissue situated at the entrance of nasopharyngeal duct. This represents an important component of mucosal lymphoid tissue in the rodents. It bears striking morphologic and functional resemblance to other central lymphoid tissues, such as GALT or BALT. The nasopharyngeal lymphoid tissue (NALT) appears to have better developed lymphoid follicles, with marked intraepithelial infiltration by lymphocytes. The follicular areas are organized into B cells and intrafollicular (T cell) areas of approximately similar size. The rodent NALT contains a wealth of DC. The lymphoid follicles are covered by ciliated epithelium containing few goblet cells and numerous M cells. The NALT M cells appear to be identical with those in Peyer's patches and BALT and are involved in similar immunological functions, including antigen uptake and subsequent mucosal immune responses to specific antigens. It is not clear if the functional role of Waldeyer's ring in humans is identical to the NALT in rodents. However, there is increasing evidence to suggest that human tonsillar and adenoidal tissues are important components of mucosal immunity and function in a manner similar to those of GALT. It has been proposed that NALT may represent a more important inductive site than BALT for mucosal immune response in the upper airway.

Mucosal Selection of Pneumococcal Capsular Serotypes by the Conjugate Vaccine and by Cystic Fibrosis

David E. Briles, Marilyn J. Crain, Susan K. Hollingshead

University of Alabama at Birmingham, Birmingham, Ala., USA

Pneumococcal conjugate vaccine is recommended for prevention of invasive pneumococcal disease in children ≤5 years of age. The 7 capsular serotypes selected for the first pneumococcal conjugate vaccine (PCV) covered 85% of the strains causing disease prior to its introduction in 2000. PCV 7 is effective against disease and colonization by capsular types present in the vaccine. Since PCV 7 licensure, the frequency of disease caused by serotypes not included in the vaccine has increased thereby reducing the efficacy of the vaccine. In 2010, a new 13-valent vaccine (containing 6 additional capsular types) was introduced in an effort to reduce the gaps left by the first vaccine. At present, our studies of pneumococcal strains in Alabama indicate that ≥50% of invasive and noninvasive isolates are not covered by the new 13-valent vaccine. In fact, from 2008 to 2010 (prior to use of the new vaccine) the frequency of strains covered by PCV 13 has continued to decrease ($p = 0.04$). This may be due to the fact that strains of a large number of different capsular types are continuing to crowd into the niche left by the original 7 capsular types. Our results and similar findings by others suggest that conjugate vaccines may need to become much more complex, if they are to continue to be able to control pneumococcal disease in children. We have observed that pneumococci in the sputum of cystic fibrosis (CF) patients have a markedly higher frequency of highly mucoid phenotypes than do pneumococci from the sputum from non-CF patients. Mucoid *Pseudomonas aeruginosa* infection is also frequently seen in CF sputum late in the course of disease. In vitro studies with *Streptococcus pneumoniae* indicate that highly mucoid pneumococci become more frequent in long-term pneumococcal biofilms. These results suggest that bacterial biofilms may exist in the CF lung where they are able to affect the characteristics of the pneumococci as well as the *P. aeruginosa* that live in/infect in the CF lung.

Mucosal Immunity and Bacterial Infections of the Upper Airways: Are Mucosal Vaccines the Answer?

Timothy F. Murphy

University at Buffalo, State University of New York, N.Y., USA

The human respiratory tract is susceptible to a variety of bacterial infections. Many of these infections, including otitis media and sinusitis, affect the mucosal surface and are primarily mucosal infections. Two important pathogens in this setting are nontypeable *Haemophilus influenzae* (NTHI) and *Moraxella catarrhalis*. In view of the observation that these upper airway infections are primarily mucosal infections, a strategy of mucosal immunization is potentially promising. A challenge for vaccine development for NTHI is genetic and antigenic heterogeneity of surface antigens among strains. To assess the major outer membrane protein P2 of NTHI as a mucosal vaccine, groups mice were immunized mucosally or systemically with purified recombinant P2, and the resulting antibody responses were evaluated. Interestingly, while systemic immunization induced strain specific antibody responses, mucosal immunization induced antibodies that recognized surface exposed epitopes in multiple strains of NTHI. Thus, the route of immunization is a critical determinant of the characteristics of the immune response, including the strain specificity of potentially protective antibodies. *Moraxella catarrhalis* is a common cause of otitis media and vaccine development for *M. catarrhalis* otitis media has lagged behind that of other bacterial pathogens. Using a genome mining approach, novel conserved surface proteins of *M. catarrhalis* have been identified. Mucosal immunization of mice with purified recombinant surface proteins induces potentially protective immune responses in the mouse pulmonary clearance model. These observations have important implications in understanding mucosal immune responses to upper respiratory tract pathogens and also suggest that mucosal immunization may be a viable and effective strategy for vaccine development for upper respiratory tract bacterial infections.

Mucosal Vaccines for Paramyxovirus Infections: Targeting the Host or the Pathogen?

Roberto P. Garofalo

Department of Pediatrics, University of Texas Medical Branch, Galveston, Tex., USA

The *Paramyxoviridae* family includes enveloped, negative-sense, single-stranded RNA viruses, which are major and ubiquitous disease causing pathogens of humans and animals. Among them are respiratory syncytial virus (RSV) and human metapneumovirus (hMPV). Vaccines for RSV and hMPV have not been developed yet and a major hurtle to their development is the understanding of the complex interaction between virus-specific proteins and host immunity. Indeed, genetics and environmental modulation of innate immune genes that affect host response to RSV and hMPV are critical in shaping the immune response in the upper and lower airways, both in naturally acquired infections and after vaccination. Viral proteins, both in the RSV in the hMPV genome, have been shown to inhibit components of the innate and adaptive immunity, thus interfering with an effective immune response following infections. The same inhibitory pathways should therefore be considered when designing new potential vaccines for such pathogens. Some examples of the innate immune genes that have been shown to affect the response to RSV and hMPV are those encoding the Toll-like receptors (TLRs), a family of evolutionary conserved pattern recognition receptors. We and other have recently shown the role of certain TLRs and downstream signaling molecules in inducing type I interferon production as well as shaping adaptive immune response against RSV and hMPV. We have also discovered that certain viral proteins are able to inhibit TLR-mediated cell signaling in important immune cells such as macrophages and dendritic cells. Other host genes that appear to be affected (inhibited) by RSV and hMPV infections are those encoding critical anti-oxidant proteins, leading to oxidative-mediated airway injury that seems to favor viral replication and pathology. This presentation will review some of the major components of the innate immune system in the airways that control and/or are affected by human paramyxovirus proteins.

CPG-DNA Induces CD274 Expression on Human B Cells

Seita Kubo, Takechiyo Yamada, Shigeharu Fujieda

Department of Otorhinolaryngology, University of Fukui, Fukui City, Japan

Background: B cells accounting for about 60% of tonsil lymphocytes not only produce immunoglobulin but also present antigens to T cells. T cell activity is regulated by co-stimulatory molecules that interact with its ligands on antigen presenting cells and act in synchrony with the T cell receptor signaling to inhibit (co-inhibition) or enhance (co-stimulation) immunity. **Objective:** We investigated the effect of CpG-ODN on human B cells in vitro. The expression of co-stimulatory molecule of B cells and its function were analyzed. **Method:** CD19 microbeads were used for the separation of B cells from tonsillar cells or PBMC. The B cells and human B lymphoma cell line Ramos 2G6 was maintained and cultured in complete RPMI 1640. The cells were stimulated with various conditions and the expression levels of CD274 (PD-L1, B7-H1) and B7.RP1 were detected by real time PCR and Western blotting. We also investigated the effect on cytokine-production from antigen-stimulated human CD4+ cells when ODN 2006-treated B cells and CD4+ cells were co-cultured. **Conclusion:** ODN 2006 (B type CpG ODN) increased PD-L1 expression while it suppressed B7.RP1 expression in human B cells. ODN 2216 had no effect on the expression of PD-L1 and B7-RP1. ODN 2006-treated B cells decreased IL-5 production from antigen-stimulated human CD4+ cells by 40%. The addition of PD-1-Ig, chimeric molecule of PD-1 and immunoglobulin, reversed its reduction of IL-5 from antigen-stimulated CD4+ cells. These results suggested that the treatment of B type CpG-DNA suppressed antigen-specific IL-5 production via PD-1–PD-L1 ligation.

Natural Killer Cells in the Upper Respiratory Immune System

Kazunari Okada[a], Shintaro Sato[b], Ayuko Sato-Kimura[b], Il-Gyu Kong[b], Tatsuya Yamasoba[a], Hiroshi Kiyono[b]

[a]Department of Otorhinolaryngology-Head and Neck Surgery, Graduate School of Medicine and [b]Division of Mucosal Immunology, Institute for Medical Science, University of Tokyo, Tokyo, Japan

Natural killer (NK) cells are known as a main character of host defense, for its antitumor and antiviral function. In spite of its importance, little is known about NK cells in the upper respiratory immune system. NKp46 (CD335) is a newly identified member of NCR receptor family, encoded by Ncr1 gene. Unlike other markers ever used, NKp46 is specific to NK cells, independent of the strain or maturation status. Recently, some groups reported about unique population of gut NKp46+ cells, which have special role in regulation of gut immune system. Here we would like to show some data about NK cells in murine nasal passage and submandibular gland, using Ncr1-GFP knock-in mice (gifted from Dr. Mandelboim, Israel), which reveal the difference between gut and upper respiratory immune system. We also adopt nasal influenza virus infection model, to find the importance of NK cells in the nasal passage.

Pneumococcal Peptidoglycan-Polysaccharides (PGPS) Regulate Toll-Like Receptor 2 (TLR2) in Human Tracheal Epithelial Cells

Masahiro Komori[a], Yoshihisa Nakamura[b], Masamitsu Hyodo[a], Jizhen Lin[c]

Departments of Otolaryngology, [a]Kochi University, School of Medicine, Nangoku-shi, and [b]Nagoya City University, School of Medicine, Nagoya, Japan; [c]Department of Otolaryngology, University of Minnesota School of Medicine, Minn., USA

Objective: Toll-like receptor 2 (TLR2) plays a key role in Gram-positive bacteria and their cell wall envelope components. However, little is known about the expression of TLR2 in the middle ear under otitis media (OM) conditions and its role in the persistent otitis media with effusion, characterized by a low profile of inflammation in the middle ear mucosa for a prolonged period of time. **Methods:** All human specimens and human tracheal epithelial cells (NL-20) were used in this study. Immunohistochemistry and ELISA for TLR2 and luciferase assays of the nuclear factor-κB (NF-kB) were performed. **Results:** The pneumococcal cell wall component, peptidoglycan-polysaccharides (PGPS), activated the expression of TLR2 in the middle ear epithelial cells through NF-kB-cytokine signaling pathway in a positive regulatory manner. While I kappa B alpha mutant (IkB α M), a dominant negative inhibitor of NF-kB, abrogated the expression of TLR2 induced by PGPS and disrupted the positive regulatory loop. **Conclusion:** This study suggests that the existence of residual PGPS in the middle ear cavity sensitizes the activity of inflammatory reaction in the middle ear mucosa via upregulation of TLR2, which may maintain a low profile of cytokine production in the middle ear mucosa and thus contribute to the pathogenesis of OME.

Roles of Eotaxin and Interleukin-17A in the Eosinophil Accumulation and Mucosal Remodeling in Chronic Rhinosinusitis with Nasal Polyps Associated with Asthma

Katsuhisa Ikeda

Department of Otorhinolaryngology, Juntendo University Faculty of Medicine, Tokyo, Japan

We reported that enhanced eotaxin family production by eosinophils resulted in the recruitment of eosinophils into the tissue by a self-amplifying process [Laryngoscope 2009;119:1053–1059]. IL-17A is a highly inflammatory cytokine with a robust effect on stromal cells in many tissues. Although IL-17A is known to be associated with inflammatory lung disorders by triggering an accumulation of neutrophils, the effect of IL-17A on the upper airway is still uncertain. The expression of IL-17A and its role were investigated in the nasal polyps of chronic rhinosinusitis associated with asthma. IL-17A was detected by immunohistochemistry and quantitative real-time RT-PCR. The cellular source of IL-17A was examined by double staining with EG2, CD4 and neutrophil elastase. The tissue remodeling of the nasal polyps was evaluated by assessing the epithelial damage and basement membrane thickness. Both the immunoreactivity and mRNA of IL-17A was significantly detected in the nasal polyps in comparison to control normal sinus mucosa. The localization of IL-17A expression predominantly coincided with eosinophils and CD4-positive lymphocytes. Furthermore, the number of IL-17A-positive cells correlated with tissue eosinophils, but not with neutrophils. The degree of epithelial damage and basement membrane thickness was dependent on the number of infiltrated IL-17A-positive cells. The present study suggests, for the first time, that IL-17A combined with eotaxin plays an important role in the eosinophil accumulation and the remodeling of the nasal polyps of chronic rhinosinusitis associated with asthma.

Expression of Trefoil Factor Family in the Human Nasal Mucosa

Nobuyuki Miyahara, Takashi Kono, Keishin Go, Takashi Ishino, Sachio Takeno, Katsuhiro Hirakawa

Department of Otorhinolaryngology, Head and Neck Surgery, Hiroshima University, Hiroshima, Japan

In the airways and gastrointestinal tract, the mucins have been important proteins to maintain epithelium of a mucous membrane. MUC5AC and MUC5B in chronic airway diseases such as chronic sinusitis, allergic rhinitis, asthma, and cystic fibrosis, are increased compared with those in normal sinus mucosa. In addition to these mucins, peptides called as trefoil factor family (TFF) were reported in late years. TFF peptides are secretory products of many mucous cells and have a close association with mucins. These peptides appear to be important in mucosal healing processes and in neoplastic. In human, three trefoil factor peptides, TFF1 (pS2), TFF2 (formerly spasmolytic polypeptide, SP), TFF3 (intestinal trefoil factor, ITF or hP1.B) are detected. TFF peptides have been detected in gastrointestinal tract, hypothalamus and pituitary, conjunctiva, uterus, breast, and also in mucosal surfaces of the human respiratory tract. Before now, the expression of TFF1 and TFF3 was observed in the human respiratory tract. However, the role of TFF peptides in nasal mucosa is still not completely understood. The aim of this study was to investigate an association with TFF peptides and mucins, and the role of TFF peptides in human inferior turbinate. The localization of TFF1 and TFF3 immunoreactively showed similar pattern in epithelial goblet cells, ciliated cells, submucosal glandular cells. In the double-staining study, TFF1 and TFF3 were extensively colocalized with MUC5AC in the epithelium. TFF1 and TFF3 were colocalized with MUC5B in the epithelium and the submucosal glandular cells. RT-PCR analysis revealed that the levels of TFF3 and MUC5B in allergic mucosa were significantly increased compared with those in non-allergic mucosa. These results suggest that TFF1 and TFF3 have an association with MUC5AC and MUC5B in nasal mucosa, and upregulation of TFF3 and MUC5B may play important roles in the clinical condition of nasal mucosa.

Cooperative Activation of Eotaxin-3 Expression by dsRNA and IL-4 in Human Nasal Epithelial Cells

So Watanabe[a, d], Jiyun Wang[c], Satoshi Matsukura[b], Harumi Suzaki[a]

[a]Department of Otorhinolaryngologyand [b]Division of Respiratory and Allergy, Department of Internal Medicine, Showa University School of Medicine, Tokyo, Japan; [c]Department of Otorhinolaryngology, Ningbo No. 2 Hospital, Ningbo, China; [d]Department of Surgery, Section of Otolaryngology – Head and Neck Surgery, University of Chicago, Chicago, Ill., USA

Background: The exacerbation of chronic rhinosinusitis is usually caused by viral infection. Virus appears to make the respiratory tract vulnerable to secondary inciting events, such as antigen challenges. Allergen challenge performed after rhinovirus inoculation showed a significantly greater increase in the nasal output of eosinophil peroxidase when compared with that performed before inoculation. These suggest enhanced functions of eosinophils after virus infection. **Objectives:** The aim of this study was to reveal the mechanism activating eosinophils during and after viral infection of the nasal epithelium, using a model of viral infection. **Methods:** A synthetic double-stranded RNA, poly inosinic-cytidyric acid (poly (I:C)), was used to stimulate a human nasal epithelial cell line RPMI 2650, to mimic a viral infection. The expression of chemokines after the stimulation was investigated by real-time PCR. **Results:** The stimulation of poly (I:C), alone, didn't affect the eotaxin-3 expression of the cells. However, the stimulation of poly (I:C) prior to IL-4 stimulation enhanced eotaxin-3 expression. **Conclusions:** These results suggest that viral airway infection might sensitize the nasal epithelial cells and enhance allergen-induced response, which might result in airway eosinophilia.

Arachidonate 5-Lipoxygenase Establishes Adaptive Humoral Immunity by Controlling Primary B Cells and Follicular B Helper T Cells

Tsutomu Nagashima[a, b], *Shingo Ichimiya*[b], *Shigeru Koshiba1*, *Hiroshi Matsumiya*[a, b], *Shihoko Ara*[a, b], *Terufumi Kubo*[b], *Noriyuki Sato*[b], *Tetsuo Himi*[a]

Departments of [a]Otolaryngology and [b]Pathology, Sapporo Medical University School of Medicine, Sapporo, Japan

Arachidonate 5-lipoxygenase (Alox5) was a key enzyme to produce lipid mediators like leukotrienes and lipoxins, but the function of Alox5 in humoral immune responses is unclear. In this study, we reported the unique role of Alox5 in the regulation of specific humoral immune responses. We have previously established L22 mAb specifically reacting to primary resting B cells of mantle zones of human tonsils. By employing LC-MS/MS analysis, we identified Alox5 as a L22 antigen. Quantitative RT-PCR and immunoblot analyses demonstrated high expression of Alox5 in both naïve and memory B cells. Interestingly, when the BCRs of tonsil-derived B cells were stimulated, the cells could secrete leukotrienes, including leukotriene B_4 and cysteinyl leukotrienes. To investigate the role of Alox5 in humoral immune responses in vivo, we immunized *Alox5–/–* mice with sheep red blood cells (SRBCs). *Alox5–/–* mice exhibited weak antibody responses specific to foreign antigens at both the initial and recall phases. According to flow cytometry analysis of freshly isolated spleen cells, *Alox5–/–* mice demonstrated a significantly decreased number of follicular B cells which play an important role in antibody production in a T cell-dependent manner. When investigating the features of follicular B cells of *Alox5–/–* mice, after examination of various molecules related to antibody production the expression levels of the IL-21 receptor of the cells were profoundly reduced. So far, weak antibody responses of *Alox5–/–* mice were probably attributable to the low number of follicular and memory B cells as well as the functional loss of IL-21-mediated responses of follicular B cells. Moreover, *Alox5–/–* mice could not fully foster the development of follicular B helper T (Tfh) cells even after immunization with foreign antigens. Our results illustrate the novel role of Alox5 in adaptive humoral immunity by managing primary B cells and Tfh cells in vivo.

Role of Infection in the Development of Adenoids

Elena P. Merkulova, Anna R. Savdon

Belarusian State Medical University, Minsk, Belarus

Introduction: The diseases of the lymphopharyngeal ring organs take a leading place among the pediatric population of the Republic of Belarus. Chronic foci of infection present an important problem in pediatric practice. **Aim:** To establish the role of infection in the etiology of hypertrophy and chronic inflammation of pharyngeal tonsils in children of various age. **Materials and Methods:** The comparative analysis of microbiological examination results of removed adenoids (n) and peculiarities of the clinical picture of pharyngeal tonsil pathology in 98 children at the ages from 2 to 18 years (N). **Results:** The analysis of microbiological examination of removed adenoids testifies to a high incidence of pathogenic flora (64%; n = 62/98), in 95% the coccous flora is revealed (n = 59/62). *Staphylococcus aureus* prevails among cocci –71%, *Streptococcus pyogenes* –16%. Allergic anamnesis is aggravated in 16.3% of the children (n = 16/98). The dependence of the pathogenic flora incidence on age and clinical picture of the disease has been established. In the group of children aged under 5, the percentage of pathogenic flora is lower than in children over 5 years (63–86.4%, $p< 0.05$); also in the group of children without adenoiditis, pathogenic flora occurs less frequently than in the group with clinical manifestations of adenoiditis (58.8–78.7%, respectively; $p < 0.05$). **Conclusions:** (1) Pathogenic microflora plays an important role in the etiopathogenesis of adenoids in children of various ages and occurs in 64% of cases. (2) The comparative analysis of the pathogenic flora incidence depending on clinical picture and age of children revealed that pathogenic microflora prevails authentically more often in the group of children over 5 years and in the group of children with clinical manifestations of adenoiditis.

M-Like Cells of Human Adenoids in vivo and in vitro

Ken-ichi Takano[a], Takashi Kojima[b], Noriko Ogasawara[a], Mitsuru Go[a], Shin Kikuchi[c], Takafumi Ninomiya[c], Makoto Kurose[a], Jun-ichi Koizumi[a], Ryuta Kamekura[a], Norimasa Sawda[b], Tetsuo Himi[a]

Departments of [a]Otolaryngology, [b]Pathology and [c]Anatomy, Sapporo Medical University, Sapporo, Japan

The human adenoid epithelium forms a continuous barrier against a wide variety of exogenous antigens. In this study, to elucidate the structures of the epithelial barrier in the human adenoid, including M cells, we identified M cells using an anti-cytokeratin 20 (Ck20) antibody and investigated expression of tight junction proteins in human adenoid epithelium in vivo and in vitro. In human adenoid epithelium and primary cultures, mRNAs of occludin, junctional adhesion molecule-A, ZO-1, and claudin-1, claudin-4, claudin-7, and claudin-8 were detected by reverse transcription-polymerase chain reaction, whereas claudin-2 and claudin-9 were expressed in vitro. In the epithelium in vivo, some Ck20-positive cells were randomly observed and indicated pocket-like structures, whereas Ck7 was positive in almost cells. Transmission electron microscopy revealed that Ck20-associated gold particles could be identified in M-like cells which had short microvilli and harbored the lymphocyte in the pocket-like structure. In primary cultures in vitro, Ck20-positive cells were also detected and had a function to take up fluorescent microparticles. In Ck20-positive cells in vivo and in vitro, expression of occludin, ZO-1, claudin-1 and claudin-7 were observed at the cell borders. These results indicate that the epithelial barrier of the human adenoid is stably maintained by expression of tight junction proteins in the epithelium including Ck20-positive M-like cells.

Morphological Changes of Olfactory Neurons after Bulbectomy

Tomoyuki Nomura[a], Tatsuo Ushiki[b], Sugata Takahashi[a]

Departments of [a]Otolaryngology and [b]Microscopic Anatomy and Bio-Imaging, Niigata University Faculty of Medicine, Niigata, Japan

Background: Morphological changes in olfactory cells after bulbectomy are largely unknown. In this study, we histologically examined time-dependent changes in the microstructure of olfactory cells after bulbectomy. **Methods:** Male ddY mice were used. Normal mice and their bulbectomized counterparts at 2–270 days after bulbectomy were perfusion-fixed with 2% glutaraldehyde, and the nasal mucosa was removed. A part of each removed specimen was embedded in epoxy resin, and semi-ultrathin sections were cut, stained with toluidine blue, and examined under a light microscope. The remaining part was processed by a combination of the KOH-collagenase digestion method and microdissection technique, and the olfactory epithelial and nasal surfaces were observed by scanning electron microscopy. **Results:** In the normal mice, various cells composing the olfactory epithelium were identified. In contrast, at 2 days after bulbectomy, degenerating cells with hollow of varying size were observed in the upper layer of the olfactory epithelium. At 5 days after bulbectomy, many olfactory cells had disappeared, resulting in a decrease in the thickness of the olfactory epithelium. At 7–14 days after bulbectomy, immature olfactory cells at various stages were observed in the epithelium, and large cells apparently representing dividing cells were present in the basal layer. At 30 and 60 days after bulbectomy, the epithelium had increased in thickness, and mature and apparently immature olfactory cells were identified in the intermediate and lower layers, respectively. However, from the 120th day after bulbectomy, the epithelial thickness decreased again, and the number of olfactory cells was very small. Very few dividing cells were observed, and supporting cells were seen to phagocytose degenerating olfactory cells. These finding were compared with the light-microscopic findings to clarify the processes of degeneration, differentiation, and maturation.

Expression and Function of Tight Junctions in the Crypt Epithelium of Human Palatine Tonsils

Mitsuru Go[a], Takashi Kojima[b], Ken-ichi Takano[a], Makoto Kurose[a], Tsuyoshi Ohkuni[a], Tomoyuki Masaki[a], Ryuta Kamekura[a], Atsushi Kondo[b], Noriko Ogasawara[a], Tetsuo Himi[a], Norimasa Sawada[b]

Departments of [a]Otolaryngology and [b]Pathology, Sapporo Medical University School of Medicine, Sapporo, Japan

The human palatine tonsils have surface and crypt stratified epithelium and may be initiated via the epithelium to mount immune responses to various presenting antigens. Here we investigated the expression and function of tight junctions in the epithelium of human palatine tonsils from patients with tonsillar hypertrophy or recurrent tonsillitis. Occludin, ZO-1, JAM-1, and claudin-1, claudin-3, claudin-4, claudin-7, claudin-8, and claudin-14 mRNAs were detected in tonsillar hypertrophy. Occludin and claudin-14 were expressed in the uppermost layer of the tonsil surface epithelium, whereas ZO-1, JAM-1, and claudin-1, claudin-4, and claudin-7 were found throughout the epithelium. In the crypt epithelium, claudin-4 was preferentially expressed in the upper layers. In freeze-fracture replicas, short fragments of continuous tight junction strands were observed but never formed networks. In the crypt epithelium of recurrent tonsillitis, the tracer was leaked from the surface regions where occludin and claudin-4 disappeared. Occludin, ZO-1, JAM-1, and claudin-1, claudin-3, claudin-4, and claudin-14, but not claudin-7, mRNAs were decreased in recurrent tonsillitis compared with those of tonsillar hypertrophy. These studies suggest unique expression of tight junctions in human palatine tonsillar epithelium, and the crypt epithelium may possess an epithelial barrier different from that of the surface epithelium.

Pretreatment of Epithelial Cells with Poly(I:C) Enhances the Adherence of *Streptococcus Pneumoniae*

Masaki Kawabata, Yuichi Kurono

Department of Otolaryngology, Head and Neck Surgery, Kagoshima University Graduate School of Medical and Dental Science, Kagoshima, Japan

Introduction: Upper respiratory tract infectins with virus are often followed by secondary bacterial infections. *Streptococcus pneumoniae* are commensal microoraganism and are also major causative bacteria of acute otitis media (AOM) and paranasal sinusitis. However, the mechanisms how commensal bacteria can be a pathogen of those infectious diseases are not completely understood. Recently, several studies have revealed the potential for respiratory viral infections to enhance *S. pneumonia* infections in lower respiratory epithelial cells. In the present study, we examined the impact of pretreatment with viral agent, Poly(I:C), in the adherence of *S. pneumoniae*. **Materials and Methods:** Detroit 562 cells (ATCC CCL-138), a human pharyngeal carcinoma cell line, were pretreated with Poly(I:C) and *S. pneumoniae* were added to the culture. Adherent FITC-labeled *S. pneumoniae* were counted visually with a phase microscope. **Results:** Pretreatment of Detroit 562 cells with Poly(I:C) enhanced the adherence of *S. pneumoniae*. **Conclusions:** These results suggest that enhanced adherence of *S. pneumoniae* may be one of the reasons commensal bacteria can be a pathogen of infectious diseases.

Measurement of Electrical Potential Differences on Human Pharyngeal Mucosa

Masato Miwa, Kensuke Watanabe

Dokkyo Medical University Koshigaya Hospital, Koshigaya, Japan

Introduction: The mucosal barrier function of the upper airways is critical to the host defense. The measurement of electrical potential differences (PD) of the skin had been proven to be an important noninvasive method for assessing the efficiency of the diagnosis for cystic fibrosis. PD has also been demonstrated in nose precisely in relation to allergic rhinitis. We have already detected the alteration of PD on the human nasal mucosal after nasal pollen challenge. The measurement of PD had been proven to be an important method for assessing the efficiency of the nasal epithelium as an electrical barrier. The aim of this study is to demonstrate the electrical feature of the human pharyngeal mucosa by measuring PD. **Methods:** PD of the posterior wall of the human pharyngeal mucosa was measured by using a high impedance voltage/current amplifier (DVC1000, WPI, Sarasota, Fla., USA) in accordance with the method previously described in experiments of human nose. We examined the effect of several test solutions on PD after nontraumatic application of 1-ml solutions of physiological saline, 0.01N HCl (and $ZnCl_2$ (0.1%), respectively, using laryngeal injector on the mucosal surface for 5 min. **Results:** We could examine PD of the posterior wall of the human pharyngeal mucosa. After application of HCl, PD was decreased compared with the basal state. After application of $ZnCl_2$, PD was significantly increased compared with the basal state. **Conclusion:** We make the first demonstration of PD through the human pharyngeal mucosa. These data should contribute to our understanding of the pathogenesis of the upper airway diseases caused by rupture of the barrier function like laryngopharyngeal reflux disease.

Sublingual Administration of Lactobacillus Inhibits Th2-Dependent Allergic Responses via the Upregulation of PD-L2 on Dendritic Cells

Ayako Inamine, Shigetoshi Horiguchi, Syu-ji Yonekura, Yoshitaka Okamoto

Department of Otolaryngology, Graduate School of Medicine, Chiba University, Chiba, Japan

Background: Lactic acid bacteria (LAB) have potential in immunomodulatory therapy, but their clinical efficacy is unclear and the underlying mechanisms have yet to be understood. **Objective:** To clarify the anti-allergic immune responses induced by lactic acid bacteria. **Methods:** The influence of lactic acid bacteria on immune responses was examined in dendritic cells (DCs) derived from murine bone marrow in vitro and in a mouse model of ovalbumin (OVA)-sensitized allergic rhinitis. **Results:** LAB influenced OVA-induced production of cytokines and expression of costimulatory molecules in mature DCs, but these patterns varied among strains. The Lactobacillus KW3110 strain increased IL-12 production, CCR-7 levels, and PD-L2 expression in DCs, and strongly inhibited IL-5 and IL-13 production in a coculture with Th2-skewed CD4+ T cells from DO11.10 mice. Sublingual administration of low doses of KW3110 to OVA-sensitized mice selectively suppressed Th2 cytokines in cervical lymph nodes and serum IgE levels, as well as improving nasal symptoms after OVA provocation. Treatment of DCs with neutralizing antibodies to PD-L2 abrogated the anti-allergic effects observed in KW3110-treated OVA-sensitized mice. **Conclusion:** KW3110 accelerates migration of DCs and inhibits production of Th2 cytokines through enhancement of CCR-7 and PD-L2 expression. Sublingual administration of KW3110 may be effective for reduction of allergic inflammation.

Production of IL-17 by Splenocytes of Offspring Delivered from PspA-Immunized Mother Mice

Masamitsu Kono, Muneki Hotomi, Akihisa Togawa, Shinji Tamura, Noboru Yamanaka

Department of Otolaryngology, Head and Neck Surgery, Wakayama Medical University, Wakayama, Japan

Background: Pneumococcal polysaccharide and polysaccharide-protein conjugate vaccines have not been ideal. These vaccines are not protective against strains with capsular types/groups not present in the vaccines. Furthermore, these vaccines have low immunogenicity against children younger than 2 years old due to the age-related immaturity of immune responses. Pneumococcal surface protein A (PspA) is a promising candidate for the development of a cost-effective protein-based pneumococcal vaccine. We have revealed the protection against pneumococcal carriage and infections to offspring by maternal immunization with PspA. In this study, we further evaluated the cytokine productions by splenocytes of mother mice and offspring, with special emphasis on IL-17A. **Method:** BALB/c bjy mice, 4-week-old female, were intranasally immunized with PspA. They were mated after the final immunization, and offspring were obtained. On day 10 days after the birth, splenocytes of offspring and mother mice were cultured with stimulation of PspA. The production of IL-4, IL-17A and IFN-g were evaluated by ELISA. **Results:** IL-17A was produced in a dose-dependent manner in PspA-immunized mother mice. The PspA- immunized mother's splenocytes produced IFN-g, but not IL-4. In offspring delivered from PspA-immunized mother and breast fed by PspA-immunized mother, the splenocytes produced IL-17A and IFN-g but not IL-4. **Discussion:** Although immunity to pneumococcal diseases has long been assumed to depend mainly on the humoral immunity, some reports have recently shown antibody-independent immunity mediated by Th17 subset in a mouse model of pneumococcal colonization. In this study, offspring delivered from PspA-immunized mother have immune responses mediated by IL-17A.

CD133/EpCAM Double-Positive Population Is a Candidate of Cancer Stem Cells in Squamous Cell Carcinoma of the Head and Neck

Hiroaki Kanaya, Wataru Konno, Hideki Hirabayashi, Shin-ichi Haruna

Department of Otorhinolaryngology, Head and Neck Surgery, Dokkyo Medical University, Tochigi, Japan

Background and Objectives: Discovery of a rare population of cancer stem cells (CSCs) has created a new focus in cancer research. Recently CD133 has been reported to be a CSCs marker in several solid tumors. The objective in this study was to evaluate the frequency of CD133 cells in head and neck cancer, and their biological behavior including tumorigenicity and tolerance to anticancer drugs in vitro. **Methods:** To detect CD133-positive cells in surgically resected pharyngeal squamous cell carcinoma (SCC), immunohistochemical examination was performed. Flow cytometric analysis of established SCC cell line (DHN1 cell) originated from tongue was also performed to evaluate actual incidence of CD133-positive cells. Subsequently, CD133-positive cells were isolated from DHN1 cell line using indirect microbeads kit. Tumorigenicity and tolerance to anticancer drugs (mitomycin C and cisplatinum) were compared between CD133 positively selected cells and bulk cells. **Results:** An immunohistochemistry showed only a small number of CD133 positive cells in resected SCC specimen. The incidence of CD133-positive cells in cultured SCC cell line was less than 0.2% by flow cytometric analysis. Enriched CD133-positive cells were successfully obtained using microbeads, and purity was up to 80%. Most of those cells were also positive for epithelial cell adhesion molecule (EpCAM), which was considered as a diagnostic marker of SCC. CD133-positive cells isolated from the DHN1 cell line possessed higher colony-forming efficiency and proliferative potential in vitro. In Annexin V-FITC staining, CD133 positive cells were not going to apoptosis and/or necrosis in media containing anti-cancer drugs. **Conclusions:** We herein reported that a very small number of tumorigenic CD133/EpCAM double positive cell is candidate of CSCs in SCC of head and neck. The identification of CSCs could provide new insight into tumorigenic process, relapsing and metastasizing lesion of SCC.

Changes in Levels of Nasal IgA and Serum IgG Antibodies against Influenza Virus Antigen in Patients with Natural Influenza Infection

Chisa Fujimoto[a], Hiroshi Kido[b], Miyoko Yamaguchi[b], Atsushi Matsunaga[c], Ayako Sawada[c], Takeshi Tanaka[d], Noriaki Takeda[a]

[a]Department of Otolaryngology, University of Tokushima School of Medicine and [b]Division of Enzyme Chemistry, Institute for Enzyme Research, University of Tokushima, Tokushima, [c]Ohkita Medical Clinic, Osaka, and [d]Mino Tanaka Hospital, Tokushima, Japan

Changes in levels of nasal IgA and serum IgG antibodies against influenza virus antigen were examined in patients with natural infection of influenza A virus during the 2007/2008 and 2008/2009 flu seasons, when H1N1 subtype of influenza A was prevalent in Japan. IgG levels in the serum and IgA levels in the nasal washing against influenza virus antigen were measured by ELISA. Nasal washings were taken by the nasal spray and aspiration method [Fujimoto C, et al: Auris Nasus Larynx 2009;36:300–304]. The levels of both serum IgG and nasal IgA antibodies against A/H1N1 antigen were significantly elevated in the patients after natural infection by influenza A virus. They reached maximum about 10 days after infection and then gradually decreased over a year. Although the H3N2 subtype of influenza A virus was a minor epidemic during the flu seasons, the levels of nasal IgA, but not serum IgG, antibodies were significantly elevated in the patients. Since most patients suffered from the H1N1 subtype of influenza A virus infection, these findings demonstrated that IgA antibodies against A/H1N1 antigen induced in the nasal cavity of the patients were able to cross-react with A/H3N2 antigen. On the contrary, it was also shown that IgG antibodies induced in the serum of the patients specifically reacted with A/H1N1 antigen. The currently available influenza vaccines administrated subcutaneously induce a predominantly IgG-mediated protection. Recently, we developed a nasal influenza HA vaccine adjuvanted with human pulmonary surfactant to induce antiviral IgA antibodies in the nose, in addition to antiviral IgG antibodies in the serum. The present findings that nasal IgA antibodies against A/H1N1 induced by infection of H1N1 subtype of influenza A virus crossreact with other subtype of A/H3N2 antigen suggested that nasal influenza vaccine induce antiviral IgA antibodies in the nasal cavity with wide cross protection activity in the airway.

New Therapeutic Strategies, a Chimeric Human-Cat Fusion Protein Inhibits Allergic Reactivity

Tetsuya Terada, Ryo Kawata, Hiroshi Takenaka

Department of Otorhinolaryngology, Osaka Medical College, Osaka, Japan

Since co-aggregation of FceRI with FcgRIIb, blocks FceRI-mediated reactivity of human mast cells and basophils, we proposed that an engineered allergen that would co-crosslink FcgRIIb to allergen specific IgE bound to the FceRI would block allergen specific reactivity and at the same time function as an immunotherapy that would not induce acute allergic reactivity. To test this concept, we created a novel chimeric fusion protein composed of the human IgGg Fc fused to the major cat allergen (GFD) and evaluated its ability to block IgE-mediated reactions in mice allergic to Fel d1. Balb/c mice were sensitized to Fel d1 by intraperitoneal injection of Fel d1 plus alum. Mice treated with three subcutaneous injections of GFD (5 mg ×3) at days 7, 14 and 21 also showed inhibition of systemic reactivity to IT challenge at days 28 and 42. Notably GFD itself failed to induce systemic allergic reactivity in animals actively sensitized to Fel d1. GFD was also tested for its effects on passive cutaneous anaphylaxis (PCA) to Fel d1 in human FceRIa transgenic mice. GFD blocked PCA in these mice. By itself, systemically GFD did not induce PCA in FceRIa transgenic mice. These results indicate that the Fcg-Fel d1 chimeric fusion protein could effectively block Fel d1 induced IgE mediated systemic reactivity while not induced mediator release on its own. GFD may provide a new and safer therapeutic approach for immunotherapy in IgE-mediated disease.

Nasal Vaccination with DNA Plasmid Encoding P6 Outer Membrane Protein of Nontypeable *Haemophilus Influenzae* (NTHi) Enhances NTHi Clearance in the Nasopharynx

Satoru Kodama, Takashi Hirano, Masashi Suzuki

Department of Otolaryngology, Oita University Faculty of Medicine, Yufu, Japan

DNA vaccines represent a new approach to the control of infectious diseases. DNA vaccine technology is a simple concept based on relatively simple design and production technology, and another advantage of DNA vaccines over conventional protein vaccines is the low cost of producing a highly purified product. Currently, nasal vaccination is the most effective regimen for the induction of antigen-specific immune responses in the upper respiratory tract, and the development of nasal vaccine is considered an important public health goal. In the present study, we examined the efficacy of nasal DNA vaccine on upper respiratory infections. P6 outer membrane protein is the common antigen among all nontypeable *Haemophilus influenzae* (NTHi) strains and is a candidate for a mucosal vaccine. A DNA plasmid encoding P6 was constructed, and then mice were immunized intranasally with DNA plasmid and immunostimulatory complex (ISCOM), which is a new vaccine delivery system and acts as an adjuvant. P6-specific immune responses were examined. In addition, live NTHi challenges were performed and the level of NTHi was quantified in nasal washes. DNA vaccination induced an increase in the number of dendritic cells in nasal-associated lymphoid tissue. P6-specific nasal wash immunoglobulin (Ig)A and serum IgG titers were elevated significantly after nasal immunization. The specific IgA-producing cells markedly increased in the nasal mucosa. In addition, enhanced NTHi clearance from the nasopharynx was also observed. The effect of nasal vaccination was prolonged for a long term. Thus, we have developed a successful DNA vaccination protocol for generation of in vivo immune responses against NTHi. These findings suggest that nasal vaccination with DNA vaccine and ISCOM might be an effective regimen for the induction of NTHi-specific protective immunity in the upper respiratory tract.

IgA Nephropathy

Role of Tonsillar B Cells in the Pathogenesis of IgA Nephropathy

Hitoshi Suzuki[a], *Yusuke Suzuki*[a], *Junichiro Nakata*[a], *Daisuke Satou*[a], *Hidenori Yokoi*[b], *Katsuhisa Ikeda*[b], *Jan Novak*[c], *Yasuhiko Tomino*[a]

[a]Division of Nephrology, Department of Internal Medicineand [b]Department of Otorhinolaryngology, Juntendo University Faculty of Medicine, Tokyo, Japan; [c]Department of Microbiology, University of Alabama at Birmingham, Birmingham, Ala., USA

IgA1 in circulating immune complexes and in the glomerular deposits of patients with IgA nephropathy (IgAN) is aberrantly glycosylated. However, the origin of this galactose-deficient IgA1 (Gd-IgA1) is unknown. Upper respiratory tract infections and/or tonsillitis are frequently associated with clinical presentation and exacerbation of IgAN. There is evidence that tonsillectomy with or without steroid pulse therapy prevents IgAN progression for certain patients. We hypothesized that tonsillar B cells may represent one of the sources of Gd-IgA1 in IgAN. In this study, we immortalized tonsillar B cells from IgAN patients (n = 21) and disease controls (n = 11; patients with chronic tonsillitis or sleep apnea but no renal disease) with Epstein-Barr virus and measured Gd-IgA1 secreted by these cells. Also, we measured serum levels of Gd-IgA1 and urinary IgA and Gd- IgA1 in the patients with IgAN before and after tonsillectomy. Although production of IgA did not differ between the two groups, only the immortalized tonsillar B cells from IgAN patients secreted Gd-IgA1 with oversialylated O-glycans. Expression of *β1,3- galactosyltransferase* was lower and that of *α2,6-GalNAc-sialyltransferaseII* was higher in the immortalized tonsillar B cells from IgAN patients compared to the cells from disease controls. Furthermore, we found that serum Gd-IgA1 levels and urinary excretion of IgA and Gd-IgA1 decreased in IgAN patients after tonsillectomy combined with glucocorticoid therapy. These results together suggest that tonsillar B cells may represent one of the potential sources of Gd- IgA1 in patients with IgAN.

Correlation among Tonsillar TLR9 Expression, *TLR9* SNP and Clinical Outcomes of Tonsillectomy with Steroid Pulse Therapy

Daisuke Sato[a], *Yusuke Suzuki*[a], *Tatsuya Kano*[a], *Hitoshi Suzuki*[a], *Hidenori Yokoi*[b], *Satoshi Horikoshi*[a], *Katsuhisa Ikeda*[b], *Yasuhiko Tomino*[a]

[a]Division of Nephrology, Department of Internal Medicine and [b]Department of Otorhinolaryngology Juntendo University Faculty of Medicine, Tokyo, Japan

Background: IgA nephropathy (IgAN) patients often show aggravation with macroscopic hematuria after tonsillar infections. Our recent report demonstrated that mucosal Toll-like receptor 9 (TLR9) activation has an important role in the pathogenesis of murine IgAN. We also found a significant association between *TLR9* single nucleotide polymorphism (SNP) (rs352140) and pathological severity in patients with IgAN. Based on these findings, the present study was intended to investigate correlations among tonsillar TLR9 mRNA expression, genotype of *TLR9* SNP and clinical outcomes of tonsillectomy with steroid pulse therapy in IgAN patients. **Methods:** Tonsillar TLR9 mRNA expression in IgAN (n = 49) and control (chronic tonsillitis and obstructive sleep apnea syndrome) (n = 15) patients who had undergone tonsillectomy were analyzed. Correlations among the expression level of TLR9 in tonsil, genotypes of *TLR9* SNP and clinical outcomes including hematuria, proteinuria and serum IgA level after the tonsillectomy with steroid pulse therapy were examined. **Results:** High expression of tonsillar TLR9 (> mean + SD) was observed in about 23% of IgAN patients. These patients showed higher and earlier remission of hematuria and proteinuria than patients whose TLR9 expression were low (< mean + SD). Patients with TT genotype of rs352140 SNP had severe renal damages. In patients who showed a more than average decrease of serum IgA level after tonsillectomy, cumulative remission rate of proteinuria were higher than in the rest of the patients. Interestingly, CC/CT genotypes were dominant and tonsillar TLR9 expressions were high in these patients. **Conclusion:** In patients with IgAN, high levels of tonsillar TLR9 expression and CC/CT genotype of *TLR9* were well correlated with treatment response of tonsillectomy with steroid pulse therapy.

Different Disease Phenotypes by Activation of TLR9 on Dendritic Cells and B Cells in Murine IgA Nephropathy

Tadahiro Kajiyama, Yusuke Suzuki, Masao Kihara, Hitoshi Suzuki, Satoshi Horikoshi, Yasuhiko Tomino

Division of Nephrology, Department of Internal Medicine, Juntendo University Faculty of Medicine, Tokyo, Japan

Background and Purpose: Pathological roles of dendritic cells (DC) and B cells in mucosal immunity have been discussed. On the other hand, we recently demonstrated that Toll-like receptor 9 (TLR9), especially in mucosa, has a crucial role in the pathogenesis of both human and murine IgA nephropathy (IgAN) [J Am Soc Nephrol 2008;19:2384–2395]. In the present study, we examined whether activation TLR9 on mucosal DC and B cells induces different disease phenotypes of murine IgAN by using different cell-specific types of CpG-ODN, which is a ligand of TLR9. **Methods:** For this study, we used three CpG-ODN, types A, B and C, which bind to TLR 9 on DC, B cells and both cells, respectively. Each 10 μg of types A, B and C CpG-ODN was nasally challenged to IgAN-prone mice (gddY) (4 weeks of age) at weekly intervals for 8 consecutive weeks. Blood and urine samples were collected before and after each administration. At 8 weeks after the mucosal immunization, kidney samples were also collected and evaluated histopathologically. **Results:** Urinary protein was aggravated after each administration of CpG-ODN in all mice. Serum elevation of IgA-IgG2a immune complexes was found in mice treated with types A and C, while serum IgA was increased in mice treated with type B. Interestingly, mice treated with type A showed mesangial proliferative glomerular lesions, while sclerotic glomerular damage mainly with sclerotic lesions was observed in those with type B, suggesting that different disease phenotypes were induced. **Conclusion:** It appears that the mucosal activation of TLR9 on DC and B cells may induce different types of glomerular damage in murine IgAN.

Image Analysis of Immune Complexes in Renal Deposits in IgA Nephropathy by Confocal Microscopy

Lea Novak[a], Hitoshi Suzuki[b], Bruce A. Julian[c], Jan Novak[b]

Departments of [a]Pathology, [b]Microbiology and [c]Medicine, Microbiology, and Surgery, University of Alabama at Birmingham, Birmingham, Ala., USA

IgA nephropathy (IgAN), the most common primary glomerulonephritis in the world, is characterized by IgA1-containing mesangial immune deposits, typically with complement C3 co-deposits. Onset of the disease frequently occurs after an episode of an upper respiratory tract infection. It has been speculated that the glomerular deposits originate from the circulating immune complexes containing aberrantly glycosylated IgA1. These glomerular immune deposits have not been well studied in terms of the composition and colocalization of the components. Frozen renal biopsy specimens from 12 IgAN patients containing IgA and C3 were double-stained with Cy3-conjugated anti-IgA and Cy5-conjugated anti-complement C3 fluorescent antibodies. The distribution, size and shape of immune complexes in the mesangium and glomerular capillaries were examined with a laser scanning confocal microscope. Colocalization of IgA and C3 in glomeruli was analyzed using image analysis software IP Lab and expressed as Pearson's coefficient (Pc = 1 indicates maximal co-localization). Moreover, lines were drawn through diameters of 10 immune complexes in each specimen to determine line intensity profiles. The mesangial immune complexes had irregular surface and variable size, up to 25 um, whereas capillary immune complexes were linear with smooth surfaces and variable in length. Furthermore, immune complexes in the mesangium exhibited two types of IgA and C3 intensity profiles: predominant IgA (n = 7) and predominant/co-dominant C3 (n = 5). An IgA-predominant profile with a higher co-localization value (mean Pc = 0.67) was observed for specimens from patients with severe renal tissue injury; specimens with a C3-predominant/codominant profile and a lower co-localization value (mean Pc = 0.50) indicated a mild injury. Most of capillary immune complexes showed IgA predominant intensity (n = 11) and there was no correlation with the degree of injury. In summary, these preliminary results suggest that confocal microscopy is a useful tool for analysis of the immune deposits in IgAN.

Immunological Study of the Tonsils in the Patients with IgA Nephropathy

Hanako Takechi[a], Koji Hozawa[b], Hiroshi Nagura[b], Takashi Oda[c], Hiroo Kumagai[c], Takeshi Matsunobu[c], Akihiro Shiotani[c], Osamu Hotta[b]

[a]Japan Self Defense Force Sendai Hospital and [b]Sendai Shakaihoken Hospital, Sendai, and [c]National Defense Medical College, Tokorozawa, Japan

The relationship between IgA nephropathy (IgAN) and the immunological abnormalities of tonsils has attracted attention in recent years. The purpose of this study was to investigate the mechanism of participation in the onset of IgAN from the standpoint of immunity of tonsils. The 209 patients with IgAN participated in this study. Tonsillectomy was performed in all of those patients. We examined histological change and immunohistochemical staining (CD8, HLA-DR, T cell, B cell) of tonsils. A phenotypic analysis was also performed using flow cytometry. The clinical data, especially the duration from the appearance of abnormalities in urinalysis to tonsillectomy, was compared with immunological data. The follicles and interfollicular areas were irregular and the border of follicle was unclear in IgAN, and these findings were the characteristics of tonsils of IgAN. HLA-DR+ T cells form nodules, and the number of nodules was significantly increased in tonsils of IgAN as compared with tonsils of chronic tonsillitis. We call these nodules T cell nodules (TCN). Tonsils removed at an earlier time (<4 years) from the appearance of the abnormalities in urinalysis showed increased TCN. The characteristics of IgAN such as irregular follicles and interfollicular area were not obvious. In contrast, tonsils removed at a later time (>4 years) appeared to have obvious characteristics of IgAN. The number of TCN was decreased. The increase of CD8+DR+ cell counts in the entire area of tonsils was correlated with the reduction of the number of TCN. These observations suggest that highly active T cell nodules in the tonsils of IgAN patients cause the overproduction of B cells which may release aberrant IgA, resulting in the onset of IgAN. In addition, immunological abnormalities, such as inappropriate T to B cell interaction, associated with reconstruction of tonsil may play a role in the progression of IgAN.

Expression of Bcl-2 Protein in Palatine Tonsil of IgA Nephropathy Patients

Hiroshi Sunaga[a], Shigeharu Fujieda[b]

[a]Department of Otorhinolaryngology, Maizuru Kyosai Hospital, Kyoto, and [b]Department of Otolaryngology, Head and Neck Surgery, Fukui University, Fukui, Japan

IgA nephropathy (IgAN) is the most common form of primary glomerulonephritis, and is recognized as a tonsil-related disease since it often gets worse after acute tonsillitis and the disease progression is often prevented by tonsillectomy. However, the molecular and cellular mechanisms between IgAN and palatine tonsil remain largely unknown. Mesangial IgA deposition seems to be the final step resulting from different genetic and immunological abnormalities of IgAN. Increased levels of circulating IgA1 and IgA plasma B cells are common immunological abnormalities observed in patients with IgAN. A lot of studies have reported that IgA1 derive from diseased IgAN have a reduced pattern of galactosylation. Marquina shows in F1 mice which defects in the regulation of B cell apoptosis, as a result of the overexpression of hBcl-2, lead to the development of IgA hypergammaglobulinemia and IgAN. The levels of galactosylation and sialylation of serum IgA in the F1 mice are reduced, thereby promoting their glomerular deposition. We have studied the immunohistochemical expression of Bcl-2 protein in human palatine tonsil of IgAN patients and non-IgAN patients. The Bcl-2 expression in tonsil of IgAN patients was significantly higher than non-IgAN patients. Furthermore, the apoptosis in the germinal center of tonsil of IgAN patients was significantly lower than in non-IgAN patients.

Impact of Nasopharyngitis as a Latent Role of 'Focal Infection' in the Pathogenesis of IgA Nephropathy

Mitsuhiro Sato, Osamu Hotta, Toshinobu Sato, Yoshio Taguma

Department of Nephrology, Sendai Shakaihoken Hospital, Sendai, Japan

We previously reported that clinical remission (CR: disappearance of hematuria and proteinuria) could be obtained by the treatment using tonsillectomy with steroid pulse (TSP) in IgA nephropathy (IgAN) [Hotta O, et al: Am J Kidney Dis 2001;38]. Also, we recently found that treatment for nasopharyngitis was effective for the patients who did not obtain CR even by the treatment using TSP. To clarify the influence of the nasopharynx on the pathogenesis of IgAN, we investigated the immunological characteristics of the nasopharyngeal cell (NC) in IgAN. 32 patients with IgAN without pharyngitic symptoms participated in this study. A phenotype analysis of the NC in IgAN was performed using flow cytometry comparing the mononuclear cell (MC) in peripheral blood of IgAN (n = 7), the removed tonsils of IgAN (n = 25), the NC of the patients suffering from pharyngitis without nephropathy (n = 8), and the NC of healthy controls (n = 9). There were numerous MCs at the surface of the nasopharynx even in healthy controls and they mainly consisted of activated lymphocytes (DR+). As compared with the peripheral blood lymphocytes subset, the following profiles were observed in the nasopharynx lymphocytes subset: (1) the percentage of B cells was increased; (2) the ratio of CD4+ T cell/CD8+ T cell was high, and (3) both the ratio of CD4DR+/total CD4 cells and the ratio of CD8DR+/total CD8 cells were high. These profiles were similar to those of the removed tonsils. Moreover, the ratio of CD4DR+/total CD4 cells, CD8DR+/total CD8 cells, and CD19+CD5+/total CD19 cells in the NC of the patients with IgAN and the patients with pharyngitis were significantly higher than those of the healthy controls. ($p < 0.01$), and the ratio of CD4DR+/total CD4 cells was positively correlated with the ratio of CD19+69+/total CD19 cells in the NC of the patients with IgAN ($r^2 = 0.181$, $p < 0.05$). These results indicate that nasopharynx has immunological characteristics like tonsil and that the NC of the patients with IgAN is more similar to that of the patients with pharyngitis than to that of healthy controls. The patients with IgAN have silent nasopharyngitis, which may play a latent role of 'focal infection'.

Increased Expression of IL-5 in Tonsils of Patients with IgA Nephropathy

Kozue Kodama, Akihiro Shinnebe, Hiromi Kanazawa, Takeharu Kanazawa, Yukiko Iino

Saitama Medical Center, Jichi Medical University, Saitama, Japan

Background: Tonsillectomy for IgA nephropathy (IgAN) has recently become the gold standard in Japan. It has been suggested that the effectiveness of tonsillectomy may be due to inhibition of the production of IgA and related cytokines in tonsils. **Objective:** To clarify the pathogenesis of IgAN, we measured the concentration of immunoglobulins and cytokines in the excised tonsil homogenates and carried out immunohistochemical studies of the tonsil specimens to demonstrate the expression of cytokines. **Patients and Methods:** Tonsil specimens were obtained from 14 patients with IgAN and from 9 patients with chronic tonsillitis (controls) at the time of operation. The tonsil homogenates were subjected to the measurement of IgG, IgA, IgE, IL-4, IL-5, IL-6, IL-8, IL-10, INF-γ and TGF-β. The tonsil specimens were also subjected to the immunohistochemial study and in situ hybridization of IL-4 and IL-5. **Results:** In IgAN patients, a significantly higher IL-5 concentration was detected in tonsil homogenates than in control patients, and the IgA concentration tended to be higher in IgAN patients than in control patients. Immunohistochemically, the numbers of cells positive for IL-5 tended to be higher in IgAN patients than in control patients. In addition, IL-5 mRNA positive cells were observed in the tonsil specimens obtained from IgAN patients. From these results, local IL-5 production occurs in the tonsils of IgAN. **Conclusion:** Locally produced IL-5 play a crucial role in the pathogenesis of IgAN. Some antigenic materials stimulate Th2 cells to produce IL-5, resulting in the production of IgA by B lymphocytes in tonsils of IgAN patients.

Planned Tonsillectomy before Renal Transplantation in Patients with IgA Nephropathy

Toshiya Hiroyoshi, Yoshihiro Kanaokam, Koki Fujikawa, Koichi Uchiyama, Masahiro Tsuchida, Hideyasu Matsuyama

Department of Urology, Graduate School of Medicine, Yamaguchi University, Ube, Japan

Background: IgA nephropathy is the most common chronic glomerulonephritis in Japan. It is a major disease in renal transplantation recipients. The recurrence rate of IgA nephropathy after renal transplantation is as high as Floege reported in 2004. The effective treatment of IgA nephropathy is unclear and has not yet been established. However, it is reported that treatment by tonsillectomy combined with steroid therapy is effective in IgA nephropathy. Thus, we tried planned tonsillectomy before renal transplantation in patients with IgA nephropathy. **Methods:** Forty-eight renal transplants were performed in our institution from January 2004 to December 2009. IgA nephropathy was confirmed by needle biopsy of native kidneys, taken before transplantation from 8 recipients. Planned tonsillectomy was performed in these 8 recipients before renal transplantation. Microscopic hematuria, proteinuria, renal function (serum creatinine), and the results of a 1-year-protocol biopsy of transplanted kidneys were studied in these patients. **Results:** The pathological finding showed chronic tonsillitis in all 8 recipients. The follow-up period was 7–52 months (average 36.2 months) for each recipient. Two of 8 (25%) recipients showed microscopic hematuria. No recipients showed proteinuria. Renal function was stable in all the recipients. The recurrence of IgA nephropathy was not observed in the 1-year-protocol biopsy of transplanted kidneys. **Conclusions:** The planned tonsillectomy before renal transplantation in patients with IgA nephropathy may be effective in preventing the recurrence of IgA nephropathy after renal transplantation.

Clinical Efficacy of Modified High-Dose Intravenous Methylpredonisolone Therapy Combined with Tonsillectomy in Patients with IgA Nephropathy

Kazuhito Takeda, Tomoharu Ueno, Hiroshi Kimura, Satsuki Nakashita, Atsuhiro Maeda, Shuhei Miura

Kidney Center and Nephrology, Aso-Iizuka Hospital, Iizuka City, Japan

IgA nephropathy (IgAN) is now recognized as the most common form of primary glomerulonephritis worldwide and is the major cause of end-stage renal disease. As reported, the renal survival rate is 61% at 20 years and the renal prognosis of this disease is relatively poor on long-term observation, hence various protocols have been attempted to control this disease. At Iizuka Hospital, a prospective study of tonsillectomy with high-dose methylprednisolone therapy (HD-MPL) was performed for the treatment of patients with IgAN from August 2002. We reviewed the clinical efficacy of our protocol. From August 2002 to December 2008, 31 patients whose IgAN was demonstrated by percutaneous renal biopsy were administered our regimen. In our study, 32 patients had an observation period of more than 24 months. Our protocol consisted of tonsillectomy with only one course of HD-MPL. Methylprednisolone at a daily dose of 1,000 mg for 3 consecutive days followed by oral steroid at the daily dose of 20 mg, was gradually tapered, and discontinued 1 year later. All of the patients were administered angiotensin-converting enzyme inhibitors or angiotensin receptor blockers with favorable control of hypertension. The mean observation period for the 32 patients with IgAN was 50.6 months. The mean age at renal biopsy was 38 ± 12 years. The male-female ratio was 15:16. At the renal biopsy in our hospital, mean creatinine value (M-SCr) was 1.1 ± 0.4 mg/dl, mean creatinine clearance (M-CCr) was 64.6 ± 48.4 ml/min, and the mean urinary protein and urinary creatinine ratio (M-UP/Cr) was 1.57 ± 1.6. After 24 months, the M-SCr was 0.97 ± 0.4 mg/dl, the M-CCr was 72.3 ± 42.7 ml/min, and the M-UP/Cr was 0.66 ± 0.7. The urinary remission rate was 62.0%. On our protocol, mean length of the hospital stay was 10.5 ± 2.0 days. Our prospective study showed that our regimen in IgAN appears to be beneficial for urinary remission and contribute to a short hospital stay.

Clinical Efficacy of Tonsillectomy in Patients with IgA Nephropathy

Koichiro Yamada

Department of Otolaryngology, Head and Neck Surgery, Kurashiki Central Hospital, Okayama, Japan

Background: Immunoglobulin A nephropathy (IgAN) is the most common chronic kidney disease in Japan. Recently, several reports have suggested that tonsillectomy could be effective to prevent progress of renal dysfunction. We performed a retrospective case-control study of 107 patients with IgAN to investigate clinical efficacy of tonsillectomy. **Methods:** 41 patients underwent tonsillectomy within three years after renal biopsy (group A), and 66 patients did not (group B). These patients were followed up for more than 5 years after renal biopsy. Stable renal function rate and renal survival rate were evaluated by Kaplan-Meier analysis. Additionally, clinical remission rate, stable renal function rate, and renal survival rate after 5 years of follow-up were compared between these two groups. **Results:** 1 (2.4%) patient in group A and 16 (24.2%) patients in group B had poor renal function (χ^2 test, $p = 0.0027$). Among these patients, 1 (2.4%) patient in group A and 6 (9.1%) patients in group B finally required dialysis therapy (χ^2 test, $p = 0.1673$). Kaplan-Meier analysis showed significant difference between groups A and B in stable renal function rate (log-rank test, $p = 0.026$), whereas no significant difference was shown in renal survival rate (log-rank test, $p = 0.889$). At the time after 5 years from biopsy, clinical remmision rate was 58.5% in group A and 27.3% in group B (χ^2 test, $p = 0.0012$). Stable renal function rate was 97.6% in group A and 92.4% in group B (χ^2 test, $p = 0.2615$). Renal survival rate was 100% in both group A and group B. **Conclusion:** Stable renal function rate in IgAN patients with tonsillectomy was significantly higher than that in patients without tonsillectomy. Though, statistical difference was not found in renal survival rate. At the time after 5 years from biopsy, the clinical remmision rate in IgAN patients with tonsillectomy was significantly higher than that in patients without tonsillectomy.

Effect of Tonsillectomy Combined with Steroid Pulse on Patients with IgA Nephropathy

Nobuo Ohta, Tomoo Watanabe, Tsukasa Ito, Toshinori Kubota, Masaru Aoyagi

Department of Otolaryngology, Yamagata University School of Medicine, Yamagata, Japan

Background: IgA nephropathy is the most common form of glomerular disease in the world. However, standard therapy is currently not established. To achieve clinical remission, tonsillectomy combined with steroid pulse is performed for IgA nephropathy recently. To clarify this point, renal function and urinary examinations were examined before and after tonsillectomy combined with steroid pulse. **Methods:** From March 1999 to February 2010, 60 of the patients with IgA nephropathy who were treated with tonsillectomy combined with steroid pulse or conventional therapy in our department. Renal function and urinary examinations were performed before and after surgery. **Results and Conclusions:** The decreases of creatinine, hematuria, proteinuria were observed after treatments. These results indicate that tonsillectomy combined with steroid pulse is potentially great value for IgA nephropathy.

Persistent Hematuria after Tonsillectomy Plus Steroid Pulse Therapy is a Significant Predictor of Poor Renal Outcome in Patients with IgA Nephropathy

Naoki Haruyama[a], Taihei Yanagida[a], Ataka Kawabata[b], Jyoji Haratake[c], Chikao Yasunaga[a]

[a]Kidney Center, [b]Department of Otolaryngology and [c]Department of Pathology Unit, Saiseikai Yahata Hospital, Fukuoka, Japan

Introduction: Tonsillectomy and steroid pulse (TSP) therapy for IgA nephropathy (IgAN) had been widely accepted in Japan. From April 1999 to December 2007, 143 patients with IgAN were received TSP therapy in our hospital, and complete remission rate at 1, 3 and 5 years was 74.4, 84.8 and 88.9%, respectively. Several prognostic factors of IgAN were reported, but not much is known whether persistent hematuria after TSP therapy affects renal prognosis. **Materials and Methods:** The treatment protocol was as follows: within 6 months after tonsillectomy, all patients received intravenous methylprednisolone 500 mg for 3 consecutive days followed by daily 0.5 mg/kg oral prednisolone, which was tapered gradually in a year. Complete remission was defined as disappearance of urinary abnormalities. When the urinary protein/creatinine ratio increased to more than 1.0 after complete remission, it was defined as disease recurrence. Continued hematuria even after TSP therapy and recurrent hematuria after complete remission are defined as persistent hematuria. We enrolled 68 subjects in this study. They were divided into three groups; complete remission group, disease recurrence group and nonremission group. Each group were compared in the rate of decline in estimated GFR from baseline. To consider the influence of persistent hematuria, log-rank analysis was used between persistent hematuria group and nonpersistent hematuria group. The primary end point was 25% decrease in estimated GFR from the baseline. **Results:** In the complete remission group, the mean rate of decline in eGFR at 5 years was 11.3%, while in the disease recurrence group, it was 4.4%. However, in the nonremission group it was 22.5%. Between the persistent hematuria group and the nonpersistent hematuria group, the rate of primary end point at 7 years was significantly different (22.2 vs. 92.3%, $p < 0.001$). **Conclusion:** Persistent hematuria after TSP therapy is a significant prognostic factor of poor renal outcome in patients with IgAN.

Tonsillectomy and Steroid Pulse Therapy for IgA Nephropathy Is Effective Regardless of Histological Classification or Duration of Disease

Yasuhide Nishio, Kana Noshiro, Tomoki Kawasaki, Ayako Yokotani, Hiromi Kihira, Manabu Haneda

Department of Internal Medicine, Tokyo Metropolitan Tama Medical Center, Tokyo, Japan

Object: There have been reports on the efficacy of tonsillectomy and steroid pulse therapy for treatment to IgA nephropathy. We examined whether the disease duration and histological classification is related to the remission rate. **Method:** We studied 21 patients who had tonsillectomy and steroid pulse therapy for IgA nephropathy from April 2006 to December 2008 in our hospital. Rate of remission on hematuria and proteinuria were retrospectively compared in the setting of disease duration and the histological classification. The duration was defined from the onset of the disease to the tonsillectomy. Histological classification was made according to the criteria proposed by the Japanese society of nephrology which classifies the disease in 4 grades of pathological severity. **Result:** In all patients who received the treatment rate of remission on hematuria was 77% in 6 months, and 92% in 1 year after the initial treatment. Rate of remission on proteinuria was 17% in 6 months, and 78% in 1 year. There was no significant difference in the rate of remission on hematuria in 1 year between histological classification of grades 1 and 2 (100%) and grades 3 and 4 (90%). In terms of disease duration, there was no significant difference in the rate of remission on both hematuria and proteinuria between patients who had treatment more than 24 months after the onset of the disease or less than that. **Conclusion:** We had good outcome on tonsillectomy and steroid pulse therapy for IgA nephropathy regardless of disease duration and histological classification. Our findings suggest that we can apply this treatment to more patients including those who had severe pathological finding or were diagnosed more than 2 years ago.

Efficacy of Adenotonsillectomy in Pediatric IgA Nephropathy

Atsuko Nakano

Division of Otolaryngology, Chiba Children's Hospital, Chiba, Japan

We reviewed the clinical course of 18 patients diagnosed with IgAN who received tonsillectomy for the treatment of IgAN in childhood at Chiba Children's Hospital between 1991 and 2008. IgAN patients who were nonresponsive to medication or who had relapsed were considered to need tonsillectomy and adenoidectomy. Most of the patients received tonsillectomy and methylpredonisolone pulse therapy. The patients included 10 males and 8 females ranging in age from 5 to 18 years old (median 12 years 5 months) at the time of surgery. The disease duration prior to tonsillectomy ranged from 3 months to 7 years and 2 months (median 10.5 months). Nine patients had recurrent tonsillitis prior to tonsillectomy and some of them had macroscopic hematuria in addition to tonsillitis. Most of the tonsils had pus at the time of the operation, even in the patients who had not been clinically diagnosed with recurrent tonsillitis. The clinic followed up the patients by administering a monthly urine examination and/or renal biopsy when advisable until they had been in remission for over 1 year. 12 of the 18 patients (66.7%) achieved remission of hematuria and 13 patients (72.2%) achieved remission of proteinuria. We could confirm some improvements in the findings from renal biopsy after tonsillectomy in 2 patients with persistent hematuria or proteinuria. After more than 10 years, the renal function in these 2 patients was still working. These results indicate that tonsillectomy for IgAN is effective especially in the early stage and that tonsillectomy and methylpredonisolone pulse therapy may be effective in the progressive stage of IgAN in childhood.

Efficacy of Tonsillectomy Alone and Combined with Steroid Pulse Therapy in Patients with IgA Nephropathy

Naoki Nakagawa[a], Maki Kabara[a], Takayuki Fujino[a], Tomoya Hirayama[b], Nobuyuki Sato[a], Naoyuki Hasebe[a]

[a]Department of Internal Medicine, Asahikawa Medical College, and [b]Department of Internal Medicine, Kitasaito Hospital, Asahikawa, Japan

Background: Tonsillectomy and steroid pulse therapy was proposed as a curative treatment for IgA nephropathy (IgAN) in Japan. However, in the clinical setting, we encounter sometimes patients who reject the steroid pulse therapy because of the possible side effects of steroids. **Purpose:** The present study aimed to examine the efficacy of tonsillectomy alone and combined with steroid pulse therapy for IgAN with urinary abnormalities. **Methods:** Data on 35 IgAN patients (12 males and 23 females, mean age of 39 ± 14 years) diagnosed by renal biopsies between 2002 and 2008 in Asahikawa Medial College Hospital, who presented glomerular haematuria and proteinuria at baseline, were analyzed. We examine associations between therapy and subsequent clinical remission (CR), defined as negative proteinuria by dipstick and urinary erythrocytes of less than 5/high-power field. **Results:** The mean serum creatinine, estimated glomerular filtration rate (eGFR), proteinuria by dipstick, and urinary erythrocytes were 0.92 ± 0.60 mg/dl, 74.1 ± 25.3 ml/min/1.73 m^2, +1.0 ± 0.8, and 19.8 ± 14.0/high-power field at baseline in all patients, respectively. During a median follow-up of 30 months, we observed CR in 13 of 21 patients (62%) in tonsillectomy alone and 7 of 14 patients (50%) in tonsillectomy combined with steroid pulse therapy at final observation point.

In comparing data from patients in the non-CR and CR subgroups, a significant difference was observed in eGFR in both therapies. **Conclusion:** Tonsillectomy alone and combined with steroid pulse therapy shows promise as a treatment that can bring about CR of urinary abnormalities, and the average CR rate is more than 50% after treatment. The present study suggests that patients with either early-stage or mild to moderate IgAN easily achieve CR following both tonsillectomy alone and combined with steroid pulse therapy, whereas patients with late-stage or severe disease are prone to these therapy resistance.

Effects of Tonsillectomy and High-Dose Corticosteroid Combination Therapy for IgA Nephropathy Patients

Mitsuaki Kaizuka[a], Yasuhiro Fujino[a], Hideaki Yamabe[b]

[a]Cardiology Division, Aomori Prefectural Central Hospital, Aomori, and [b]Hirosaki University School of Health Sciences, Hirosaki, Japan

Objective: We studied the effects of tonsillectomy and high-dose corticosteroid combination therapy for IgA nephropathy patients. **Patients and Methods:** Sixteen patients (ages 16–60 years, mean age 39 years) were studied. Eight male and 8 female patients were included in the study. All patients were diagnosed as IgA nephropathy by renal needle biopsy. Examination of tonsils was performed by Otolaryngologists and whether patients have tonsillitis or not, tonsillectomy was performed. About one week later of tonsillectomy corticosteroid therapy was launched. Three days of methylprednisolone 500 mg intravenous infusion and thereafter 4 days of oral prednisolone 30 mg administration were defined as one course. Three courses of this therapy were repeated. Thereafter, oral prednisolone 30 mg was administered every other day. The dose of prednisolone was reduced by 5 mg every other month and terminated after 1 year. Delay times from disease onset to therapy start varied widely between individuals (2–304 months). Serum creatinine levels, the amount of proteinuria and hematuria were compared before and after the therapy. Second renal biopsy was performed on some of these patients and histological changes were examined. **Results:** Tonsillectomy and high dose corticosteroid combination therapy in IgA nephropathy patients reduced the amount of proteinuria and hematuria. Serum creatinine level did not show a marked change, but tonsillectomy could cause a temporary serum creatinine increase. Histological improvement of the renal biopsy specimen was confirmed. Delay time from disease onset to the start of combination therapy and initial serum creatinine level might affect the effectiveness of this therapy.

Outcome of Tonsillectomy Combined with Steroid Pulse Therapy for IgA Nephropathy

Miha Kunii, Takamichi Matsui, Masakazu Ikeda, Ryo Suzuki, Koichi Omori

Department of Otolaryngology Fukushima Medical University, Fukushima, Japan

IgA nephropathy is one of the most chronic glomerular nephritis in Japan and since the 1980s it has been considered one of the tonsil-related diseases. In recent years, tonsillectomy combined with steroid pulse therapy is assumed to be effective for long term prognosis, but the evidence for this prognosis is not established. In our current study, in 119 cases of IgA nephropathy for which tonsillectomy and steroid pulse therapy were performed at Fukushima Medical University Hospital, we report 43 cases (adult: 37, children: 6) with observation of 36 months or more. The results of kidney examination and postoperative complications will be presented. Thirty-six months after the therapy, 32 of 43 patients (74.4%) were free from hematuria. Twenty-one patients (49%) kept the urinary condition and the kidney function at the reference value. Eight of 119 patients (6.7%) with IgA nephropathy had postoperative bleeding. A procedure to control postoperative bleeding under general anesthesia was required in 3 patients (2.5%). In contrast, 13 of 156 patients (8.3%) without IgA nephropathy experienced bleeding post-tonsillectomy. Six patients (1.9%) needed to control bleeding under general anesthesia. Tonsillectomy combined with steroid pulse therapy was considered to be effective for IgA nephropathy.

Combination of Tonsillectomy and Corticosteroid Suppresses Recurrence of Urinary Protein or Occult Blood in Patients with IgA Nephropathy, Compared with Corticosteroid Alone

Hirotsugu Iwatani[a], *Atsushi Takahashi*[a], *Ryohei Yamamoto*[a], *Yasuyuki Nagasawa*[a], *Arata Horii*[b], *Tadashi Kitahara*[b], *Hidenori Inohara*[b], *Atsushi Yamauchi*[c], *Enyu Imai*[a], *Hiromi Rakugi*[a], *Yoshitaka Isaka*[a]

[a]Geriatric Medicine and Nephrology and [b]Otolaryngology, Osaka University Graduate School of Medicine, Suita, and [c]Nephrology, Osaka Rosai Hospital, Sakai, Japan

Background: Approximately 30–40% of patients with IgA nephropathy (IgAN), the most common primary glomerulonephritis in the world, progressed to end-stage renal disease over a period of 20 years. Several recent studies have suggested that combination therapy of corticosteroid and tonsillectomy (TLX+CS) exerts more renoprotective effects on IgAN than corticosteroid alone (CS). **Aim:** To compare the rate of recurrence between TLX+CS and CS. **Methods:** We retrospectively reviewed medical records of 59 IgAN patients who received TLX+CS and 37 patients who underwent CS therapy between 2000 and 2007 in two major nephrology centers in Osaka, Japan. Outcome measures were time from initiation of TLX+CS or CS to disappearance (– or ± by dipstick) and recurrences of urinary protein (UP) or occult blood (UOB). Cumulative incidence rate of outcomes in TLX+CS and CS were estimated and compared using Kaplan-Meier method and Log-rank test. **Results:** No significant difference between TLX+CS and CS groups was observed in baseline characteristics before treatment, including age (median 31 (interquartile range 24–40) months in TLX+CS vs. 34 (25–45) in CS, p = 0.24), gender (male 46 vs. 43%, p = 0.81), urinary protein/creatinine ratio (0.64 (0.39–1.38) vs. 0.78 (0.48–1.45), p = 0.58), eGFR (77 (58–88) vs. 72 (56–86) ml/min/1.73 m^2, p = 0.83), and systolic blood pressure (116 (105–130) vs. 114 (107–123) mm Hg, p = 0.37). Cumulative remission rates of UP and UOB were not significantly different between TLX+CS and CS (UP 64 vs. 64% at 24 months, p = 0.73 for log-rank test, and UOB 62 vs. 40%, p = 0.10). On the contrary, cumulative recurrence rates of UP and UOB were significantly lower in TLX+CS than in CS (p = 0.007 and 0.002, respectively). **Conclusions:** Tonsillectomy with corticosteroid is more effective than corticosteroid alone in preventing recurrence of IgA nephropathy.

Relation between the Efficacy of Tonsillectomy and Renal Pathology in Patients with IgA Nephropathy

Tsutomu Nomura[a], *Yoshimi Makizumi*[b], *Tsuyoshi Yoshida*[c], *Tatsuya Yamasoba*[b]

[a]Department of Otolaryngology, JR Tokyo General Hospital, [b]Department of Otolaryngology and Head and Neck Surgery, Faculty of Medicine, University of Tokyo, and [c]Department of Otolaryngology, Takeda General Hospital, Tokyo, Japan

Introduction: In Japan, IgA nephropathy (IgAN) is the most common form of chronic glomerulonephritis with IgA deposits present mainly in the mesangial areas. The purpose of this study was to evaluate the influence of tonsillectomy as a treatment for IgA nephropathy in relation with pathological findings. **Materials and Methods:** We performed a retrospective review for eleven patients with IgAN referred from nephrology department. Eleven patients (4 males and 7 females) underwent tonsillectomy. Renal biopsy findings were classified for prognosis as good (grade I), relatively good (grade II), relatively poor (grade III) and poor (grade IV) with the criteria of the Committee of IgA Nephropathy, the Special Study Group of Progressive Glomerular Disease, the Ministry of Health, Labor and Welfare of Japan. Pre- and postsurgical serous IgA level, urine protein, urine creatinine and extent of hematuria were reviewed. **Results:** The age at tonsillectomy was 29 years on average, ranging from 13 to 65 years. In terms of renal biopsy, 4, 2, 1 and 4 patients were classified as grades I, II, III and IV, respectively. Improvement of the hematuria was seen in 2, 1 and 1 patient in groups I, II and IV, respectively. Score of urine protein/urine creatinine was reduced in 1, 2, 1 and 2 patients in groups I, II, III and IV, respectively. **Conclusion:** Although tonsillectomy has been recommended for patients exhibiting grade I–III in renal biopsy, this study suggested that some improvement of the extent of urine protein can be achieved in patients with grade IV.

Study on Perioperative Changes in Urinary Findings in Patients with IgA Nephropathy

Doi Akira[a], Tamura Kozo[a], Kozakura Kenichi[a], Yamamoto Miki[a], Shimamoto Kumiko[a], Ayu Ogawa[b], Matsuoka Takashi[b], Tuchiyama Yoshinori[b], Hiroshi, Uchida[c], Akagi Hirofumi[d], Nishizaki Kazunori[e], Masuda Yu[c]

[a]Division of Otolaryngology, [b]Division of Nephrology, Kochi Health Sciences Center, Kochi, [c]Department of Otolaryngology, Mizushima Kyodo Hospital, Kurashiki, [d]Department of Otolaryngology, National Hospital Organization Minami-Okayama Medical Center, and [e]Department of Otolaryngology, Head and Neck Surgery, Okayama University Graduate School of Medicine – Dentistry, Okayama, Japan

Subjects and Study Items: The subjects were 26 patients with IgA nephropathy who received TE at our department between July 2006 and January 2008 and underwent perioperative, 6 months postoperation and 2 years postoperation follow-ups. Study items to be measured during the perioperative period were measured on the day of operation and at days 1 and 3 postoperation. Subjects with exacerbations of uric blood (UB) and uric protein (UP) were classified as positive. Furthermore, the positive group was classified into the day 1 group (i.e. subjects who were found positive from day 1 postoperation) and the day 3 group (i.e. those who were found positive only on day 3 postoperation). Subjects without UB/UP exacerbation were classified as nonresponders. Prognosis was assessed based on the results of urinalysis conducted at 6 months and 2 years postoperation. UB and UP were assessed and classified into 4 categories: remission (negative), improvement, no change and aggravation. **Conclusion:** Urinary findings at 2 years postoperation indicate that positive status at day 3 post-operation is an indicator of good prognosis. Positive status at day 1 postoperation and being a nonresponder seem to be indicators of poor prognosis in cases who already had deteriorated renal function.

Tonsillectomy in Combination with Steroid Pulses Exerts Additive Antiproteinuric Effect to Steroid Pulses Alone in Patients with IgA Nephropathy

Keita Hirano, Yasunori Utsunomiya, Masato Ikeda, Makoto Ogura, Tetsuya Kawamura, Tatsuo Hosoya

Division of Nephrology and Hypertension, Jikei University School of Medicine, Tokyo, Japan

Aim: Pozzi's group [JASN 2004] demonstrated that in patients with IgA nephropathy (IgAN), treatment with glucocorticoids for 6 months improved renal survival and proteinuria for 10 years of follow-up. Since the degree of reduction in proteinuria may influence the renal outcome of IgAN, increasing attention has been drawn to tonsillectomy in terms of inducing clinical remission. Here, we performed a retrospective study to examine whether tonsillectomy has an additive antiproteinuric effect when combined with glucocorticoid therapy of Pozzi's protocol (GTPP). **Methods:** Of patients diagnosed as IgAN from June 2004 through May 2008 in four affiliated hospitals of Jikei University School of Medicine, those who received GTPP with or without tonsillectomy were enrolled in this study. At 1 year after treatment, 'improvement of proteinuria' was defined as having proteinuria less than 0.5 g/day, or 'clinical remission' defined as having both proteinuria <0.2 g/day and urinary RBC sediments <5/HPF was determined as renal outcome. Independent prognostic value of tonsillectomy was examined in a logistic regression model with adjustment for age, disease period, blood pressure, creatinine clearance and renal pathological findings which include rate of global sclerosis, focal segmental sclerosis, celluar crescents and adhesion at baseline. **Results:** A total of 77 patients with IgAN were included and 37 patients (48%) were treated with tonsillectomy in addition to GTPP. Improvement of proteinuria was significantly associated with tonsillectomy (OR 17.86, 95% CI 1.66–507.50, $p < 0.05$). In contrast, clinical remission was not associated with tonsillectomy (OR 2.09; 95% CI 0.54–8.38, $p > 0.1$). **Conclusion:** Under the limitation of a short-term follow-up, our results indicated that tonsillectomy in combination with GTPP exerts an additive antiproteinuric effect to GTPP alone in patients with IgAN.

Effect of Tonsillectomy and Steroid Pulse Therapy on Patients with Advanced IgA Nephropathy at Our Hospital

Yoshihiro Yamamoto[a], Koichiro Yamamoto[a], Shigehisa Koide[a], Kazutaka Murakami[a], Kunihiro Nabeshima[a], Makoto Tomita[a], Midori Hasegawa[a], Satoshi Sugiyama[a], Yoshiyuki Hiki[b]

[a]Department of Nephrology Fujita Health University, and [b]School of Health Sciences, Fujita Health University, Toyoake, Japan

Tonsillectomy and steroid pulse (T-SP) therapy were conducted on 10 patients (7 males, 3 females) with advanced IgA nephropathy in accordance with their wishes for the therapy. These cases were diagnosed as IgA nephropathy by renal biopsy during a period from September 2003 through August 2007. All of the patients had eGFR under 50 ml/min at the time of renal biopsy and more than 1 g/day (or g/g Cr) of proteinuria. They were 34.9 years of age on average with the following clinical profile (mean values): serum Cr of 1.58 mg/dl, eGFR of 41.2 ml/min, and urinary protein of 1.38 g/g Cr. Pulse therapy was done by giving 4 courses of 500 mg of methylprednisolone (mPSL)/day over 3 successive days every 2 months. Completion of the therapy brought about significant improvement of the parameters (mean values): serum Cr of 1.38 mg/dl, eGFR of 46.5 ml/min, and urinary protein of 0.473 g/Cr ($p < 0.05$). Oral administration of PSL was started with a dose of 20 mg/day after the initial pulse therapy and the dose was tapered down to null over 2 years. At the end of oral PSL intake, the mean levels of serum Cr, eGFR, and urinary protein were 1.35 mg/dl, 47.5 ml/min, and 0.438 g/Cr, respectively, indicating significant improvement of urinary protein ($p < 0.01$). Hematuria disappeared in 6 cases. **Conclusion:** These results suggested that even cases with advanced IgA nephropathy could benefit from T-SP therapy due to its promising suppressive effect on disease progress. It would therefore be worthwhile to give consideration to individual cases as possible indications for therapy.

Impact of Annual Urinalysis System on Obtaining Clinical Remission in Patients with IgA Nephropathy Treated with a Tonsillectomy and Steroid Pulse Therapy

Norio Ieiri, Osamu Hotta

Department of Nephrology, Sendai Shakaihoken Hospital, Sendai, Japan

Background: Because of the well-established annual urinalysis system in Japan, the duration of nephropathy (DN) can be estimated in more than half of all patients with IgA nephropathy (IgAN). Treatment using a combination of tonsillectomy and steroid pulse (TSP) therapy has been recognized as an effective method of obtaining clinical remission (CR), which was defined as negative hematuria and proteinuria, in Japanese IgAN patients. However, the correlation between the CR rate and the DN in IgAN patients treated using TSP therapy has not been elucidated. **Methods:** We retrospectively investigated 830 IgAN patients who were followed up for 81.6 months after TSP therapy. The DN could be estimated in 495 of the 830 patients. **Results:** The CR rate among patients whose DN was 36 months or less was 87.3% (295/338 patients). The CR rate among patients whose DN was between 37 and 84 months was 73.3% (63/86 patients), while that among those whose DN was 85 months or more was 42.3% (30/71 patients); the CR rate among the remaining 335 patients whose DN could not be estimated because of missing annual urinalysis results was 43.6% (146/335 patients). A multivariate Cox regression model using data from the 495 patients showed that a DN of 36 months or less had a significant impact on the CR (hazard ratio 1.839; 95% CI, 1.410–2.398; $p < 0.001$). **Conclusions:** A shorter DN is associated with a better chance of obtaining clinical remission in IgAN patients treated with TSP therapy.

Tonsil-Associated Skin Diseases

Impact of Tonsillectomy on Patients with Chronic Psoriasis

Helgi Valdimarsson[a], Ragna H. Thorleifsdottir[a], Andrew Johnston[d], Sigrun L. Sigurdardottir[a], Jon H. Olafsson[b], Bardur Sigurgeirsson[b], Hannes Petersen[c]

Departments of [a]Immunology, [b]Dermatology and [c]ENT Surgery,Landspitali, University of Iceland, Reykjavik, Iceland; [d]Department of Dermatology, University of Michigan, Ann Arbor, Mich., USA

Background: Psoriasis can be associated with streptococcal throat infections, and cross-reactive T cells that respond to short peptides that are common to streptococcal M-protein and skin keratins have been detected in the blood of psoriasis patients. We are therefore studying the impact of tonsillectomy (TX) on psoriasis. **Methods:** 30 patients with chronic psoriasis were recruited and 15 were tonsillectomized. They are followed for 2 years and monitored by PASI score, quality of life (QoL) questionnaires and enumeration of blood T cells that respond by IFN-γ or IL-17 production to short homologous M-protein or keratin peptides. **Results:** Two patients dropped out of the study, 1 TX patient and 1 control. After 2, 6 and 12 months, a mean PASI reduction of about 40% has been observed in the TX group ($p = 0.012$) but no consistent changes were noted in the controls ($n = 12$). The improvement of the TX patients has generally coincided with a marked decrease in the frequency of circulating cross-reactive CLA+CD8+ T cells and this decrease has persisted for at least 12 months. A corresponding decrease has not been observed in the controls. The data obtained after 24 months are currently being analyzed. **Conclusion:** TX has at least a temporary beneficial effect on chronic psoriasis, and is associated with a reduction in the frequency of circulating skin homing CD8+ T cells that are specific for peptides with amino acid sequences that are present in both streptococcal M-proteins and human keratins.

Assessment on the Quality of Life of Patients with Palmoplantar Pustulosis Using Skindex-16 and GHQ-28

Yukari Okubo, Kae Usui, Shoko Natsume, Ryoji Tsuboi

Department of Dermatology, Tokyo Medical University, Tokyo, Japan

Objective: Recently, much attention has been given to the quality of life (QoL) of patients suffering from skin diseases. The aims of this study are to evaluate the QoL of patients with palmoplantar pustulosis (PPP) and their level of satisfaction with the current treatment. **Methods:** The patients were asked to complete the Skindex-16 and GHQ-28 (General Health Questionnaire – 28) questionnaires and the VAS scale (Visual Analogue Scale rating itching, nail lesions, joint pain and stress experienced while applying ointment), and to report the specific times at which they applied ointment, and their degree of satisfaction with the treatment. **Results:** Patients with PPP at Tokyo Medical University Hospital reported a decrease in their QoL, as indicated by Skindex-16. The results of the QoL ratings using GHQ-28 indicated that half of the patients apparently suffered from some form of nonpsychotic, psychological disorders. A number of the patients reported impaired QoL despite mild skin symptoms, while patients who spent over 30 min in applying topical ointments reported feeling a significantly greater degree of stress. Sixty percent of patients, including first-time patients, reported feeling 'satisfied' or 'moderately satisfied' with their treatment. The number of PPP patients who claimed to have nail-related and joint-related complaints was significantly higher in comparison with the psoriasis patients. The resulting trend was generally similar to that of the QoL evaluation of the psoriasis patients reported previously, except that the PPP patients reported greater dissatisfaction in the social activity category. Many of these patients reported deterioration in their QoL despite low PPPASI scores. Owing to the fact that the lesions which develop on the hands and feet of PPP patients tend to severely impact everyday functioning, the choice of treatment should be based on the evaluation not only of the severity of the lesions but also of the QoL of the patient.

Surface Molecules on Tonsillar T Cells in Patients with Psoriasis

Sigrun L. Sigurdardottir[a], *Andrew Johnston*[c], *Ragna H. Thorleifsdottir*[a], *Hannes Petersen*[b], *Hannes Hjartarson*[b], *Helgi Valdimarsson*[a]

Departments of [a]Immunology and [b]ENT Surgery, Landspitali, University of Iceland, Reykjavik, Iceland; [c]Department of Dermatology, University of Michigan, Ann Arbor, Mich., USA

Background: Psoriasis, a chronic inflammatory skin disease, is often associated with streptococcal throat infections and psoriasis patients have a markedly increased occurrence of such infections. We hypothezise that psoriasis patients have dysregulated innate immune responses in their tonsils which leads to upregulation of the various molecules that may be relevant in psoriasis. **Methods:** Mononuclear leukocytes were isolated from psoriatic tonsils (PST, n = 11–17) and recurrently infected tonsils (RT tonsils, n = 10–15) and stained for various cell-surface receptors and their phenotype analyzed by FACS flow cytometry. The frequency of streptococcal throat infections was comparable in both groups of patients. Student's t test was performed to evaluate statistical significance ($p < 0.05$). **Results:** Tonsillar T cells from patients with psoriasis expressed significantly more of the skin homing molecule CLA than T cells from the RT tonsils. There was also an increased frequency of CCR6+ T cells in tonsils from psoriasis patients. In contrast, T cells from RT tonsils expressed significantly more CCR5, CD69 and CD25. **Conclusion:** The results are consistent with the hypothesis that innate immune responses in PST tonsils are dysregulated. The increased expression of CLA and CCR6 is of particular interest as CLA is important for skin homing and CCR6 is specific for TH17 cells which play a key role in the formation of psoriatic plaques. The frequency of T1 and T17 cells are currently being compared in the PST and RT patients as well as the histological features of the tonsils.

Case of Anaphylactoid Purpura with Nephritis Possibly Associated with Tonsillitis

Takeo Shiga, Kimiko Nakajima, Masahito Tarutani, Shigetoshi Sano

Department of Dermatology Kochi Medical School, Nankoku, Japan

A 41-year-old woman presented at our hospital with complaints of purpura over the entire body, fever, general malaise, and leg edema. A number of palpable purpuric papules were presented on the extremities, trunk and face. Ecchymotic macules were found in the oral mucosa and tongue. Legs, fingers, dorsum manus showed an intense edema. She had severe arthralgia in the knees and wrists. The laboratory data had no abnormality in the renal function, and the increase of the immunoglobulins was not seen. MPO-ANCA, PR3-ANCA was negative. Histologic findings from a purpura in the right leg revealed a leukocytoclastic vasculitis with perivascular infiltrates of neutrophils and lymphocytes in the superficial dermis through subcutaneous tissue. Since she was diagnosis of anaphylactoid purpura, we treated her with oral prednisolone 30 mg/day and antibiotics, which made no satisfactory progress. A few days later, hematuria and oliguria developed. Examination with renal biopsy revealed mesangial nephritis stage II with IgA and fibrin deposition in the glomerulus, by which we diagnosed of purpura nephritis. We conducted steroid pulse therapy followed by oral administration of the prednisolone, DDS (75 mg/day) and CyA (150 mg/day), all of which gave partial remission. Edema and tenderness of the legs recurred 8 months later. Although her pharyngeal tonsils were not swollen, we performed provocation test, which showed a positive response with an emergence of purpura on her foot. Finally, we performed tonsillectomy and steroid pulse therapy, which resulted in a complete remission. We suspected that she had anaphylactoid purpura and nephritis because of the latent bacterial infection in the tonsils.

Case Report of Henoch-Scholein Purpura Nephritis Treated with Tonsillectomy Combined with Steroid Pulse Therapy

Yoshiharu Muto, Hideyuki Mukai, Hiroshi Okuda, Masahide Furusho, Satsuki Nakashita, Shuhei Miura, Atsuhiro Maeda, Hiroshi Kimura, Hideki Kondo, Kazuhito Takeda

Iizuka hospital, Iizuka-city, Fukuoka, Japan

Background: We can find several reports about favorable results of tonsillectomy combined with steroid pulse therapy for IgA nephropathy. On the other hand, some reports suggest effectivity of the combination therapy for Henoch-Scholein purapura nephritis (HSPN), which has identical renal pathologic feature with IgA nephropathy, but no randomized control study supporting the hypothesis has been done. We report an adult case of HSPN with chronic renal failure successfully treated with tonsillectomy combined with steroid pulse therapy. **Case Presentation:** A 67-year-old male with hypertension and chronic kidney disease (Cr 1.2 mg/dl) suffered from rhinitis, fever, systemic edema and purpura had been admitted to our hospital in March 2009. He had a past medical history of acute glomerulonephritis remitting spontaneously at the age of 64. His blood test showed as follows: Hg 13.1 g/dl, Cr 1.5 mg/dl, TP 6.1 g/dl, albumin 3.1 g/dl, ASO 908U/ml, RF 9U/ml, IgG/IgA/IgM 1,250/238/38 mg/dl, C3/C4 134/30 mg/dl, CH50 56 U/ml and negative for antinuclear antibody. His urine drip test revealed occult blood (3+) and proteinuria (4.97 g/day). Renal biopsy revealed IgA nephropathy with moderate mesangial proliferation. Based on these findings, he is diagnosed with HSPN. After admission his serum creatinine level rapidly elevated. He was started with oral prednisolone but his urine protein did not reduce. He underwent tonsillectomy followed by corticosteroid pulse therapy (intravenous methyl-prednisolone 1,000 mg/day, 3 days) in addition to hemodialysis (HD). The therapy resulted in a dramatic decrease in proteinuria and his creatinine level quit rising at around 4 mg/dl. HD was withdrawn within 2 weeks. After discharge, his renal function has been maintained without dialysis for about a year. **Conclusion:** We thought tonsillectomy combined with steroid pulse therapy might be indicated for HSPN associated with nephritic syndrome and renal dysfunction despite conventional therapy.

Questionnaire Survey of Opinions Regarding the Treatment of Palmoplantar Pustulosis Including Tonsillectomy

Satomi Kobayashi

Division of Dermatology, Seibo International Catholic Hospital, Tokyo, Japan

Pustulosis palmaris et plantaris (PPP) is a chronic recurrent dermatosis characterized by sterile intraepidermal pustules associated with erythematous scaling on the palm and sole. Some patients have skeletal involvement, and the pain that is experienced is sometimes very severe. Although an average of 5–7 years of symptomatic therapy is required for any improvement, tonsillar and dental focal infections are well known to be largely involved in the onset of PPP, and rash and joint symptoms are often improved rapidly after a tonsillectomy or the treatment of dental focal infections. However, the opinions of dermatologists and otolaryngologists regarding the treatment of focal infections for PPP vary, and the fact that the treatment of PPP performed is not consistent among dermatologists is problematic. Therefore, a questionnaire survey about the treatment of PPP was sent to dermatologists and otolaryngologists working at university hospitals throughout Japan. Regarding the efficacy of symptomatic treatment such as topical ointment, smoking cessation, phototherapy, biotin intake, intake of antibiotics, etretinate, both dermatologists and otolaryngologists answered that most treatments were effective but did not cure patients, or that the effects were variable. In contrast, some percentages of physicians answered that patients were effectively treated or cured within 1–2 years in more than 70% of cases in which dental treatment or a tonsillectomy was performed. Although 63% of the otolaryngologists and 14% of the dermatologists answered that focal infections are involved in PPP in more than 70% of cases, more than half of dermatologists answered that they are involved in less than 50% of cases, the opinion was conflicting. Regarding the indications for a tonsillectomy, large differences were observed between otolaryngologists and dermatologists.

A Case of Behçet's Disease Deteriorating with Tonsillitis

Rei Akashi[a], *Aya Osada*[a], *Makoto Kawashima*[a], *Satomi Kobayashi*[b]

[a]Department of Dermatology, Tokyo Women's Medical University, and [b]Division of Dermatology, Seibo International Catholic Hospital, Tokyo, Japan

A 29-year-old woman was admitted to our hospital with a 1-week history of oral aphta, tender erythematous subcutaneous nodules on the extremities and arthralgia in August 2006. Laboratory examination revealed a WBC count of 8,700/μl (neut 79.4%) and serum CRP of 9.98 mg/dl. Serum tests for antinuclear antibody, rheumatoid factor and HLA B51 were negative. Histological findings in the biopsies obtained from the subcutaneous nodules revealed septal panniculitis with neutrophilic and lymphocytic infiltration. New lesions continued to appear, but without ocular symptoms, therefore, a diagnosis of incomplete type Behcet's disease was made. Oral prednisolone (PSL) at the dose of 20 mg resulted in resolution of the symptoms. PSL was tapered to 3 mg by degrees. In December 2006, all of the symptoms recurred along with the appearance of genital ulcers ten days after the patient suffered from an episode of tonsillitis. Serum CRP was elevated to 20.32 mg/dl. Increase of the PSL dose again to 20 mg, along with antibiotic administration, resulted in improvement. In July 2007 and in May 2008, the third and the fourth episodes occurred, and the patient again gave histories of tonsillitis 3–4 days prior to the appearance of the mucocutaneous lesions. Subsequently, the patient administered antibiotics for the precursor sign of sour throats resulted in the minimum recurrences of erythema nodosum without increase of the PSL dose over 5 mg. Behcet's disease is a syndrome characterized by recurrent aphthous stomatitis, genital ulcers, erythema nodosum and pustules, along with eye involvement. There is a genetic background, with a high prevalence in people from the Mediterranean region, the Middle East, China, and Japan, and a particularly strong association has been shown with HLA B51. Even though rare, our experience revealed that Behcet's disease or Behcet's syndrome can be precipitated by tonsillar focal infection, with no relation to HLA B51, in Japanese patients.

Two Cases of Cutaneous Vasculitis Successfully Treated by Tonsillectomy

Shigetsuna Komasu, Shin Iinuma, Hajime Iizuka

Department of Dermatology, Asahikawa Medical College, Asahikawa, Japan

Case 1: A 54-year-old woman was referred to our hospital because of painful nodules on her lower legs, which was accompanied by hematuria. Skin biopsy disclosed leukocytoclastic vasculitis with IgA and C3 deposition on her deep skin vessels. Renal biopsy disclosed IgA nephropathy, which was confirmed by immunofluorescent analysis. **Case 2:** A 67-year-old man was referred to our hospital because of urticarial edematous erythema accompanied by proteinuria and hematuria. Skin biopsy disclosed leukocytoclastic vasculitis consistent with urticarial vasculitis. Neither immunoglobulin (IgG, IgA, IgM) nor C3 was detected on his skin blood vessels. However, IgA nephropathy was confirmed by renal biopsy with positive renal IgA deposition. In both cases serum IgA level was increased, and tonsillectomy resulted in a quite favorable response.

Bacterial and Viral Infection

Role of Colonization in Otitis Media

Howard Faden

State University of New York, Buffalo, N.Y., USA

Acute otitis media (AOM) is an extremely common infection in childhood; more than 50% of children have at least 1 episode by 2 years of age. *S. pneumoniae* (SP), *H. influenzae* (HI), and *M. catarrhalis* (MC) cause most AOM. All 3 pathogens are part of the normal nasopharyngeal (NP) flora. Colonization with these pathogens begins early in life. Age, household members, school contacts, diet and antibiotics may increase colonization with SP, HI and MC. In contrast, colonization with non pathogens such as viridians streptococcus reduces colonization with SP, HI and MC. Approximately 5–10% of children become colonized with SP, HI, and MC early, repeatedly or persistently and they become prone to repeated AOM. Otitis prone children fail to mount normal systemic and local immune responses to SP, HI, and MC. The basis for the immunologic defect is unknown. Thus, colonization appears to be the key to the prevention of AOM. Since immunization with SP is limited by the numbers of SP types that can be included in a conjugated vaccine and the probability of the development of vaccines against HI and MC seems unlikely in the near future, an effort to reduce colonization with the three pathogens by other means seems reasonable and desirable. Three potential solutions to the problem include selective use of antibiotics, intranasal immunization and re-colonization with normal flora. The latter two approaches are medically attractive because they will not result in increased antibiotic resistance. However, it remains to be seen if the group at greatest risk, i.e. the otitis prone children, will respond appropriately to immunizations.

Are Palatine Tonsils a Market Place for Herpes Viruses?

David Nadal

Division of Infectious Diseases and Hospital Epidemiology, University Children's Hospital of Zurich, Zurich, Switzerland

The Waldeyer's ring designates a functional unit of lymphoid tissue within the pharynx including the adenoids and tonsils. Tonsils and the other lymphoid tissues of the Waldeyer's ring act as gatekeepers at the intersection of the respiratory tract and the gastrointestinal tract, and, since herpes viruses may use this anatomical site as portal of entry and exit, tonsils are involved in the infection process. Given that the hallmark of herpes viruses is the establishment of latency to reside in the host for a lifetime following primary infection, tonsils may function as anatomical reservoir for herpes viruses. This lecture will review published data on the eight human herpes viruses known to date in tonsils and also focus on potential viral exploitation of host tissue characteristics as well as on potential interactions between the single herpes virus species. In addition, gaps to be filled by future research will be identified as tonsils may serve as unique organs to study interactions between herpes viruses and the role of and the effects on the immune system in these processes. Gaining insights into the mechanisms involved will contribute to a better understanding of human herpes viral infection biology and the risks in and for immunocompromized hosts.

Clonal Spread of Beta-Lactamase-Producing, Amoxicillin-Clavulanate-Resistant Strains of Nontypeable *Haemophilus influenzae* (BLPACR) among Young Children Attending a Day Care Center in Japan

Makoto Ito, Risa Kato, Yumiko Maruyama, Tomokazu Yoshizaki

Department of Otolaryngology, Head and Neck Surgery, Kanazawa University, Kanazawa, Japan

Background: Resistant strains of non typeable *Haemophilus influenzae* (NTHi) is one of the principal causes of recurrent acute otitis media, rhinosinusitis, and pneumonia in young children. Beta-lactamase, nonproducing, ampicillin-resistant (BLNAR) strains are particularly common in Japan, and beta-lactamase-producing amoxicillin-clavulanate-resistant (BLPACR) strains are now emerging. We investigated the nasopharyngeal carriage status of these resistant strains among children attending same day care center during the ten years period. **Methods:** From 1999 to 2008, we obtained nasopharyngeal swab specimens from young children attending a same day care center in central Japan and examined the incidence of resistant strains of NTHi. Antimicrobial resistances of NTHi were identified based on polymerase chain reaction analysis of mutation of the penicillin-binding protein (PBP) genes. Pulsed-field gel electrophoresis (PFGE) was performed to examine the clonal relationship of each resistant strain. **Results:** The prevalence of genetically BLNAR (gBLNAR) among the children attending day care has been significantly increased during the past 10 years. In addition to the gBLNAR, genetically BLPACR (gBLPACR) strains have dramatically increased since 2007. Most of the children in day care seen recently had resistant strains with PBP gene mutations in their nasopharynx. PFGE analysis demonstrated that all gBLPACR strains were clonally identical. This represents the first report of the apparent clonal dissemination of the gBLPACR strain of NTHi occurred in a certain condition such as day care. **Conclusions:** A rapidly increasing prevalence in resistant strains, especially gBLPACR in day care, may predict the high incidence of these resistant bacteria from clinical isolates in the near future and the serious medical problems worldwide.

Influence of Epstein-Barr Virus-Encoded Latent Membrane Protein-1 on the Potentiation of Cε mRNA Expression in Human Tonsil-Derived Cells

Shigeto Ohta[a], Kazuhiko Hanashiro[b], Masanori Sunagawa[b], Mikio Suzuki[b], Tadayoshi Kosugi[b]

[a]Department of Otorhinolaryngology, Head and Neck Surgery, and [b]Department of Physiology, Unit of Physiological Science, Faculty of Medicine, University of the Ryukyus, Nishihara, Okinawa, Japan

The aim of our study was to investigate a possible correlation between Epstein-Barr virus (EBV) infection status, including its latent gene expression, and expression of allergy-related genes in human tonsil derived cells. In the tonsil-derived cells from the patients undergoing routine tonsillectomies for palatine tonsil hypertrophy or tonsillar focal infection, the presence of EBV DNA and mRNA expressions of latent membrane protein (LMP)-1, Cε chain, and activation-induced cytidine deaminase (AID) were detected by PCR and RT-PCR analysis, respectively. Of all the 12 patients, PCR products amplified from EBV DNA *Bam*HI W fragment were detected in the tonsils from the 10 patients (83.3%). LMP1 mRNA expressions were confirmed in 6 patients (50%). Both LMP1 mRNA expressions and EBV DNA were detected in 5 patients. EBV DNA, but not LMP1 mRNA expression, was detected in 5 patients. LMP1 mRNA expression, but not EBV DNA, was detected in one patient. In one patient, neither EBV DNA nor LMP1 mRNA expression was confirmed. Cε mRNA expressions were confirmed in all the 12 patients along with AID mRNA expressions. The degree of Cε mRNA expression, however, varied according to the patient. Fisher's exact probability test revealed a statistically significant correlation between LMP1 and Cε gene expressions, indicating that Cε mRNA expression level was significantly higher in the LMP1-positive samples than in the negative samples. On the other hand, there was no significant correlation between AID and LMP1 mRNA expressions. Thus, EBV infection is a notable factor capable of exacerbating allergic inflammation.

Characteristics of the Tonsil and Upper Airway Mucosa during Viral Infection

Keiko Yoda

Department of Otorhinolaryngology Tokyo Women's Medical University Medical Center East, Tokyo, Japan

This presentation demonstrates the tonsil and upper airway mucosal lesions during viral infection in adult cases encountered in our department. Aphtha, ulcer, erosion, vesicle, exudation, white patches, petechial hemorrhagic lesion, and gingivitis were commonly found. Aphtha, erosion, ulcer and vesicle in oropharynx arise due to herpes simplex (HSV) or varicella zoster virus (VZV) infection. Primary HSV infection is characterized by the presence of multiple, small and painful aphthae or ulcers, located in the oral cavity, in front of the pharynx, and generally on the gingiva, lips, tongue, buccal mucosa and palate (herpes gingivostomatitis). Herpes zoster as a reactivation of VZV is characterized by aggregated vesicles and exudative erosions in the unilateral oropharynx. These vesicles immediately rupture and turn into irregular exudation and erosions causing severe pain. Trigeminal herpes zoster presents ipsilateral vesicles and pustules on the lip, chin and cheek, or the external ear. Glossopharyngeal herpes zoster appears as exudation on tonsil. The lesion could be distinguished from exudation of tonsillitis because it is located in the unilateral tonsil and complicated by erosions of the palate, buccal mucosa and tongue on the same side. Exudative tonsillitis occurs in HSV, Epstein-Barr virus (EBV) or adenovirus infection. Petechial hemorrhagic lesions are sometimes seen in EBV tonsillitis. An adult case of measles demonstrates widespread white spots in the oropharynx. Redness, swelling and erosion of the gingiva are found in HSV and EBV infections. We reconfirmed that viral infections with HSV, VZV, EBV, adenovirus, and measles show characteristic features involving the tonsil, upper airway mucosa and surrounding structures.

A Case Resembling Infectious Mononucleosis in a 40-Year-Old Father

Yumiko Maruyama[a], *Makoto Ito*[b], *Tomokazu Yoshizaki*[b]

[a]Department of Otolaryngology Kurobe City Hospital, Kurobe, Toyama, and [b]Division of Otolaryngology,Head and Neck Surgery, Kanazawa University Graduate School of Medical Science, Kanazawa, Ishikawa, Japan

We have experienced a case resembling infectious mononucleosis (IM) in a 40-year-old male, who was the father of 2 children. He visited our hospital with aggravating throat pain and high grade fever. He had trismus and swelling of bilateral paratoglossal arch. His blood sample showed leukocytosis, atypical lymphocytosis (22%), hepatic insufficiency, first infectious pattern of Epstein-Barr virus (EBV), that is EB-VCA IgG+, VCA IgM+, EA IgG+, EA IgM–, EBNA–. CT scan showed multiple low-density areas with ring enhancement of a bilateral peritonsillar lesion. Incision to abscess lesion of the bilateral peritonsil led drainage and plural bacteria including fusobacterium were detected by cultivation. He recovered and was discharged on the 5th day. EBNA antibody still retained negativity 4 months after discharge and a blood sample from his wife was revealed to be already infected with a pattern of EBV. There were some reports which showed complicated bacterial infections with IM, such as sepsis by fusobacterium species, infectious endocarditis, pyomyositis, toxic shock syndrome, and peritonsillar abscess. Confusion of the host immune system is thought to cause the complication of bacterial infection and to make it grave. It is reported that about 80% of 3-year-old children have been already infected with EBV, and almost adults are infected with it. But we have experienced some other fathers or mothers whose EBNA antibody revealed negative and/or who showed progress like first infection progress of EBV. There is, however, the possibility that there might be some cases that trace an unusual course of antibody production around the EBV infection.

Phosphorylated Ezrin Is Associated in Nasopharyngeal Carcinoma with EBV Latent Membrane Protein 1 and Induces Cell Migration

Kazuhira Endo, Satoru Kondo, Tomokazu Yoshizaki

Division of Otolaryngology Kanazawa University, Kanazawa, Japan

Tumor metastasis is a complex phenomenon that is the culmination of effects of numerous cellular factors. We have shown that the EBV oncoprotein, latent membrane protein 1 (LMP1), is capable of inducing a wide range of such factors in cell culture, expression of which is also elevated in the LMP1-expressing tumor, nasopharyngeal carcinoma (NPC), a highly invasive neoplasm. Recently, the membrane-crosslinker protein ezrin has been implicated in tumor cell metastasis and malignant progression. In this study, we evaluated the possible role of LMP1 and ezrin in the pathophysiology of NPC. We show that C-terminal phosphorylation of ezrin is increased by expression of LMP1 in nasopharyngeal (NP) cells through a protein kinase C (PKC) pathway. LMP1 enhances organization of a ternary complex of CD44, ezrin and F-actin which is a prerequisite for ezrin phosphorylation. In NPC tissues, expression of phosphoezrin and LMP1 is directly correlated. Silencing of endogenously expressed ezrin suppresses LMP1-induced cell motility and invasiveness. Moreover, inhibition of ezrin phosphorylation by PKC inhibitor suppresses migration and invasion of NP cells. These data demonstrate that phosphorylation of ezrin and its recruitment to the cell membrane linked to F-actin and CD44 is a process required for LMP1-stimulated cell motility and invasion of NP cells.

Prevalence of Human Papillomavirus DNA in Patients with Squamous Cell Carcinoma in Waldeyer's Tonsillar Ring

Zeyi Deng, Masahiro Hasegawa, Asanori Kiyuna, Sen Matayoshi, Mikio Suzuki

Department of Otolaryngology- Head and Neck Surgery, Faculty of Medicine, University of the Ryukyus Okinawa, Japan

Background: Human papillomavirus (HPV) has been shown to be etiologically related to development of uterine cervical cancers, but their roles in head and neck cancers remain unestablished. This study was undertaken to investigate the frequency of HPV DNA in squamous cell carcinoma in Waldeyer's tonsillar ring. **Materials and Methods:** DNA was extracted from frozen tissue of 39 SCCs in Waldeyer's throat ring including nasopharynx (n = 10), tonsillar fossa (n = 21), and base of tongue (n = 8). The DNA was screened for HPV sequences by polymerase chain reaction (PCR) with three sets of consensus primers, one to a conserved region in the E1 gene (CP-I/CP-II), and the other two to a conserved region in the L1 gene (GP5+/GP6+ and MY09/MY11). The PCR products were run on agarose gels and were visualized by ethidium bromide staining. HPV types were determined by direct sequences. **Results:** According to the tumor localization, the frequency of HPV positive lesions was 30% for nasopharynx, 52.4% for tonsillar fossa and 12.5% for base of tongue. HPV type16 DNA was detected in 80% of the HPV-positive specimens. As a control group, 47 tumor free tonsils were analyzed. Only 1 of the control specimens (2.1%) had HPV sequences. The incidence of HPV infection rate in either patients with tonsillar or nasopharyngeal carcinoma was significantly higher than in patients with tumor free tonsil ($p = 0.015$ and $p < 0.001$, respectively). **Conclusions:** Our study shows the HPV genomes, especially HPV type16, are highly located in the cancer cells of Waldeyer's tonsillar ring.

A Clinical Study of Tonsils in Carcinoma

Yohei Kawasaki, Kohei Honda, Omi Eigo, Sinsuke Suzuki, Takashi Sito, Koji Kudo, Teruyuki Sto, Yasufumi Omori, Kazuo Ishikawa

Department of Otorhinolaryngology, Akita University School of Medicine, Akita, Japan

We retrospectively analyzed 87 cases of the oropharyngeal squamous cell carcinoma (OPSCC) treated at Akita University Hospital from 1999 to 2009. When those cases were classified into four groups according to their primary sites, 42 cases had arisen from anterior wall, 25 from lateral wall, 11 from upper wall and 9 from posterior wall, respectively. Overall 5-year survival rate was 67.3%. With regard to primary site specific survival rate of those OPSCC patients, those from anterior was 64.0%, lateral 72.0%, upper 43.6, and posterior 77.8%, respectively. Among the OPSCC patients arisen from lateral wall, those from the tonsils had fairly better prognosis than those from the other site. One of 17 patients of OPSCC appeared at the tonsil was stage I or II, and all the others were stage III or IV. Those patients received either a primary surgical resection or a radical concurrent chemoradiation. As a result, their disease-specific 5-year survival rate was 100%. Thus, the prognosis of the OPSCC arisen from the tonsil was significantly better than those from any other site. To clarify the reason for such a favorable prognosis of OPSCCs of the tonsils, various immunohistochemical analyses results will also be shown.

Human Papillomavirus Frequency in Oropharyngeal Squamous Cell Carcinoma in Japan

Takatsugu Mizumachi, Satoshi Kano, Naoya Inamura, Toshihiro Hara, Fumiyuki Suzuki, Seigo Suzuki, Akihiro Homma, Nobuhiko Oridate, Satoshi Fukuda

Department of Otolaryngology, Head and Neck Surgery, Hokkaido University Graduate School of Medicine, Sapporo, Japan

Background: In recent years, there has been mounting epidemiologic and experimental evidence of a role for human papillomavirus (HPV) as the etiologic agent of a subset of head and neck cancers. In this study, we estimated the frequency of HPV in squamous cell carcinoma (SCC) at different subsites of the oropharynx in Japan. **Methods:** The presence of HPV was analyzed using multiplex PCR from paraffin-embedded tissue of 76 patients diagnosed with oropharyngeal SCC at Hokkaido University Hospital, Japan, between 1998 and 2009. **Results:** In total 20/76 (26%) tumors were HPV-positive, and the majority of these were HPV-16-positive. HPV was detected in the following tumor subsites: 17 of 28 (61%) in the tonsil, 0 of 16 in the tonsil fossa and tonsillar pillar, 2 of 16 (13%) in the base of the tongue, 0 of 1 in the vallecula, 0 of 4 in the posterior wall, 1 of 9 (11%) in the soft palate, and 0 of 2 in the uvula. **Conclusions:** In the oropharynx, HPV-associated SCC had site specifity in the tonsil in Japan.

Acute Pharyngotonsillitis: Microbiology and the Predictive Signs Value

Leandro A. de Camargo, Luiza H. Endo, Eulalia Sakano, Juliana M.A.C. Bertoncello, Ulysses M. Oliveira

Universidade Estadual de Campinas- UNICAMP, Campinas, Brazil

Pharyngotonsillitis is a very usual disease in children and adults. The diagnosis has to be done with great accuracy, to prevent rheumatic disease that is frequent in some countries. The rapid test for detection or the culture of group A streptococcus (GAS) is expensive to be done routinely in our country. **Aim:** This study was done, in order to obtain the frequency of GAS pharyngotonsillitis and the relationship with predictive symptoms and signs of these acute infections. **Study Design:** Prospective observational study. **Patients and Method:** Patients complaining of classic clinical features of GAS infection included sudden onset of sore throat, fever, pharyngeal exsudate, and/or anterior cervical lymph nodes, with or without signs of viral infections, were submitted to a swabbing of both tonsils surface and posterior pharynx. The symptoms and signs were recorded to determine the relationship between the results of the culture. This data was submitted a statistical analysis. **Results and Conclusion:** Eighty patients were enrolled in our study, culture of 37 cases (46.2%) were positive and 43 cases (53.7%) were negative for *S. pyogenes*. We studied the relationship between the number of signs and the age of the patients and we found that when they are less than 15 years old and have 3 or 4 signs they have a high sensitivity to have *S. pyogenes*. This kind of sensitivity does not occur in patients older than 16 years. The presence of erythema with pus or exudates presents high sensitivity and specificity with significant relationship to the presence of *S. pyogenes*. Our study demonstrated that the diagnosis, of GAS pharyngotonsillitis can be done with accuracy in patients with sore throat under the age of fifteen where the four signs: fever higher than 38.5°C, erythema with pus or erythema with exudates, cervical tender lymph nodes and without upper airway respiratory viral signs were present.

Clinical Efficacy of Garenoxacin (GRNX) for Adult Acute Pharyngitis and Tonsillitis – Pharyngo-Tonsillitis Study Group (PHATONS) Surveillance

Yorihiko Ikeda, Akihisa Togawa, Kouzou Inui, Muneki Hotomi, Shinji Tamura, Noboru Yamanaka

Department of Otolaryngology, Head and Neck Surgery, Wakayama Medical University, Wakayama, Japan

Aim: Garenoxacin mesylate hydrate (GRNX) is a novel oral fluoroquinolone with potent antimicrobial activity against common respiratory pathogens, including resistant strains. We have organized Pharyngo-Tonsillitis Study Group (PHATONS) to examine causative pathogens and appropriate antimicrobial use for acute pharyngitis and tonsillitis. The aim of this study was to evaluate clinical efficacy of garenoxacin for adult acute pharyngitis and tonsillitis by a scoring system. **Methods:** The patients with acute pharyngitis and tonsillitis were evaluated for causative pathogens and were assessed clinical symptoms and pharyngotonsillar findings by a clinical scoring system. We evaluated difficulties in a daily life, sore throat, and fever as symptoms and scored erythema and swelling of pharyngotonsillar mucosa and the presence of exudates or plugs in tonsils grading from 0 (none) to 2 (marked). Severities of the diseases were classified into three groups according to total scores. Patients with total scores more than 9, 4–8 and less than 3 were assigned into the severe, moderate and mild groups, respectively. **Results and Conclusion:** A total 106 adult patients (55 male, 51 female, average age 36.4) were enrolled in our study. Major causative pathogens were *S. pyogenes*, 15%, *H. influenzae*, 3%, and *S. pneumoniae*, 2%. The numbers of total white blood cells (WBC) and the levels of C-reactive protein (CRP) rapidly improved after garenoxacin treatments, and the clinical scores also markedly improved in moderate cases and severe cases. In concluson, our results clearly indicate that the clinical scoring system is very useful to assess the severity of acute pharyngitis and tonsillitis and to select the appropriate treatment. Garenoxacin is the choice of antimicrobial agent for severe cases of adult acute pharyngotonsillitis.

Risk Factors for Nasopharyngeal Carriage of Potential Pathogens in Infancy: Birth Cohort Study in Sado Island

Taketo Otsuka[a], Yasuhiro Syoji[a], Jun Nirei[a], Takeshi Ono[a], Kou Matsui[a], Atsushi Iwaya[b], Minoru Okazaki[b]

[a]Sado General Hospital and [b]Ryotu Hospital, Sado, Japan

Background: To reduce the spread of drug-resistant pathogens, appropriate use of antibiotics (Abs) is an indispensable measure. Following the guidelines for use of Abs, we reduced 87% of Abs prescription in Sado Island, Japan. **Methods:** We conducted a birth cohort study, the SADO (Sado Island, Abs, Day-care attendance, Older siblings) -study in Sado Island to evaluate risk factors for nasal carriage of *Streptococcus pneumoniae*/*Haemophilus influenzae* and their resistance in infants. The study was undertaken before the introduction of routine use of PCV-7 and Hib vaccine. Nasopharyngeal cultures were obtained from subjects born in 2008, at 3–4, 6–7, and 9–10 months health checkups. Medical history of the subjects was obtained from patient records during their first 1 year of life. Demographic data, duration/exclusiveness of breastfeeding, and attending a day-care center (DCC) were evaluated using a questionnaire. **Results:** A total of 349 newborns in 2008 were enrolled (95.9% of those eligible). The average visit-based Abs prescription rate was 39 per 1,000 hospital visits in this study. Altogether, 1,009 nasopharyngeal cultures (341, 334, and 334 samples at 3–4, 6–7, and 9–10 months health checkups, respectively) were obtained. These included 248 (24.6%) *S. pneumoniae* and 120 (11.9%) *H. influenzae*. 118/248 (47.6%) of the *S. pneumoniae* isolates were resistant to penicillin and 59/120 (49.2%) of the *H. influenzae* isolates were resistant to ampicillin. Living with older sibling(s) (39.6 vs. 9.5%, $p < 0.01$) and DCC attendance (69.6 vs. 33.8%, $p < 0.01$) were significantly associated with nasal carriage of the two pathogens; however, these two factors did not correlate with resistant rates. Abs prescriptions, aged individual(s), and breastfeeding did not correlate with nasal carriage of any of the two pathogens or drug resistance. **Conclusions:** Our data indicated that decreasing prescriptions of Abs alone could not achieve elimination of resistant pathogens in a semi-closed area with controlled Abs usage. Strategies to control transmission at DCCs or from older sibling(s) are also essential.

Concordance of Isolated Bacteria from Middle Ear and Nasopharynx of Acute Otitis Media

Kenji Suzuki, Toshiyuki Fujisawa, Ichiro Kato, Mayuki Nakashima, Atsusi Nakayama, Seiichi Nakata

Department of Otolaryngology, Second Hospital, Fujita Health University School of Medicine, Nagoya, Japan

Background: To study the differences of detected bacteria from the middle ear and the nasopharynx of an acute otitis media patient. **Objective:** To investigate a genetic difference of mainly isolated bacteria species from the middle ear and the nasopharynx of an acute otitis media patient. **Methods:** By using pulse-field electrophoresis, genetic concordances of isolated bacteria species from the middle ear and the nasopharynx of patients. We investigated 17 patients (34 strains) with *Staphylococcus aureus*, 49 patients (98 strains) with *Streptococcus pneumoniae*, 10 patients (20 strains) with *Moraxella catarrhalis*, and 55 patients (110 strains) with *Haemophilus influenzae*, respectively. **Results:** Concordant rate of *S. aureus* was 94.1%, *S. pneumoniae* was more than 77.6%, *M. catarrhalis* was 100%, and *H. influenzae* was more than 78.2%, respectively. **Conclusion:** When we detect *S. pneumoniae, H. influenzae*, and *Streptococcus pyogenes* from nasopharyngeal fluid, we decide those isolates as causative bacteria of an acute otitis media even if we are not be able to detect any bacteria from the middle ear, whereas when we detect *S. aureus* and coagulase-negative *Staphylococcus*, we should consider the possibility of contamination from the external ear canal.

Math1 Drives the Differentiation of Middle Ear Epithelial Cells into Mucous Cells in vitro

Yoshihisa Nakamura[a], Masahiro Komori[b], Shingo Murakami[a]

[a]Department of Otolaryngology, Nagoya City University School of Medicine, Nagoya, and [b]Department of Otolaryngology, Kochi University School of Medicine, Kochi, Japan

Introduction: Under inflammatory conditions, mucous cell numbers are dramatically increased by differentiation from epithelial cells (mucous cell metaplasia). Mucous cell metaplasia results in the hyperproduction of mucous in the middle ear and chronicity of otitis media. We hypothesized in this study that Math1, a transcription factor for the initial differentiation of goblet cells in the mouse intestine, is an important molecular switch for mucous cell differentiation in the inflammatory setting. **Methods:** Mouse middle ear epithelial cells (mMEECs) were cultured in a chamber slide for 2 weeks in the presence of retinoic acid (RA) and TNF-α to induce mucous cell differentiation. Mucous cell differentiation was evaluated as the percentage of AB-PAS (specific stain for mucin)-positive cells. To investigate the role of Math1, sense and anti-sense Math1 vector, and empty vector transfected cells were compared. Math1 activation pathway by RA and/or TNF-α was also investigated. **Results:** Transfection of mMEECs with s-Math1 significantly induced the AB-PAS positive cells in the presence of RA and TNF-α compared with empty vector. Blockage of Math1 with as-Math1 abrogated mucous cell induction. Transfection of s-Math1 alone (in the absence of RA or TNF-α) induced just a few AB-PAS-positive cells. Concerning the activation of Math1, not TNF-α but RA treatment for 12 h obviously increased the Math1-positive cell expression. A specific inhibitor for EGFR tyrosine kinase, AG1478, abrogated RA-induced Math1 expression. **Conclusion:** Math1 collaborated with RA (differentiation factor) and TNF-α (inflammatory cytokine) to promote the differentiation of middle ear epithelial cells into mucous cells. RA acted to strengthen the expression of Math1 via EGFR tyrosine kinase. The results are suggesting that Math1 is a therapeutic target for mucous cell metaplasia in otitis media.

to the middle ear compared to the transparent variant. The observation of phase variation in surface structure suggested a potential significance for this phenomenon in the pathogenesis of pneumococcal infection.

Phase Variation of *Streptococcus Pneumoniae* Isolated from Middle Ear Fluid and Nasopharynx of Children with Acute Otitis Media

Jun Arai, Muneki Hotomi, Masashi Ogami, Masamitu Kono, Shin Takei, Yorihiko Ikeda, Kazuma Yamauchi, Akihisa Togawa, Shinji Tamura, Noboru Yamanaka

Otolaryngology, Head and Neck Surgery, Wakayama Medical University, Wakayama, Japan

Background: *Streptococcus pneumoniae* is a leading cause of acute otitis media (AOM). The pathogen undergoes spontaneous intra-strain phase variation in colony morphology depending on the capsular synthesis. The transparent variant is more efficient in colonizing the nasopharynx while the opaque variant exhibits greater virulence on systemic infections. However, there is little information about the pneumococcal phase variations of both middle ear isolates and nasopharyngeal isolates. In this study, we investigated phase variation of *S. pneumoniae* isolated from middle ear fluid and nasopharynx of children with acute otitis media. **Materials and Methods:** Middle ear fluids and nasopharyngeal swabs were collected from pediatric patients with acute otitis media before the antimicrobial treatments. The serially diluted specimens were plated on the trypticase soy agar (TSA) plates with 6,300 U/plate catalase. After the 16 h incubations at 37°C with 5% CO_2 atmosphere, the pneumococcal phase variations were determined under the phase-contrast microscopy. The present study was designed to investigate from the nasopharynx to middle ear transmission of *S. pneumoniae* with AOM utilizing restriction fragment length polymorphism analysis by PFGE. **Results:** All of the middle ear isolates were classified into the opaque variant, while the pneumococcal phase variation of nasopharyngeal isolates showed phase variations with transparent and opaque variants. We evaluated clinical isolates from three cases with acute otitis media regarding to the phase variation and clonality of strains isolated from middle ear fluids and nasopharyngeal swabs. We observed an identical PFGE pattern on the strains showing different phase variation patterns in the middle ear fluid and in the nasopharynx. **Discussion:** Our results suggest that the opaque variant of *S. pneumoniae* is highly adapted

Minimal Biofilm Eradication Concentration of Antimicrobial Agents against *Haemophilus influenzae* Isolated from Otitis Media

Shin Takei, Muneki Hotomi, Satomi Moriyama, Akihisa Togawa, Noboru Yamanaka

Department of Otolaryngology, Head and Neck Surgery, Wakayama Medical University, Wakayama, Japan

Introduction: For antimicrobial susceptibility testing, the minimal inhibitory concentration (MIC) has long been the standard measurement. The MIC measures the antimicrobial activity against planktonic organisms. Nontypable *Haemophilus inlfuenzae* (NTHi), one of the leading causative pathogen for acute otitis media (AOM) and acute rhinosinusitis, has been reported to form a biofilm. The antimicrobial susceptibility would be different between planktonic and biofilm-forming conditions. In this study, the MIC and minimum biofilm eradication concentration (MBEC) were compared to determine changes in the pattern of antimicrobial susceptibility of NTHi from the planktonic to the biofilm phase. **Methods:** The MIC and MBEC of cefems, penicillins, macrolides and quinolones were evaluated against NTHi isolates obtained from pediatric patients with AOM. The 96-pin replicator assay produces 96 equivalent biofilms for the antimicrobial susceptibilities. MBEC was defined as the minimal concentration of antibiotic agents at which no bacteria growth was seen on a chocolate agar plate. At the same time, Cristal violet stain was performed to evaluate biofilm inhibition effect quantitatively. **Results:** Every antimicrobial agent reduced the amount of biofilms in a concentration-dependent manner, but did not extinguish biofilms completely even at very high concentrations. The antimicrobial susceptibility of biofilms was significantly lower than that of planctonic bacteria. Some antimicrobial agents seemed to be effective to eradicate NTHi in the biofilm in clinical concentration. MBEC of LVFX was low enough. In the clinical setting, FOM and OFLX are frequently used in high concentration as ototopical drugs; therefore, they seem to eradicate organisms in biofilms at clinical concentrations. **Conclusion:** It is clear that the antimicrobial susceptibilities of planktonic populations are not necessarily applicable to effective treatment of the same organism in biofilms. The MBEC will be essential for the appropriate selection of antimicrobial agents against microbial biofilms and for the screening of new effective antimicrobial agents.

Evaluation of the Clinical Efficacy of Antibiotics Using a Scoring System for Acute Pharyngo-Tonsillitis

Nobuyuki Bandoh[a], Miki Takahara[b], Tomoki Yoshizaki[b], Seigo Ueda[b], Yoshiya Ishida[b], Kan Kishibe[b], Takashi Goto[a], Tatsuya Hayashi[b], Yasuaki Harabuchi[b], Noboru Yamanaka[c]

Departments of Otolaryngology, Head and Neck Surgery, [a]Hokuto Hospital, Obihiro, [b]Asahikawa Medical College, Asahikawa, and [c]Wakayama Medical University, Wakayama, Japan

Acute pharyngo-tonsillitis is one of the most common upper respiratory tract infectious diseases. We have shown that a clinical scoring system consisting of symptoms and local findings in tonsils with a total score of 12 points reflected the disease severity accurately in each patient. However, the clinical efficacy of antibiotics using the scoring system has not been analyzed yet. In this study, the clinical efficacy of antibiotics was assessed by two methods we originally developed. First, when the clinical scores were reduced by equal or more than 3 points in moderate cases and by equal or more than 4 points in severe cases, the patient was regarded as effective. The percentage of patients assessed as effective in each antibiotic-treated group was defined as efficacy rate. Second, the improvement rate in each patient was calculated as folllows: {(clinical score on day 0)-(clinical score on day 3–5)}/(clinical score on day 0) ×100 (%). The average improvement rate in each antibiotic-treated group patient was calculated. A total of 214 patients were analyzed. In moderate cases, AMPC, CFPN, CPDX, and LVFX were given orally to 17 (16.9%), 37 (36.6%), 11 (10.9%), 5 (4.9%) and 18 (17.8%) of 101 patients, respectively. There was no difference in the efficacy and improvement rate between each antibiotic-treated group. In severe cases, AMPC, CFPN and LVFX were given orally to 8 (15.1%), 5 (9.4%) and 12 (22.6%) out of 53 patients respectively. CTRX and FMOX were intravenously injected to 12 (22.6%) and 5 (9.4%) patients, respectively. There was no difference in the efficacy rate, but improvement rates with CFPN, LVFX and CTRX were significantly higher than those with FMOX. A clinical scoring system for acute pharyngo-tonsillitis is a simple, easy and useful diagnostic with which to evaluate the clinical efficacy of antibiotics. The improvement rate can be one of the indicators of the clinical efficacy of antibiotics.

Eustachian Tube Status and Pharingeal Ring Disease

Elena P. Merkulova, Konstantin N. Ustinovich

Belarusian State Medical University, Minsk, Belarus

Introduction: Otolaryngologists have no unique opinion regarding the role of various pathologies of pharyngeal tonsils in etiopathogenesis of persisting exudates from the eardrum cavity of children. The task of our investigation is studying of the impact of pathology varieties of pharyngeal tonsils on functional condition of eustachian tubes (ET). **Materials and Methods:** The method of acoustic impedansometry before surgical treatment was used to examine 154 children. Three groups were revealed: (1) patients with adenoids (n = 103); (2) patients with hypertrophy of palatal and nasal tonsils (n = 33), and (3) children with chronic tonsillitis (n = 18) who were admitted for tonsillectomy. Statistical processing of tympanograms (n = 308) was conducted using the χ^2 test. **Results:** Dysfunction of ET with registration of tympanograms of type 'B' was marked in 57.7% (n = 119/206) of children admitted for adenomectomy. Functional impairment of an ET occurs more often if the enlargement of all tonsils is marked, as registrations of tympanograms of 'B' type in this group before operation is noted in 81.8% (n = 54/66) of cases. Tympanogram of 'A' type is accordingly registered in 24.8% in the first and 12.1% in the second groups. Chronic tonsillitis rarely causes functional impairment of an ET (n = 2/36). The difference is authentic in comparing these three groups by χ^2 test, p = 0.0463 (comparison of groups 1, p = 0.0044; groups 1–3, p < 0.0001; groups 2–3, p < 0.0001). **Conclusions:** (1) The size of pharyngeal tonsils plays an important role in the etiopathogenesis of dysfunction of ET in children. (2) Children with hypertrophy of all tonsils of the pharynx are at the main risk group of developing chronic dysfunction of the acoustic tubes. (3) In chronic inflammation of the palatal tonsils, impairments of ventilation of the eardrum cavity appear to be rare.

Two Cases of Pediatric Retropharyngeal Abscess

Kunihiro Sato, Akio Tsuchiya, Naotaka Aizawa, Sugata Takahashi

Department of Otorhinolaryngology, Niigata University Faculty of Medicine, Niigata, Japan

Retropharyngeal abscess occurring due to lymph node suppuration in the retropharyngeal space requires prompt, precise diagnosis and treatment, but has yet to have a standard of care established, especially for the necessity of surgical drainage. We report 2 cases of pediatric retropharyngeal abscess. **Case 1:** A 2-year-old boy had an abscess in the retropharyngeal and right parapharyngeal space. He underwent surgical management without suppuration following 5 days of intravenous antibiotic administration, recovering with postoperative antibiotic administration. **Case 2:** A 4-year-old boy's CT findings demonstrated a well-enhanced lesion in the retropharyngeal space. His condition was improved by intravenous antibiotic therapy alone without requiring surgical drainage. Decisions on retropharyngeal abscess treatment must thus consider the possibility of improvement with intravenous antibiotic alone. However, surgical drainage should be performed in the case of having either extended inflammation, airway stenosis or thrombophlebitis.

Peritonsillar Abscess in Children

Masashi Yamamoto[a], Yuko Sasaki[b], Mamiko Yasuda[b], Mayumi Kobayashi[b], Sachiko Omae[b], Humiyo Shimura[b], Yutarou Ida[b], Hideo Matsuno[b], Hideo Edamatsu[b]

[a]Toho University School of Medicine and International Friendship Hospital, Tokyo and Yokohama, and [b]Toho University School of Medicine, Tokyo, Japan

Preface: Peritonsillar abscess is a serious complication after acute tonsillitis, which needs both quick surgical treatment and strong antibiotic therapy. The disease is often seen in adults but is very rare in children. The general condition in children with peritonsillar abscess, however, may rapidly worsen and so it is becomes a serious emergency ENT disease. Therefore, fast diagnosis and careful treatment in children are very important. **Cases:** Nine cases of children with peritonsillar abscess have been admitted to our hospital during the last 10 years (1999–2009). They were 6 boys and 3 girls, and their ages ranged from 3 to 11 years with mean of 6.7. They have had no special immunological problems or previous episodes of recurrent tonsillitis. Treatments were tonsillectomy in 5 children, puncture and drainage in 3, and no surgery in 1. Indication for surgical treatment was made by CT findings of the abscess. Pyogenesis of the bacteria was not consistent. All cases recovered well in hospitalization. **Conclusion:** Children suffer so many flu or Streptococcal infections in the tonsils, but why is a peritonsillar abscess very unusual in younger age? Immunological or anatomical differences of the tonsils between adults and children have been suggested, but no evidence has been confirmed. Surgery for infectious tonsil very easily incurs bleeding and is sometimes dangerous. Therefore, fast diagnosis of tonsillar abscess and adequate surgery are very important especially in children.

Image Analysis of Peritonsillar Abscess by Computed Tomography

Junichiro Ohori, Mizuo Umakoshi, Tamon Hayashi, Yuichi Kurono

Department of Otolaryngology, Head and Neck Surgery, Kagoshima University Graduate School of Medical and Dental Sciences, Kagoshima, Japan

Objective: Quinsy tonsillectomy is one of the effective treatments for peritonsillar abscess and is frequently performed in our hospital. Before surgery, enhanced CT scan is indispensable and provides useful information. The CT findings revealed that peritonsillar abscess is classified into two categories: intracapsular type (ICPA) mostly showing an egg-shaped abscess and extracapsular type (ECPA) mostly showing a cap-shaped abscess. In the present study, the CT findings and clinical characteristics of ICPA and ECPA are further investigated and the pathogenesis of peritonsillar abscess is discussed. **Material and Method:** A retrospective study was conducted for patients who were examined by CT scan to diagnose peritonsillar abscess at Kagoshima University Hospital between April 1, 2005 and December 31, 2009. The patients who received puncture drainage before the CT scan were excluded from the analysis. **Results:** A total of 79 patients, aged 39.8 ± 15.9 years (range 7–85) were examined with enhanced CT scan to evaluate the location of the abscess. Forty-eight (61.5%) patients were diagnosed as ICPA, 17 (21.8%) as ECPA, and 13 (16.7%) as mixed (intra- and extracapsular) type abscess. Forty-five cases (95.7%) of ICPA have egg-shaped abscesses and 14 cases (82.3%) of ECPA have cap-shaped abscesses. **Conclusions:** The location of the abscess is not identical in patients with peritonsillar abscess, and the incidence of ICPA is much higher than that of ECPA. The findings suggest that most abscesses occur in the intracapsular space, not in the extracapsular space.

Update on Mast Cells in Allergic Airway Inflammation

Ruby Pawankar

Nippon Medical School, Tokyo, Japan

Mast cells reside within tissues which interface with the external environment as well as within vascularized tissues next to nerves, blood vessels and glandular structures. Thereby they can react within minutes but also over hours to specific stimuli with local and systemic effects. Mast cells have conventionally been recognized for their role in the genesis of allergic inflammation. However, recently it is known that activated mast cells can induce and regulate much of the allergic inflammation as well as participate in innate immune responses. In allergic rhinitis and atopic asthma, mast cell numbers are increased within the airway epithelium and mast cell mediators such as histamine, leukotrienes and prostaglandins can induce eosinophil recruitment, increase vascular permeability and smooth muscle contraction while proteases can activate fibroblasts promoting collagen deposition and fibrosis. Mast cells can also induce basophil histamine release, recruit neutrophils and eosinophils, and promote the development of T cells into a T helper 2 (Th2) phenotype. Thus, mast cells may induce an immediate reaction and contribute to a late-phase reaction. Furthermore, mast cells can induce IgE synthesis in B cells and can autoactivate via the mast cell-IgE-FceRI cascade thus contributing to on-going allergic inflammation. Mast cells can play a role in antigen presentation and mast cell-epithelial cell interactions can upregulate the production of several chemokines and cytokines that regulate allergic inflammation. An increased expression of VLA-4 and VLA-5 in mast cells of patients with allergic rhinitis may contribute to nasal hyperresponsiveness. Mast cells are also increased within the airways smooth muscle (ASM) of asthmatics and can facilitate hyper-responsiveness through localized mediator release and/or direct cell-to-cell contact. Together with this, a greater number of degranulated mast cells are found in fatal cases of asthma. Furthermore, an increase in degranulated mast cells near the mucosal glands is observed in fatal and nonfatal asthma and amphiregulin produced by mast cells can upregulate mucin gene expression in epithelial cells. Moreover, mast cells can be activated by TLRs and complement receptors in addition to via the –FceRI. Taken together, mast cells are not only involved in the genesis but also in the perpetuation of on-going allergic inflammation and airways remodeling. As our molecular understanding of the mast cell evolves, novel targets for modulation are being identified with promising therapeutic potential.

IgE Production and Ig Class Switch Recombination in Allergic Diseases of Upper Airways

Takechiyo Yamada, Seita Kubo, Hiroshi Sunaga, Shigeharu Fujieda

Department of Otorhinolaryngology, Head and Neck Surgery, University of Fukui, Fukui, Japan

Allergic diseases of the airways represent a major worldwide health issue and the hallmark of disorders is increased immunoglobulin E (IgE) production. Although antibodies are secreted by plasma cells and their precursors, the plasma blasts, Ig class switch recombination to epsilon is essential for IgE production in human B cells. In previous reports, we found that the inhibitory molecules or signaling for Ig class switch recombination to epsilon in human B cells employing the established switch vector assay, digestion-circularization-PCR, RT-PCR, and real-time PCR, and these inhibitory molecules or signaling also decreased the IgE production. On the contrary, they are long-lived.

Role of Lipid Mediators on Allergic Rhinitis

Hideaki Shirasaki, Tetsuo Himi

Department of Otolaryngology, Sapporo Medical University, Sapporo, Japan

Lipid mediators such as cysteinyl leukotrienes (CysLTs), thromboxane A2 (TXA2), prostaglandin D_2 (PGD2), platelet-activating factor (PAF) have been thought the potent mediators involved in allergic rhinitis, because these chemical mediators were recovered from the nasal lavage fluid of allergic rhinitis patients after allergen provocation and these receptor specific-antagonists relief nasal allergic symptoms. In order to clarify the role of thses lipid mediators, we have investigated the expression of these receptors on human nasal mucosa by in situ hybridization and immunohistochemistry. For example, our previuous studies revealed that the major target of CysLT1 receptor antagonists are vascular bed and the infiltrated leukocytes such as mast cells, eosinophils, and macrophages, and that TXA2 receptors expressed on vascular smooth muscle cells and vascular endothelial cells.

We would like to present evidence that: (1) these lipid mediators are released during a nasal allergic response, (2) receptors for these mediators are located in the human nasal mucosa, (3) the lipid mediators are related nasal symptoms of allergic rhinitis, and (4) there is clinical efficacy of these receptor antagonists for allergic rhinitis.

Roles of Prostaglandin D_2 in the Pathophysiology of Allergic Rhinitis

Mitsuhiro Okano

Department of Otolaryngology and Head and Neck Surgery, Okayama University Graduate School of Medicine, Dentistry and Pharmaceutical Sciences, Okayama, Japan

Prostaglandins (PGs) are lipid mediators that regulate immune function. Among these, PGD_2 is thought to mediate airway inflammation. PGD_2 mediates a variety of biological activities, including vasodilation and eosinophilic inflammatin. However, the precise roles of PGD_2 in the pathophysiology of allergic rhinitis remain unclear. First, we sought to determine the expression and characterization of synthases and receptors for PGD_2. Hematopoietic-type PGD_2 synthase (h-PGDS) was selectively expressed in human nasal mucosa, and the expression of h-PGDS in allergic patients was significantly higher than in patients without mucosal hypertrophy. A variety of infiltrating cells including mast cells, eosinophils as well as constitutive cells such as epithelial cells and fibroblast expressed h-PGDS. In addition, the expression of both DP and CRTH2 was confirmed. DP was expressed in a variety of cells whereas CRTH2 was selectively expressed in infiltrating cells and some glands. The amount of CRTH2 but not DP was highly and significantly correlated with the number of eosinophils infiltrating into nasal musosa. Next, we sought to determine whether receptors for PGD_2 play a role in the pathogenesis of allergic rhinitis in vivo, and we developed a murine model of allergic rhinitis using Cry j 1, the major allergen of Japanese cedar pollinosis. CRTH2-gene-deficient mice had significantly weaker Cry j 1-specific IgE/IgG1 production, nasal eosinophilia, and IL-4 production by submandibular lymph node cells than wild-type mice. On the other hand, DP-gene-deficient mice showed a similar pathogenesis as compared with wild-type mice. These results suggest that the PGD_2-CRTH2 interaction plays a proinflammatory role in the pathophysiology of allergic rhinitis.

Proteases Induce Production of Thymic Stromal Lymphopoietin by Airway Epithelial Cells through Protease-Activated Receptor-2

Hideaki Kouzaki[a], Hirohito Kita[b], Takeshi Shimizu[a]

[a]Shiga University of Medical Science, Shiga, Japan; [b]Mayo Clinic, Rochester, N.Y., USA

Rationale: Allergen proteases may act as potent Th2 adjuvants. Production of thymic stromal lymphopoietin (TSLP) by airway epithelial cells or by skin keratinocytes is implicated in the development of Th2-type immune responses and allergic diseases. However, the triggers and mechanisms involved in TSLP production by these cell types are poorly understood. **Methods:** An airway epithelial cell line, BEAS-2B, was stimulated with authentic proteases, including trypsin and papain, with or without IL-4. Cells were also stimulated with *Alternaria alternata* extract; *Alternaria* is implicated in the development and exacerbation of human asthma. TSLP production was examined by real-time PCR and ELISA. Protease and candidate receptor participation was examined by biochemical approaches and by small interfering RNA (siRNA) treatment. **Results:** Incubation of BEAS-2B with trypsin and papain induced TSLP mRNA expression and protein production; these responses were abolished by their respective protease inhibitors, APMSF and E64. TSLP production was synergistically enhanced by IL-4. A heat-labile component(s) in *Alternaria* extract also potently induced TSLP production by BEAS-2B. This *Alternaria*-induced TSLP production was inhibited significantly by a cysteine protease inhibitor, E64 ($p < 0.05$), but not by a serine protease inhibitor, APMSF. Furthermore, suppression of the protease-activated receptor (PAR)-2 expression by siRNA inhibited *Alternaria*-induced TSLP expression by approximately 50%; suppression of PAR-1 or TLR4 showed no effects. **Conclusions:** Airway epithelial cells recognize cysteine protease activities in certain allergens, such as *Alternaria*, through PAR-2 and produce TSLP. Induction of TSLP may explain the potent Th2 adjuvant activities of allergens.

Clinical Characteristics and Pathogenesis of Eosinophilic Otitis Media

Yukiko Iino

Jichi Medical University Saitama Medical Center, Saitama, Japan

Eosinophilic otitis media (EOM) is an intractable otitis media characterized by the presence of a highly viscous yellow effusion containing eosinophils. It mainly occurs in patients with bronchial asthma and is resistant to conventional treatments for otitis media. Here we discuss the clinical features, pathogenesis and managements of EOM. EOM predominantly affects females and occurs most often in patients in their 50s. The clinical features of the middle ear in EOM are roughly divided into the (OME) type and the chronic otitis media (COM). The latter is further divided into two subtypes: simple perforation subtype and granulation tissue formation subtype. EOM is often complicated by rhinosinusitis, which is called eosinophilic sinusitis. High tone loss is more frequently found and more severe in EOM patients than in COM control patients and EOM patients sometimes become deaf suddenly. The Eustachian tube function using sonotubometry clarified that the tubal opening duration in EOM patients was significantly longer than that in the control groups, indicating the presence of patulous eustachian tubes in EOM patients. Regarding the management of EOM, systemic or topical administration of steroids is the most effective for patients with EOM. The instillation of treamcinolone acetonide, a suspension of steroids, into the middle ear is very effective for the control of eosinophilic inflammation.

Application of Rapid Test for Allergic Conjunctival Diseases to Nasal Diseases

Kei Fukushima[a], Horomi Takeuchi[a], Rie Morizane[a], Hiroya Kitano[a], Sakoda Takema[b], Tadao Enomoto[b]

[a]Department of Otolaryngology, Head and Neck Surgery, Faculty of Medicine, Tottori University, Yonago, and [b]Department of Otorhinolaryngology, Rinku General Medical Center, Izumisano Municipal Hospital, Osaka, Japan

Objective: Allergic rhinitis is a general term for nasal inflammatory diseases in which type-I allergic reactions are involved, and which have usually been diagnosed according to clinical symptoms, local detection of eosinophils from the nose, total IgE in serum, allergen-specific IgE in serum, and a skin test as a scratch or patch test. Recently, a new assay system for the rapid semiquantification of IgE antibodies in tear fluid has been established by applying the technique of immunochromatography. In the present study, we have examined if this new assay system is applicable to the diagnosis of allergic rhinitis. **Methods:** A total of 22 adult volunteers with Japanese cedar pollinosis were included in the study. They were exposed to Japanese cedar pollen in an environmental exposure unit. Eosinophil from nose, serum total IgE antibodies, Japanese cedar pollen specific IgE antibodies, local IgE antibodies from nose, and local IgE antibodies from eye were analyzed. **Results:** Statistically, local IgE antibodies from nose correlated with Eosinophil from nose. **Conclusion:** It is expected that this new assay can be useful for the clinical diagnosis of Allergic rhinitis.

Regulation and Characterization of IL-17A Expression in Chronic Rhinosinusitis and Its Relationship with Eosinophilic Inflammation

Miki Yamamoto

Okayama University Graduate School of Medicine, Dentistry and Pharmaceutical Sciences, Okayama, Japan

Background: Interleukin-17A (IL-17A) is a Th17-related cytokine that affects chronic inflammation. **Objective:** The regulation and characterization of IL-17A expression during chronic rhinosinusitis were investigated. **Methods:** Dispersed nasal polyp cells (DNPCs) were stimulated with Staphylococcal enterotoxin B (SEB) in the presence or absence of neutralizing antibodies against regulatory cytokines and COX inhibitor. IL-17A supernatant levels were then measured, and the effects of prostaglandin E2 (PGE2) on IL-17A production in DNPC were examined. Furthermore, the direct effects of IL-17A on cytokine production were measured. The expression of IL-17A in sinonasal tissues was examined via immunohistochemistry. **Results:** DNPC synthesized IL-17A in response to SEB. Neutralization of IL-12/IL-23 p40 and IFN-γ significantly suppressed and augmented production, respectively. COX inhibition also significantly reduced IL-17A production. The addition of PGE2 and EP2/EP4 receptor-selective agonists reversed these reductions. IL-17A was mainly expressed by infiltrating inflammatory cells in the sinonasal tissues. Expression in nasal polyps, especially in patients with aspirin-induced asthma, was significantly higher than control mucosa samples. The number of IL-17A+ cells positively correlated with tissue eosinophilia and radiological severity of sinusitis, and was inversely correlated with FEV1/FVC ratio. Recombinant IL-17A augmented GM-CSF and IL-6 production by DNPC. **Conclusion:** SEB-induced IL-17A synthesis in DNPC was regulated by IL-12/IL-23 p40, IFN-γ and PGE2. The pro-inflammatory effects of PGE2 on IL-17A production was mediated via coupling to EP2/EP4. Elevated expression of IL-17A may be involved in eosinophilic inflammation during chronic rhinosinusitis via the augmentation of GM-CSF and IL-6 production, and may be associated with lower airway obstruction.

OSAS and Tonsillectomy

New Surgical Method for OSAS Patients with the Circumferential Stricture Type of Soft Palate

Kenji Suzuki, Takahiro Kitanaka, Yoichi Nishimura, Toshiyuki Fujisawa, Ichiro Kato, Seiichi Nakata

Department of Otolaryngology, Second Hospital, Fujita Health University School of Medicine, Nagoya, Japan

Objective: To evaluate the efficacy of our new surgical method for the circumferential stricture type of soft palate. It has been said that the circumferential stricture type of soft palate should be treated with nasal CPAP and not with the surgical UPPP procedure because of the poor outcome after the surgical method. In this paper, we indicate the merit of our surgical method. **Patients and Methods:** Between April 2004 and December 2009, 15 OSAS patients with the circumferential stricture type of soft palate were treated with our new surgical method at the Department of Otolaryngology, Second Hospital, Fujita Health University School of Medicine, Nagoya, Japan. The mean age of the patients was 42 + 10 years (range 27–64 years; 14 males and 1 female). Apnea hypopnea index (AHI) was from 16 to 82 with a mean of 42 + 23 times per hour. Body mass index (BMI) was from 20 to 36 with a mean of 25 + 4. Our surgical method are performed by following procedures with both-side tonsillectomy and wide removal of both-side anterior palatine arch then sew up posterior and anterior palate by 3.0 Vicryl. **Results:** The efficacy rate of our new surgical method is 67% and that of the traditional method of UPPP is only 16% for the circumferential stricture type of soft palate.

3D-CT Evaluation of Upper Airway Morphology of OSAS Patients

Hirotaka Hara, Hideki Toyota, Kenji Takeno, Hiroshi Yamashita

Department of Otolaryngology, Yamaguchi University Graduate School of Medicine, Ube, Japan

Obstructive sleep apnea (OSA) is a common form of sleep-disordered breathing characterized by repetitive episodes of partial or complete upper airway obstruction. It usually causes sleep fragmentation, reduced blood oxygen levels, and excessive daytime somnolence. Cognitive deficits, impaired psychosocial well-being, reduced driving competence, cardiovascular morbidity, and mortality have been reported. Because the clinical significance of OSA is increasing, more exact diagnosis for successful treatment is required. Multiple factors like enlarged tonsils, nasal disease, body weight, age and craniofacial morphology causes OSAS. But it is well known that the breathing route affects the upper airway morphology. It has been suggested that patients with OSA have narrower pharyngeal airways than normal persons, therefore breathing with mouth open affect the upper airway morphology of OSA patients significantly compared to non-OSA patients. To assess the relationship between pattern of breathing and upper airway morphology in OSA patients, we perform 3D-CT examination and evaluate the changes of upper airway morphology with mouth open and close with DICOM viewer (Osirix). Nine patients were examined 3D-CT with breathing with mouth open and close. Even in awake, upper airway became narrow with oral breathing. It has been reported that the imaging results while awake do not necessarily reflect conditions during sleep, when tone of the upper airway dilating muscles is decreased. But on the standpoint of relationship between breathing routes and upper airway morphology, 3D-CT while awake can be a useful tool for OSA treatment.

Surgical Treatment for Obstructive Sleep Apnea in Children

Akihiro Katada, Tomoki Yoshizaki, Miki Takahara, Akihiro Katayama, Isamu Kunibe, Tatsuya Hayashi, Yasuaki Harabuchi

Department of Otolaryngology- Head and Neck Surgery, Asahikawa Medical College, Asahikawa, Japan

Obstructive sleep apnea (OSA) in children is a breathing disorder that occurs during sleep and is characterized by upper airway collapse that disrupts normal respiratory gas exchange. OSA is characterized by habitual snoring, heavy breathing, sleep-related hypoxia and arousals from sleep. Furthermore, there has been increasing evidence that pediatric OSA is associated behavioral and neurocognitive problems as well as poor school performance, failure to thrive, and poor quality of life. The pathophysiology of pediatric OSA is multifactorial, with enlargement of the lymphoid tissues of Waldeyer's ring contributing to abnormalities of craniofacial/pharyngeal structure and coordination of upper airway tone. Adenotonsillectomy is the initial treatment of choice for otherwise healthy children diagnosed with OSA. Such surgery can be expected to relieve sleep-related airway obstruction in the great majority of children. Although the actual effectiveness of adenotonsillectomy for long-term cure of OSA in children has been recently debated, the short-term benefits have been well documented with clinical improvements in sleep-related airway obstruction as well as in quality of life measures. This surgery remains the mainstay of treatment for childhood OSA. In this paper, we evaluated the efficacy of adenotonsillectomy in treating pediatric OSA. Improvement of OSA is assessed with postoperative apnea-hypopnea index (AHI), and changes if quality of life measures are assessed using questionnaire. More than 90% of the subject achieved at least partial cure in AHI score and snoring after surgery. These results indicated that adenotonsillectomy was highly effective in treating OSA in children. Furthermore, we mentioned complications of surgery and our surgical techniques for adenotonsillectomy using powered instruments.

Bipolar Scissors Tonsillectomy: Cooling of the Pharyngeal Mucosa Reduces Postoperative Pain

Arata Horii[a], Masayuki Hirose[b], Ryuichi Mochizuki[c], Keisuke Yamamoto[c], Masahiro Kawamoto[d], Tadashi Kitahara[e], Takayuki Kawashima[f], Yoshifumi Yamamoto[f], Maki Yamashita[g], Suetaka Nishiike[f], Hidenori Inohara[f]

[a]Department of Otolaryngology, Suita Municipal Hospital, [b]Department of Otolaryngology, Osaka Medical Center and Research Institute for Maternal and Child Health, [c]Department of Otolaryngology,Osaka Kaisei Hospital, [d]Department of Otolaryngology,Ikeda Municipal Hospital, [e]Department of Otolaryngology,Osaka Rosai Hospital, [f]Department of Otorhinolaryngology Head and Neck Surgery, Osaka University Graduate School of Medicine, [g]Department of Otorhinolaryngology Head and Neck Surgery, Department of Otolaryngology,Toyonaka Municipal Hospital, Osaka, Japan

Tonsillectomy is the most common surgery in otolaryngology practice. Although tonsillectomy is basically a safe procedure, two issues still remain: hemorrhage and postoperative pain. Regarding the surgical techniques for tonsillectomy, various devices and techniques including traditional cold dissection, electrocautery, ultrasonic scalpel, coblator, bipolar forceps, and bipolar scissors were developed. Among these devices, bipolar scissors have already been available in most hospitals in Japan, because they are frequently used in abdominal surgery. In the present study, bipolar scissors tonsillectomy (n = 79) was compared with traditional cold dissection tonsillectomy (n = 120), which is the commonest technique used in Japan. Although intra-operative blood loss would be expected to be small in bipolar scissors tonsillectomy, post-tonsillectomy pain due to burns might be more serious than cold dissection. Therefore, we cooled the oral mucosa with cooled saline for 10 min after bipolar scissors tonsillectomy. Main outcome measures were intra-operative blood loss and postoperative pain using a visual analogue scale. Results showed that both intra-operative blood loss and postoperative pain were significantly smaller in bipolar scissors tonsillectomy than cold dissection. It is suggested that dissection with bipolar scissors followed by cooling of the oral mucosa is a recommended method as a new surgical technique of tonsillectomy.

Roll of Antibiotics to Reducing Post-Tonsillectomy Hemorrhage in Adult Patients

Masahiro Okada[a], Hirotaka Takahashi[a], Naohito Hato[a], Kiyofumi Gyo[a], Taisuke Kobayashi[b], Koshiro Nakamura[a]

[a]Department of Otolaryngology, Head and Neck Surgery, Ehime University, Toon, and [b]Department of Otolaryngology, Head and Neck Surgery, Kochi University, Nangoku, Japan

Hemorrhage following tonsillectomy is still a major complication despite the development of new hot knives. In this study, a retrospective review of 242 adult patients who underwent tonsillectomy in the Department of Otolaryngology, Head and Neck Surgery, Ehime Prefectual Central Hospital between January 2000 and March 2007 was conducted. Post-tonsillectomy hemorrhage occurred in 56 patients (23.1%); 4 of these patients experienced hemorrhage during the first 24 h postoperatively, and the remaining 52 had delayed bleeding. Nine of 56 patients (3.7%) required a procedure to control their bleeding under general anesthesia. The hemorrhage rate in males was significantly higher than in females. There was no statistically significant difference in hemorrhage rates based on age, body mass index (BMI), duration of surgery and smoking. Patients who received antibiotics postoperatively experienced less secondary hemorrhage than those without antibiotics. In 99 patients who were administered antibiotics, patients who used cephalosporins experienced less secondary hemorrhage than those who received penicillins. These results indicate that antibiotics after tonsillectomy are effective to reduce post-tonsillectomy hemorrhage rates.

Relation of Sleep Apnea and/or Snoring and Obesity in School Children

Fumiyo Kudo, Takashi Hasegawa, Yasue Hosoyamada, Hiromitsu Inoue, Sachiko Sugizaki, Yoshie Yamauchi, Masako Yamada

Department of Nutrition, Faculty of Health Care Sciences, Chiba Prefectural University of Health Sciences, Chiba, Japan

It is said that obstructive sleep apnea (OSAS) has a close relationship with obesity in adults, however, there are a few obese children who have sleep apnea, especially in small children. The purpose of this report is to clarify the relation of SAS and obesity in children. The basic data were provided from the investigation that the 'sleep apnea syndrome research committee' of the Japanese Society of School Health (JSSH) carried out in 2007. The questionnaires were sent to 21 elementary schools nationwide, with 1,764 returned by 835 first-graders, 703 fifth-graders, and 168 sixth-graders. Their weight and height were also filled in the questionnaire by school nurses. The degree of obesity (percentage of overweight) was calculated by the ideal weight for age and height in school-age children (by Dr. Mitsunori Murata, from the Japanese Society of School Health). Children with habitual snoring (frequently or always) were extracted from the questionnaires and the degree of obesity compared with a no snoring child. In a fifth-grade boy, a significant difference ($p = 0.012$) was observed between obesity and habitual snoring (frequently or always). There was no significant difference compared with girls and other grades. We will take these results for the prevention of OSAS and obesity in school health also in adults.

Indications for Adenotonsillectomy to Treat Pediatric Obstructive Sleep Apnea Syndrome

Naotaka Aizawa, Kunihiro Sato, Akio Tsuchiya, Sugata Takahashi

Department of Otorhinolaryngology, Niigata University Faculty of Medicine Niigata, Japan

Objectives: We studied surgical indications for treating pediatric obstructive sleep apnea syndrome (OSAS) at the Otorhinolaryngology Department of the Niigata University Hospital. **Methods:** The 103 subjects under 15 years of age, seen for snoring and/orsleep apnea, were evaluated in overnight polysomnography (PSG). We clinically assessed adenoid and tonsillar hypertrophy and minimal upper airway measured using radiography, and the apnea index (AI), apnea and hypopnea index (AHI), cumulative percentage at SpO_2 below 90% (CT 90%), lowest SpO_2, and mean SpO_2 using PSG. **Results:** Thirty-four boys and six girls, of whom 28 had been first seen in our hospital before the age of 7, required adenotonsillectomy. Only 4 children over 7 years of age underwent adenotonsillectomy. Otitis media with effusion accounted for the most popular complication for pediatric OSAS, followed by allergy disease and upper respiratory illness. The incidence of the adenotonsillectomy increased significantly with the size of adenoid vegetation and tonsillar hypertrophy, but local findings alone were not enough to determine the surgical indications. AI, AHI, CT 90%, lowest SpO_2 and mean SpO_2 differed significantly between the surgical and nonsurgical groups. Subjects with AHI >5 had high adenotonsillectomy rates as did those with CT90% >1. **Conclusions:** Children with narrow upper airways easily developed sleep breathing disorder and required PSG evaluation, which was also important with other findings in determining the necessity of adenotonsillectomy.

Endoscopic Adenoidectomy with Microdebrider for Sleep Apnea Children

Shigeru Higami, Hiroya Kitano

Tottori University Faculty of Medicine, Division of Sensory and Motor Organs, Otolaryngology- Head and Neck Surgery, Yonago, Japan

Adenoidectomy is a common ENT procedure and is indicated in patients with recurrent adenoiditis, nasal obstruction or obstructive sleep apnea in hospitals. The numbers of both adenoidectomy and tonsillectomy for obstructive sleep apnea children have been increasing. Over the years, many methods have been introduced for these surgeries. There isn't any report that showed a big difference of the efficacy between the classic tonsillectomy technique and new methods. However, there are advances in the new techniques of adenoidectomy. We had been using a traditional Beckmann adenotome, and started transoral adenoidectomy using curved microdebrider-assisted intranasal endoscopy since 2004. The purpose of this presentation is to describe the technique and emphasize the advantages of this procedure over the conventional classic technique and assisted transoral endoscopy. This technique enabled us to remove even small adenoids, and gave a remarkable decrease of intra-operative bleedings, and decreased postoperative signs and symptoms of sleep breathing disorder. Adenoidectomy using both types of equipment is easy to move around the lateral band and nasal cavity and is safe to stop bleeding. The number of adenoidectomies using this technique was over 500 during this 5-years period, and we have not had any big complication.

Quality of Life after Adenotonsillectomy for Obstructive Sleep Apnea in Children under 3 Years

Jiro Aoi

Department of Otolaryngology, Kochi University, School of Medicine, Nankoku, Kochi, Japan

Object: Adenotonsillectomy is highly effective in reducing the severity of pediatric obstructive sleep apnea syndrome (OSAS), making it a good first-line therapy for OSAS. According to a systematic review study in 2009, however, only 66.3% of patients achieve an AHI <1. Children under 3 years of age are considered to be at high risk for developing complications after adenotonsillectomy. **Methods:** 66 children (24 children younger than 3 years and 42 children older than 3 years) that had undergone the surgery between April 2004 and December 2008 were included in our study. The symptoms concerning OSAS and tonsillitis and satisfaction after the surgery were answered by mail in a questionnaire. The rate of collection was 44% (66/150). **Results:** Improvement rate of the symptoms in children younger than 3 years and in children older than 3 years was 95 and 97% for apnea, 90 and 97% for snoring, and 91 and 93% for repeatable sore throat and fever, respectively. In physical development, an obvious and a small improvement was seen in 33 and 21% of children younger than 3 years, and in 39 and 20% of children older than 3 years, respectively. 95% of parents with children younger than 3 years, and 100% of parents with children older than 3 years were satisfied with the result of the surgery. **Conclusion:** Our study confirmed that adenotonsillectomy can be as effective for children younger than 3 years as for children older than 3 years.

Power-Assisted Adenoidectomy in Infants under 2 Years of Age

Tomoki Yoshizaki, Isamu Kunibe, Akihiro Katada, Tatsuya Hayashi, Yasuaki Harabuchi

Department of Otolaryngology- Head and Neck Surgery, Asahikawa Medical College, Asahikawa, Japan

Upper airway obstruction in children is most commonly caused by adenotonsillar hypertrophy. Because children, particularly infants, mainly breathe through the nose, adenoidal hypertrophy easily produces obstructive sleep apnea syndrome (OSAS). Furthermore, OSAS may be the cause of not only sleeping disorders but also of suckling disorders leading to poor growth in infants. Adenoidectomy has not been performed frequently in infants under 2 years of age. However, recent progress in anesthetic techniques and operation instruments has allowed for safer operation of infants. We are performing endoscopic power-assisted adenoidectomy as a safer technique for very young cases, especially under 2 years old. The greatest advantage of endoscopic power-assisted adenoidectomy is that it can have a good view through the endoscope and the adenoid can be shaved surely and safely. But the cost of this method exceeds the cost of the operation because the microdebrider blade is not reusable and very expensive. However, adenoidectomy for infants should be differentiated from one for older children in terms of an impact on the growth of the child and the difficulty of perioperative management. So, in the future it should be considered with an aspect of fee-for-service.

Effect of Tonsillectomy or Adenotonsillectomy on Quality of Life in Pediatric Patients with Sleep-Disordered Breathing

Hideki Toyota, Hirotaka Hara, Hiroshi Yamashita

Department of Otolaryngology, Yamaguchi University Graduate School of Medicine, Ube, Japan

It is well known that the general population of children with sleep-disordered breathing (SDB) shows dramatic improvements in the physiological parameters of sleep after surgery. However, there are few reports related to the evaluation of the changes of the quality of life for children with SDB after tonsillectomy or adenotonsillectomy in Japan. We evaluated the effect of tonsillectomy or adenotonsillectomy on quality of life (QoL) in 19 pediatric SDB patients (age range 3–12 years; median age 4.6 years) with the translated version of OSA-18, an 18-item QOL survey. Eighteen children who underwent tonsillectomy or adenotonsillectomy showed improvement in physiological parameters of sleep and QoL after those surgeries. One child with worsened physiological parameters of sleep after surgery due to re-enlargement of the adenoid did not show enough improvement in QoL after surgery. Even in Japan, the OSA-18 can be useful for the evaluation of the effect of surgical treatment on QoL in SDB children.

Relationship between Sleep and Posture in Patients with Obstructive Sleep Apnea Syndrome

Motofumi Ohki, Sota Yamaguchi, Yuuko Higuchi, Haruka Okubo, Yoshiko Ishii, Soichiro Sakurai, Toshio Ogoshi

2nd Department of Otolaryngology, Toho University School of Medicine, Tokyo, Japan

Objective: At our department, patients with obstructive sleep apnea syndrome (OSAS) are advised to sleep in the lateral position, and this is done as part of the treatment for this disorder. The objective of this study is to determine the correlation between the apnea hypopnea index (AHI) and posture during sleep, based on overnight polysomnographic recordings. **Subjects and Methods:** The study included 52 patients who visited our department with complaints of snoring and sleep apnea, and were diagnosed to have OSAS by an overnight polysomnography. Patients' posture during sleep and changes in sleep position were assessed in terms of their relationship with sleep apnea and hypopnea. For convenience, the postural change index was defined as the quotient obtained from dividing the frequency of changes in the sleep position by the sleeping hours. Nasal resistance was also measured before the sleep study. **Results:** The AHI was significantly decreased for sleep in the lateral position as related with that in the supine position ($p < 0.01$). There was also a significant correlation between the postural change index and AHI ($p < 0.01$), and the postural change index was correlated with the difference of left-right nasal airflow, although AHI was not correlated with nasal resistance. **Conclusion:** The AHI is significantly improved during sleep in the lateral position, compared to that in the supine position. It may be reasonable to assume that OSAS patients have difficulty in sleep because of repeated changes in the sleep position to alleviate upper airway obstruction.

Effects of Nasal Surgery in Obstructive Sleep Apnea Syndrome Patients Treated by Nasal Continuous Positive Airway Pressure

Misato Kasai, Akira Minekawa, Hirotomo Honma, Asami Nakazawa, Takashi Iizuka, Chieri Hayashi, Kaori Kasa, Ayako Inoshita, Katsuhisa Ikeda

Department of Otorhinolaryngology, Juntendo University School of Medicine, Tokyo, Japan

Objective: The purpose of this study was to assess the effect of nasal surgery on nasal resistance, sleep-related symptoms, nasal continuous positive airway pressure (n-CPAP) compliance and the mean ventilation pressure in patients with obstructive sleep apnea syndrome (OSAS) patients treated by n-CPAP. **Method:** Ten OSAS patients treated by n-CPAP suffering from symptomatic nasal obstruction were enrolled in the study. They underwent endoscopic sinus surgery and/or septoplasty and/or submucosal inferior turbinectomy and/or nasal mucosa laser ablation. Nasal resistance, Epworth sleepiness scale, n-CPAP compliance and the mean ventilation pressure were evaluated before and after the surgery. **Results:** Nasal resistance, Epworth sleepiness scale, and the mean ventilation pressure decreased significantly after the surgery ($p < 0.001$). N-CPAP compliance was significantly improved postoperatively ($p < 0.001$). **Conclusions:** Nasal surgery significantly improves nasal resistance, n-CPAP compliance, and daytime sleepiness in OSAS patients treated by n-CPAP.

Clinical Predictor in Obstructive Sleep Apnea Syndrome with Dynamic MRI

Aya Sakai[a], *Takaki Miwa*[b]

[a]Department of Otolaryngology, Asanogawa General Hospital, and [b]Department of Otolaryngology, Kanazawa Medical University, Kanazawa, Japan

Background: Obstructive sleep apnea/hypopnea syndrome (OSAHS) develops or occurs through local obstruction in the upper airway. Currently, this is primarily treated with nasal-continuous positive airway pressure (n-CPAP). However, because the obstructed sites are different in each case, n-CPAP does not always work effectively. In choosing a treatment, the dynamic MRI is useful for assessing the morphology of obstruction in the upper airway during sleep. **Objective:** We will report on the results of treatment of an adult OSAHS case where a dynamic MRI was used to specify the site of obstruction. **Subjective and Method:** Fifteen subjects with OSAS were administered dynamic MRI. The subjects were divided into three groups by obstructive region; tongue base swelling (n = 9), palatine tonsil swelling (n = 3) or velopharynx (n = 3). Each patient was treated with n-CPAP, tonsillectomy, coblation surgery of uvulo-palatine and/or guidance of sleep posture by the lesion of dynamic MRI. All of the subjects who had tongue base swelling pattern were treated by n-CPAP. The subjects with tonsiller swelling pattern were treated by UPPP with or without n-CPAP. Three cases with lesion of velopharynx were treated by coblation surgery, n-CPAP or guidance of sleep position, respectively. **Results:** All of the patients had an improved apnea-hypopnea index (AHI) after treatment. **Conclusion:** Our results strongly suggest that information of dynamic MRI is useful to decide the treatment strategy for OSAS.

Effect of Tonsillectomy on Sleep Disturbance of Patients with Obstructive Sleep Apnea

Nobuo Ohta[a], *Tomoo Watanabe*[a], *Tsukasa Ito*[a], *Toshinori Kubota*[a], *Masaru Aoyagi*[a], *Sawako Masuda*[b]

[a]Department of Otolaryngology, Yamagata University School of Medicine, Yamagata, and [b]Department of Otolaryngology, National Mie Hospital, Mie, Japan

Background: Sleep apnea in children is usually caused by adenoidar and tonsillar hypertrophy. Moreover, the resulting reduction of efficiency in performing daily tasks such as study and daily life is widely reported. This indicates that, due to obstructive sleep apnea, patients will experience difficulty sleeping and thus may experience a reduction in quality of life. While there is much research on the effectiveness of the initial treatment for the sufferers of obstructive sleep apnea, there has not been enough research into the effects on quality of life and sleep disturbance. To clarify this situation a survey of sufferers of obstructive sleep apnea was carried out. Symptoms, quality of life, and sleep disturbance were each investigated. **Methods:** From March 2009 to February 2010, 20 of the patients with obstructive sleep apnea who were treated with adeno-tonsillectomy in our department answered the questionnaire regarding sleep disturbance before and after surgery. **Results and Conclusions:** The sleep disturbance of obstructive sleep apnea patients was recognized before adeno-tonsillectomy. However, with surgery the ability to control the negative effects on sleep disturbance and the effectiveness of surgery were confirmed.

Clinical Analysis of Sleep Apnea Syndrome in our Department

Tomotaka Miyamura, Masayoshi Kobayashi, Kazuhiko Takeuchi

Department of Otorhinolaryngology, Head and Neck Surgery, Mie University Graduate School of Medicine, Tsu, Mie, Japan

Sleep apnea syndrome (SAS) is a critical disease and it is estimated that 2–4% of the Japanese population are suffering from this condition. We analyzed 238 patients presenting to the Otorhinolaryngology Clinic of Mie University Hospital for the past 5 years with complaints of sleep apnea and associated symptoms such as snoring. Sleep studies revealed that one half of them were suffering from obstructive SAS (OSAS) but that one third of them were snoring patients to whom SAS criteria were not applied. Male patients were greater in number than female patients. For the OSAS, the soft palate and uvula were the most responsible regions for sleep apnea, and severe OSAS patients tended to have multiple regions responsible for their sleep apnea. More than 90% of SAS patients complained of snoring and about 60% of them had excessive daytime sleepiness. Many patients had been suffering from these symptoms for more than 2 years and some for more than 20 years before presenting to our hospital. SAS patients had a history of hypertension and cardiac diseases more often than non-SAS patients. SAS patients had traffic accidents more often than non-SAS patients. Smoking and drinking were more often noted in SAS than in non-SAS patients. Lowest SpO_2 and oxygen desaturation index (ODI) correlated with the grade of SAS. Severe SAS patients had less nasal patency. The SAS patients were treated with nasal CPAP, diet, surgical therapy such as tonsillectomy, oral device, or a combination of these modalities, according to the regions responsible for sleep apnea in each individual. After the treatments, the SAS symptoms disappeared in most patients. About 90% of the patients who were introduced on n-CPAP were continuously using the n-CPAP. In conclusion, selecting appropriate treatments for individual SAS cases is important for a good prognosis. In addition, smoking and drinking should be prohibited in SAS patients.

Four Cases of Pharyngeal Flap Construction with Tonsillectomy

Seiji Horibe, Kensei Naito, Tomoko Horibe, Keishiro Nagashima, Masako Shimizu

Department of Otolaryngology, Fujita Health University, School of Medicine, Aichi, Japan

Tonsillectomy is a suitable indication of palatine tonsil hypertrophy, while we must pay attention to the indication in cleft palate children after closure operation because of the possibility of postoperative velopharyngeal incompetence. On the other hand, pharyngeal flap construction is an appropriate indication of velopharyngeal incompetence, while we must pay attention to the indication in palatine tonsil hypertrophy patients because of the possibility of obstructive sleep apnea after the flap construction. We have operated on pharyngeal flap construction in 42 velopharyngeal incompetent children in our department during the period between 1992 and 2009. We simultaneously operated on both pharyngeal flap construction and tonsillectomy in four cleft palatine children after a palatal closure operation with velopharyngeal competence accompanying prominent palatine tonsil hypertrophy of the 42. In the 4 cases, we have encountered a satisfactory postoperative course. However, we must take account of careful indication of the combination of the contradictive operation in these cases for fear of the worst results of both obstructive sleep apnea and velopharyngeal incompetence.

Efficacy of Surgical Treatment for Patients with Obstructive Sleep Apnea

Yasuhiro Miyamoto[a], Takenori Kawakami[a], Masahiko Fukasawa[a], Mitsuharu Takatsu[a], Daisuke Kuwahara[a], Naohiko Osada[b], Izumi Koizuka[a]

Departments of [a]Otolaryngology and [b]Cardiology, St. Marianna University School of Medicine, Kawasaki, Japan

Obstructive sleep apnea syndrome (OSAS) is a common sleep apnea caused by obstruction of the airway especially in the upper airway and is characterized by pauses in breathing during sleep. In obstructive sleep apnea, breathing is interrupted by physical blockage of airflow, i.e. hypertrophic tonsils, despite the effort to breathe. The most widely used current therapeutic intervention is continuous positive airway pressure (CPAP) whereby a breathing machine pumps a controlled stream of air through a mask worn over the nose or mouth or both. Additional pressure is also provided to splint or hold open the relaxed muscles. When this treatment fails, surgical treatments are considered to improve the airflow interrupted by physical blockage. Current treatment of obstructive sleep apnea (OSAS) largely consists of surgical treatments. Tonsillectomy is the most common surgical intervention for the treatment of OSAS. To determine the efficacy of tonsillectomy to treat OSAS, we retrospectively assessed the outcomes of patients with OSAS due to obstructive hypertrophic tonsils who underwent tonsillectomy at St. Marianna University School of Medicine between April 2007 and March 2009. The success rate of tonsillectomy for OSAS was measured by objective criteria based on the apnea hypopnea index (AHI). We evaluated the safety and efficacy of tonsillectomy for patients with OSAS and discussed the treatment precautions during surgical intervention for the patients with OSAS.

A Case Report: The Sudden Respiratory Failure of Newborn Baby Causing by Thyroglossal Cyst

Kaoru Takeuchi[a], *Shigeru Higami*[a], *Hiroya Kitano*[a], *Shinichi Mochida*[b]

[a]Division of Sensory and Motor Organs, Otolaryngology, Head and Neck Surgery and [b]Department of Anesthesiology and Critical Care Medicine, Tottori University Faculty of Medicine, Tottori, Japan

Thyroglossal duct cysts are common neck masses of benign lymph nodes. They originate from the primitive thyroglossal duct, so they could be located along its course. Some reports showed sudden death newborns had thyroglossal ducts in the base of the tongue, which are considered as causes of obstructive respiratory failure. A 1-month-old male infant was referred because of producing noisy breathing sounds during inspiration. First examination of endoscopic finding looked like laryngomalacia and did not show the primary tumor through the upper airway. As a first treatment, we tried a noninvasive positive airway pressure ventilation system (N-DPAP) in the ICU; however, his respiratory condition could not controlled by maximal pressure. Our decision was immediate intubation; however, ICU anesthesiologists had difficulty in doing the intubation. After intubation, secondary endoscopic examination revealed a swelling of the base of the tongue. MRI showed a circumscribed cystic lesion located in the tongue base. We tried to remove the cyst using coblation -assisted endoscopy. Histological diagnosis was thyroglossal duct cyst. After 3 days' intubation, he had no breathing disorder in ICU. After 6 months of follow-up, he has no recurrence of cyst or dyspnea.

Author Index

(A) = Abstracts

Subject Index